“The bioethics [illegible]
national and n[illegible]
bioethics. He helps the re[illegible]

looks like—not in some theoretical way far from the nitty-gritty [illegible] private and professional life, but in the lived experience of evangelical believers committed to being personally and communally faithful to their God. He goes on to show that such incarnational faithfulness is not something that properly focuses only in-house, within the church, but necessarily reaches out to join with the wider human community in the task of learning and living what it means to be human. Many will begin reading this book simply because of the unusually wide range of bioethical issues it addresses. They will finish it not merely much better informed bioethically but also inspired to put their deepest convictions and values to work on the great bioethical challenges of today and tomorrow.”

John F. Kilner, director, Bioethics Program, and Forman Chair of Ethics and Theology, Trinity International University

“Dr. Thobaben’s book offers keen insight into the complex bioethical issues facing our culture and our church. His work adds richly to our conversations about healing, death and eternal life.”

Bishop Lindsey Davis, Louisville Episcopal Area, United Methodist Church

“In this book, Jim Thobaben offers even more than the title promises. This book is not just a comprehensive Christian resource on health-care ethics, but is instead a primer in theological anthropology that then leads to profound reflections on bioethics. The book is rich at every level—biblically, theologically, philosophically and ecclesiologically. Thobaben demonstrates wide reading, mastery of a great breadth of material and precision in argumentation. One does not have to agree with every argument made in this substantial book to appreciate its significance. With this book, Jim Thobaben has established himself as a major evangelical voice in theological bioethics.”

David P. Gushee, Distinguished University Professor of Christian Ethics, Mercer University

"Jim Thobaben has provided a valuable resource for helping readers reflect on Scripture and think about the myriad moral dimensions of health care from the perspective of Christian faith. In a society where many of our definitions of 'good life' are mediated through biotechnologies and what we can do, Thobaben helps us sort through options for more faithful responsibilities and responses in order to understand what we should do to embody the gospel of Christ and serve the holistic needs of humanity. This is a very timely book for classrooms and congregations given the importance of bioethics and in light of our current social debates."

Dr. Wyndy Corbin Reuschling, professor of ethics and theology,
Ashland Theological Seminary

"Dr. Jim Thobaben has done a masterful job of weaving together a tapestry of threads, including ethical analysis, theology, biblical studies and moral practice. *Health-Care Ethics* has been written by a master teacher and practitioner resulting in a text that is not only engaging but pertinent to the lives of those who read it."

James W. Holsinger Jr., Wethington Endowed Chair in the Health Sciences,
University of Kentucky

HEALTH-CARE ETHICS

A Comprehensive Christian Resource

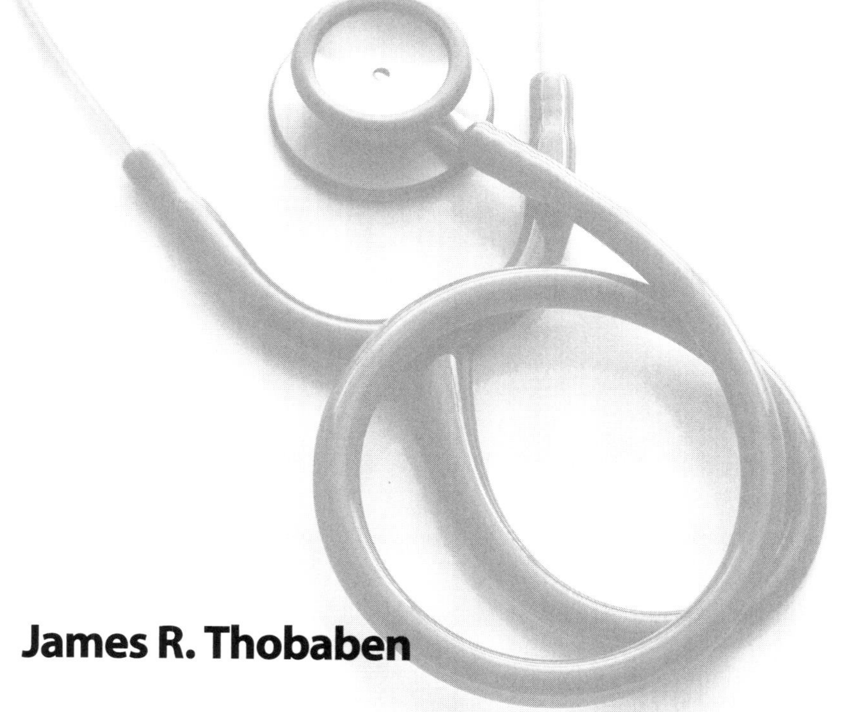

James R. Thobaben

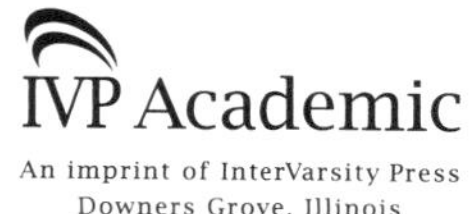

IVP Academic
An imprint of InterVarsity Press
Downers Grove, Illinois

InterVarsity Press
P.O. Box 1400, Downers Grove, IL 60515-1426
World Wide Web: www.ivpress.com
Email: email@ivpress.com

InterVarsity Press® is the book-publishing division of InterVarsity Christian Fellowship/USA®, a movement of students and faculty active on campus at hundreds of universities, colleges and schools of nursing in the United States of America, and a member movement of the International Fellowship of Evangelical Students. For information about local and regional activities, write Public Relations Dept., InterVarsity Christian Fellowship/USA, 6400 Schroeder Rd., P.O. Box 7895, Madison, WI 53707-7895, or visit the IVCF website at *<www.intervarsity.org>.*

Design: Cindy Kiple

Images: syringe: Yong Hian Lim/iStockphoto
stethoscope: David Muir/Getty Images

ISBN 978-0-8308-2673-5

Printed in the United States of America ∞

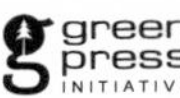

InterVarsity Press is committed to protecting the environment and to the responsible use of natural resources. As a member of Green Press Initiative we use recycled paper whenever possible. To learn more about the Green Press Initiative, visit <www.greenpressinitiative.org>.

Library of Congress Cataloging-in-Publication Data

Thobaben, James R., 1954-
Health-care ethics: a comprehensive Christian resource / James R. Thobaben.
p. cm.
Includes bibliographical references and indexes.
ISBN 978-0-8308-2673-5 (pbk.: alk. paper)
1. Medical ethics—Religious aspects—Christianity. 2. Christian ethics. I. Title.
R725.56.T46 2009
174.2—dc22

2009021604

P 22 21 20 19 18 17 16 15 14 13 12 11 10 9 8 7 6 5 4 3 2 1
Y 27 26 25 24 23 22 21 20 19 18 17 16 15 14 13 12 11 10 09

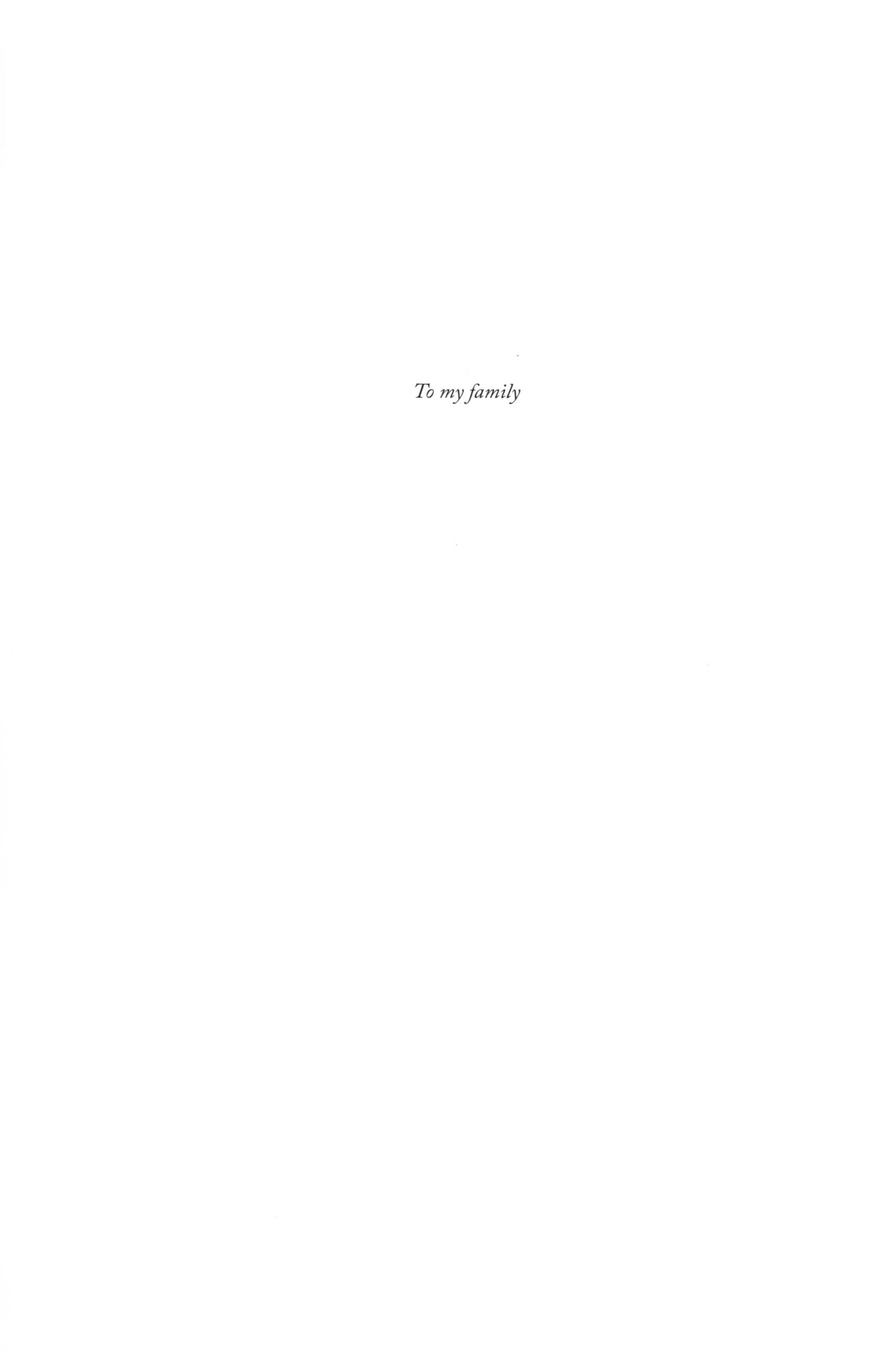

To my family

Contents

Preface

For a follower of Jesus Christ, writing a work that calls for specific moral conduct and judges the behaviors of others to be correct or incorrect is spiritually awkward. Certainly there are immature believers who presume to speak from their own purported purity and there may be the occasional prophet who proclaims particular words in particular times that are clearly from God. The latter is not a claim I make, and I hope I am not manifesting the former. In other words, regardless of how others may "feel" about ethical declaration, I have a great sense of self-consciousness. After all, I have been saved by grace, and that is not my own doing; therefore, I have nothing of which to boast except the mercy of God.

I came to God through several events in high school, college and seminary. While sitting behind my house in my early years, I intellectually concluded that it was rational, or more precisely not irrational, to believe in God. Later I discovered Pascal and others made this argument, but it was refreshing and enlightening to me. Though I had a family tradition of singing hymns and attending church, a friend who was part of the Jesus movement helped initiate my more rigorous consideration of spiritual matters. In the early 1970s he took me to a Billy Graham Crusade where I heard for the first time (or the first time I remember) that Jesus was the full *and* exclusive incarnation of God. Yet, it was not the Jesus movement counterculture but the dominant youth culture (that masqueraded as a counterculture) that was most influential morally. So, in college I held an intellectual belief in Christ, but lived fully within the baby boomer generation, holding at least some degree of genuine sociopolitical concern while indulging in self-righteous indignation and pubescent angst. My first years at college were simply an expression of irresponsibility. Then, during my junior year, I experienced an epiphany. One winter night, while walking through a building on campus, I was suddenly struck with the necessity of having Jesus as my Lord, not just an abstract representation of Christianity. This was not an experience of the "Christness of the universe" or the "mystery of God" in some generic sense, but a confrontation with the living One who had dwelt on the earth as one of us. I realized Jesus expected to be Lord of anyone who claimed to affirm him as God. And if that was the case, then so be it.

Though my behaviors did not absolutely and completely change, they were immediately altered in a manner that allowed me, by the Spirit, to discard—some quickly, some over time—inappropriate habits and tendencies. With this change, many of my friends fell away, or more precisely, I began to fall away from them. To this day, I regret never apologizing to them if my hypocritical Christian example hurt them or led them away from the One. Further, I was still so spiritually immature that I did not seek out a strong Christian community, which meant I had no significant encouragement or accountability. The only Christian community I had was the "cloud of witnesses" as I started to read various works of Jonathan Edwards, John Wesley and Søren Kierkegaard.

Soon, I realized that for me submission to God included a calling into ministry, so I applied to seminary. I chose Yale for no particular reason beyond the name. This was the hand of Providence. Though Yale had no expectation of doctrinal orthodoxy, the Yale faculty honestly noted that historical Christianity had been trinitarian and dependent on the idea that grace was dispensed through the presence of God on earth as Jesus of Nazareth (though some faculty thought it was wrong). My roommate, who was going through the same process of theological clarification, and I often discussed how to understand our faith. The result was that I (and he) became clearly doctrinally orthodox at Yale and began to self-identify as an evangelical in the Wesleyan tradition, one who asserted the need to express the relationship with God in correct understanding and in personal holiness and social service.

My doctrinal and ethical position was solidified by my marriage to a woman who had traveled from high Episcopalian through New Age religion into Pentecostal holiness Protestantism. It was further reinforced in raising children, as the values one holds are either validated or negated by how one treats, teaches and sets an example for the young over whom one is responsible. Wesleyan evangelicalism remains the position to which I adhere and is, no doubt, expressed in this book.

Nonbelievers who read this work should feel free to ascribe my religious transformation to the following sociological and psychological arguments:

- Family of origin: *I was raised in a family that was nominally Christian.*
- Cultural linguistic: *I accepted the value grammar of my "tribe."*

- Neo-Freudian: *I lost an ego integration conflict to the superego, with a seemingly excessive response to guilt and shame.*
- Reductionist humanism ("Scientism," particularly its harsher forms from Nietzsche through Thomas Huxley, Herbert Spencer, and, more recently, Richard Dawkins and Peter Singer): *My religiousness is indicative of intellectual and personal weakness that "should" be selected out evolutionarily.*
- Popular humanism: *I needed to be justified and was not able to find self-esteem.*

No doubt, there are other reasons that can be used to explain away faith.

I do not deny that some of these may have been partial factors in my life. I did have Christian models to use. I did have a moral language to use, and I have certainly attempted to teach the same to my children. I did feel guilty and I was ashamed. Further, I was too weak to do anything about it. I did believe I needed a justification—a purpose—beyond myself. And, I do deny that even if those were factors they in any way negate the reality of God.

These "explanations" elevated to the status of worldviews may partially explain away my choices and behaviors to those who find reductionist metanarratives sufficient intellectually and existentially. I do not find them compelling. Rather, the lives of those I have known—in particular those marked by humility, service, gentleness, confidence and kindness—have led me to conclude that life has purpose only if there is a Purpose-Giver, and I am not capable of filling that role for myself.

Since that epiphany and my acceptance of what in my faith tradition is labeled a *call* into ministry, I have been blessed and privileged to serve as a local pastor, as a seminary professor, and as a clinical ethicist and chaplain. To those of the various communities I have served or of which I have otherwise been a part, I offer the following apologies and declarations of appreciation:

- I know the many failures of my past and realize my potential for failing in the future. No Christian should enter into the analysis of morality, especially when dealing with nonbelievers, with any pride or arrogance. Pascal said that "true religion would have to teach greatness and wretchedness, inspire self-esteem and self-contempt, love and hate."[1] Metaphorically, then, I turn away from the altar rail and ask all those against whom I have sinned, with malice or through a lack of concern, to forgive me. If those sins are old, my hope in Christ is that they have not had any harsh impact. If those sins are recent, then I am willing to be held accountable by those

[1]Pascal *Pensées* # 450

of the faith. I am well aware of my sins of the past and beg forgiveness from any I have offended.

- I am also well aware of my current weaknesses and take responsibility for any mistakes in my ministry generally and in this manuscript in particular.
- In the work on this book, fellow believers have proved invaluable. Though my failures are my own, my successes have come, always, with the support of others.
- Specifically:
    - For years of working together on various projects, including this one, I want to thank Rev. Bruns Myers from the Mississippi Methodist Rehabilitation Center (MMRC). It has always been a blessing to have a brother in Christ with whom to work and, even on occasion, to play. Bruns can take credit for the good things in at least one chapter of this book. Specifically, Bruns and I together developed the material on the ordinal understanding of autonomy in chapter 13.
    - I want to thank my other friends at MMRC, especially Mark Adams, the C.E.O. who hired me as an "ethicist" and, *in memoriam*, Earl Wilson, the founding trustee chair, and to all who set an example of industriousness.
    - I want to thank my brothers and sisters at Asbury Theological Seminary. In particular, Joel Green for a conference he coordinated, Christine Pohl (the other professor of social ethics on the Wilmore campus) for long conversations, Joe Dongell for discussions about the personal impact of the health-care system, Jim Holsinger for hours working on the morality of financing health care, Jerry Walls for calling for philosophical precision, and Tapiwa Mucherera for copastoring and for long talks about the interface of bioethics and pastoral care. Also, to Isaac Hopper and David Lilley who helped so much with the initial proofreading.
    - Without question, I want to thank my students and administrators, especially in the various bioethics classes at Asbury Theological Seminary, Trinity International and at University of Kentucky, College of Public Health. They are too numerous to mention by name and should I attempt, I would certainly leave out someone who had been helpful.
    - The Bioethics Working Group for the 2005 meeting of the Lausanne Committee on World Evangelism. Special thanks to Brian Edgar for

the time together when he came to Asbury for sabbatical. And very special thanks to John Kilner for his leadership with Lausanne and at the Center for Bioethics and Human Dignity and for providing me the opportunity to teach at Trinity.

> The Molecular Biology Program and the Agricultural Economics Department at the University of Missouri, for the opportunity to serve as Visiting Ethics Scholar and to work on the subject of genetic modification of nonhuman organisms. Especially to Michael Roberts, Don Riddle, Mark McIntosh, Nick Kalaitzandonakes, Steve Matthews, Phil Peters, Lutine Hartley and Ginny Booker who, likely, would disagree with portions or all of this work, but still were so very gracious in conversation.

> The people of Mt. Zion—all the students and particular thanks to the "community members." You got your money's worth, or better, I hope.

> Likewise, to the people who are my Christian friends in Kazakhstan. You constantly remind me that all Christians are called to minister to the broken. Were it not for your gentle love, your ongoing witness of service would make me ashamed of myself.

> The patient people at InterVarsity Press.

> Melissa Waugh for proofreading with a legal eye and a public health perspective, though she may well not share some of the opinions herein suggested.

> As far as just "talking" about the impact of moral decision making on how we live our lives, I suppose, excepting my family, two people have had to hear more from me than any others. My friends in ministry have been a continuing source of spiritual guidance and advice about the reality of bioethical issues in the parish. I want to thank Karl Stonebraker for proofreading and for countless conversations in canoes, on hiking trails and on the Camino de Santiago. Similarly, Rod Buchanan must be thanked for proofreading and because his questions keep me thinking and his determination kept Karl and me from simply goofing around in the wilderness instead of actually traveling down the path (any spiritual metaphors are accidental). I thank them.

> I need to thank my father, my mother *(in memoriam)* and my biological brothers. Through their own injuries and illnesses and responses to the same, they introduced me to the complexity of health care and to the

importance of kindness among those who suffer. And special thanks to my father for help with the farm.

- Finally and most significantly, it would be difficult for me to overstate how thankful I am to God for my wife and children. Marcelyn is my love and my fellow sojourner on the path of holiness, which we have traveled always with joy and usually with happiness. My children, Zechariah, a pediatric dentist (and his wife, Rebekah Adele), and Anna Rebecca, an anesthesiologist (and her husband, Josh), have been a true blessing. Many fathers can say that they have always loved their children, but I can truly say I like them as friends, as equals. I also need to thank six other family members: Diana Rutiba, Tim Wingerter, Kenyon and Tierre Williams, and Kuda and Simba Kagoro. They were under our guardianship (legal or informal) for extended periods during their teenage years and they remain, to greater or lesser extents, woven into the fabric of our home.
- I need to thank and acknowledge others in the academic field of bioethics. Persons with whom I have had discussions or by whom I have been influenced through their writings are too numerous to mention. Still, I should note that academics will find commonalities with the following:
    - My tendency to distinguish strongly between Christian ethics and non-Christian ethics is paralleled in two books by T. Engelhardt.
    - My strong emphasis on the obligations of the believer, especially as patient, within and to the community of faith is not dissimilar to that described by S. Hauerwas.
    - My emphasis on American contractarian thought is in some ways similar to J. Rawls and in others to M. Walzer.
    - My understanding of the obligations of individual believers as they practice caregiving has some similarity to that described by W. May and E. Pellegrino.
    - My emphasis on the role of the local church and the necessity for non-professional ethicists within the body of believers to learn and engage society is similar to that of my friends J. Kilner and D. Hollinger.

Needless to say, these various thinkers might well disagree strongly with large portions of this work and the peculiar combination of these characteristics. Perhaps none would like my emphasis on moral learning through the sermon, which is not drawn from any other particular ethicist.

For Christians, obligations spring from receiving grace and those obligations extend beyond the faith community. I am duty-bound to serve those of the world by (1) in a small way replicating God's kindness to me, (2) witnessing and (3) advocating and serving justice and mercy, which is a component of God's character and ours as his children. Consequently, I hope, that by God's grace, some part of this work may be useful for those who follow the Christ, but also for those who want to understand why Christians (specifically evangelical Christians) respond to bioethical issues as they do.

Peace in the One who is and was and is to come.

James R. Thobaben
April 2009

Introduction

On some matters of social ethics Christians are able to provide a precise understanding of the issues based on Scripture and/or community tradition, but this is not always true when new concerns arise. In particular, with issues in bioethics, specific scriptural direction is not always to be found in the Text.[1] This is further complicated for believers when needing to "get along" with those of the world in a particular setting (that is, with those who are not Christians but fellow residents of morally complex communities). Still, for the evangelical, *bioethics* is a subset of moral living, one that can be interpreted with biblically described virtues and vices.

Sometimes believers become vulnerable to moral carelessness and want the quickest moral answer in order to either work with or conflict with those of the world. When a clear path for moral action is not readily discovered, believers may abandon Christian values because of uncertainty about application, favoring some clearer position based on supposedly more fundamental "human" principles, or social convention. At best, this is done under the assumption that standards are established by general revelation or natural law. At worst, there is an appropriation of the world's standards without serious consideration of Christian values.

It is equally problematic when some believers use simplistic rules, sometimes called a cookie-cutter approach, by imposing preexisting Christian moral categories or rules in circumstances for which they do not apply and on people for whom such categories make little or no sense. At best, this allows a

[1]Verhey notes: "There is, for one thing, the *silence* of Scripture about bioethics. Scripture simply does not speak of the new powers of medicine or the new moral problems that they pose. . . . The Bible simply does not answer many of the questions that new medical powers have forced us to ask. The authors of the Scripture, even the most visionary of them, never dreamt of these new powers, and it is folly to 'search the Scriptures' looking for them" (Allen Verhey, *Reading the Bible in the Strange World of Medicine* [Grand Rapids: Eerdmans, 2003], p. 35).

Verhey is correct in a specific sense and to this extent, the Scripture is silent directly; but, as noted in the body of this chapter, the epistemological expectations of evangelicals require that the Text be used in defining, even if only analogically, core moral issues. Verhey would likely agree, at least to some extent.

quick response at moments of crises. At worst, it eliminates needed careful analysis in emerging fields of ethics.

Believers must acknowledge that when new circumstances call for new moral considerations, they must base their final decisions on and live their lives in light of the relationship they have with God through Jesus Christ, yet with the hope that various points may be found for common action with those of the world. The Christian, in seeking the eternal good (true virtue), may be satisfied to some degree when proximate goods are obtained or earthly moral ends are met while cooperating with those of the world. The virtuosity of the Christian life should not be any different now than in the past, though the specific expressions may vary with circumstances and values of the societies in which they live.

The purpose of this work, then, is threefold:

1. To provide believers with Christian models for making decisions in bioethics and shaping behavior in life sciences and health care.
2. To assist Christians in finding language that can be used with those of the world in reaching agreement on common, proximate moral concerns.
3. To help those of the world to understand Christian, specifically evangelical Christian, morality.

The chapters of this work are arranged in a pattern not unlike the Sunday morning sermon that is addressing a specific community concern, so that

- core Christian moral understandings are drawn from Scripture;
- an evangelical Christian interpretation of a current bioethical concern is offered in light of that core understanding;
- a "translation" of this Christian position into language usable by Christians operating in the arenas of the world, and by those of the world who have to engage evangelical believers, is provided.

The first task of Christian bioethics is *not* to enter into extensive ethical discussions with those of the world, but to determine from within the Christian community what relationships define, which virtues inform, and what principles guide any moral analysis. Then the believer may draw conclusions consistent with the Christian faith regarding moral matters of health care and the life sciences. The believer can then translate those conclusions for the world for the purpose of cooperating in non-Christian settings.

Among evangelical Christians, the primary source of moral analysis and conversation is not, as might be expected by academics—the scholarly study of Barth, or Ramsey, or Schaeffer, or even Calvin or Wesley. Generally, these are not nearly as important to evangelicals as C. S. Lewis, Billy Graham, John Stott and even the devotional author Oswald Chambers. Not "pure" academics, but popularizers and pastors provide the basic moral guidance for the community through readily accessible moral analysis. This is not usually done out of intellectual laziness, but because evangelicalism is a movement that emphasizes the simplicity of the message. Protestantism generally, and evangelicalism specifically, is a leveling religion. It is to be expected, then, that the vast majority of moral analysis within the evangelical community occurs not in the classroom or in scholarly papers, but in the congregation listening to a sermon, in the small-group fellowship and between individual believers.

The closest parallel from another religious community is Rabbinic Judaism with the emphasis on Scripture distinctly understood within its own community, past voices being given precedent, but the uniqueness of contemporary concerns requiring renewed dialogue. Finally, after the community and the individual decide how to act, the individuals and community enter into conversation with those outside that community. In comparison, evangelicals are likely to cite a short story or parable of Jesus' ministry, discuss it with other believers, then draw from it specific commands or inferences for moral guidance.[2]

Admittedly, some evangelical academics construct their ethical arguments using deductive philosophical approaches. This is usually done on the basis of some principle or two, presumably thought to be found in the Text or based on natural law or general revelation, which then leads to various conclusions. However, the best reading of the Scripture is not in part, but as a whole. If the language of principles is to be used, then multiple principles should be recognized. These, which are more observations of what the story of redemption contains than principles in a philosophical sense, can be drawn together more inductively than deductively, as an expression or working out of the gospel story in the lives of individuals and communities.

Recently, perhaps in rebellion against reductionist deductive approaches, some evangelicals have asserted the need to "contextualize" using sociopsychological arguments. They claim that new understandings have emerged. Such might reasonably be claimed for bioethics, but great care must be taken

---

[2]The Jewish parallel is described well in Scott B. Rae and Paul M. Cox, *Bioethics: A Christian Approach in a Pluralistic Age* (Grand Rapids: Eerdmans, 1999), pp. 36-38.

not to assert the need for new examinations in order to justify discarding the old. Aside from the fact that this is demonstrably not consistent with the gospel that uses both the old and the new, it sometimes borders on the edge of hubris even while providing an important critique. The usefulness of such an approach is that it takes into account new issues, such as some of those in bioethics. In addition, the use of contemporary non-Christian language is useful in translating Christian values to the unbelieving world. Still, "contextualizing" is not ethically sufficient reasoning.

In actual practice the primary reasoning method used by most evangelicals is analogical. Each Sunday in virtually every evangelical pulpit, scriptural stories are read, considered in their original context and then applied to contemporary concerns—evangelistic or ethical. There is no reason for those in the evangelical community who are more seriously engaged in ethical analysis not to do the same. With bioethics this is particularly true, given the paucity of direct reference in the Text to bioethical issues and the significant disagreements about such in society at large. This primary reasoning method is not unlike that used with Hassidic storytelling or even some of Aesop's and Philo's allegories. It should come as no surprise given the approach of Christ and, in particular, his use of narrative.

The story of Jesus as the Christ uniquely explains the fundamental relationship between God and humanity, and how that relationship should come to define all other relationships. These cannot be reduced to specific worship patterns, doctrinal proclamations or ethical injunctions, but can be expressed in them. As is sometimes said among evangelicals, one does not so much make the Christ story a part of one's life as make one's life a part of the Christ story. As such, to the believer, this true story is uniquely authoritative.

The core doctrines, the worship and the morality of Christianity center on the salvation narrative. The most important creed, the Nicene Creed, is a distilled telling of the offering of Jesus Christ. When recited with "I believe . . . " or "We believe . . . ," it becomes more than a statement of historical fact, but a statement of the source of the believer's salvation. Similarly, the central rituals of Christianity are retellings of the life of Jesus Christ with the believer inserted into the story as a participant. Likewise, Christian ethics are, or should be, an adaptation of one's life to the story by acting in conformance to the life of the Lord.

Analogically, the church is like a guild to which one is drawn, and in which a convert is apprenticed in the doctrinal beliefs, the morality and the worship practices of the faith relationship. Or the convert is like an adopted child who learns the grammar of morality, the pattern of worship and the lessons of doctrine of his or her spiritual family. Or the convert is like an immigrant immersed in a new national culture, adopting with fervor the values of the new homeland that she or he had admired from afar. Or using an analogy pertinent in bioethics, the believer is like a physician who needs an internship and residence under the supervision of a more experienced practitioner to develop skills in moral diagnosis and treatment. These are only similes, metaphors and analogues for the actual process of living within *the* faith relationship.

As a simple practicality, then, Christian ethics can genuinely be expressed only from within the community of faith and, then, directed toward the world. Therefore, it is incumbent on believers, as part of the faith community, to be as informed as possible about issues they may need to address. In the West at the end of modernity, this certainly includes the arena of bioethics. Believers, then, need models that are coherent with Scripture and in accord with appropriate traditional interpretations of Scripture while being informed (but not governed) by information that is accessible to both the faithful and those of the world (i.e., "facts" of history, sociology, psychology, the natural sciences, etc.).

Using the Scripture in this way, Christians acknowledge the final inadequacy of moral constructs based on anything but Jesus Christ. What he said and what he did is the foundation of truly right and good moral action. This means that while important matters—for instance, cost, individual rights, aversion to pain and so on—may be properly taken into account, they cannot be allowed moral preeminence within the community of faith. Rather, individual believers involved in bioethical analysis—and this means everyone from family members making decisions for themselves and their loved ones, to researchers studying genetic modification of nonhuman organisms, to practitioners determining which technologies might serve both the needs of the patient and the treatment funder—must recognize that their decisions are not isolated from the community of faith, commitment to Christ and belief that he is Lord. Christianity, after all, is a religion based on relationship: first with God, then with other believers and then with all those who are made in the image of that saving God.

Three levels of analysis correspond to these three levels of relationship and are needed for Christians to engage in contemporary bioethics. Using all three allows one to remain true to the gospel and make positions understandable for constructive exchange with the world.

- Core Christian moral understandings are represented in the stories of the gospel narrative.
- Evangelical Christians can interpret these to obtain guidance about contemporary moral concerns, including those in bioethics.
- "Translation" of Christian positions can be made using the languages of the world, including philosophy and the social sciences.

For the evangelical Christian, relationships with God, other believers and those of the world are interactions of ongoing obligation. The obligations arise out of a categorical duty to God, that is, they are deontological. These relationships are shapers of virtue in that they are the pattern of imitating Christ. And they are actions that will lead to the best ultimate outcome, thus serving the utility of the divine economy.

Any number of persons can use this book, including ministers or teachers for preaching or instructing within the church and Christian laypersons involved in health care. Also, this book can assist nonbelievers to better understand how evangelical Christians tend to think about the morality of health issues. The book is structured with two broad sections. Part one, "The Theological and Ethical Nature of Evangelicals," includes chapters one through three. The second broad section addresses characteristics of all humans and how those are expressed in bioethical debates. Part two, "Characteristics of Humanity and Bioethical Debates," includes chapters four through seventeen. To be true to the ethical method, each includes three main sections: "Part One: The Text" considers the biblical passages; "Part Two: Christian Bioethics" makes observations about the Christian life and health care; "Part Three: Christian Bioethics and the World" then applies these observations in non-Christian bioethical settings. Perhaps one could call these observations principles of evangelical ethics, or core values, but the empirical process is more akin to engaging the story of the Text and then determining how it can be lived out.

Each chapter addresses specific bioethical topics. In addressing these topics, the primary purpose is to lay the foundation for approaching the moral concerns rather than to provide final resolution of those concerns. This is contrary to most bioethics works, which focus on particular topics or emphasize cases. These are appropriate approaches, but to understand evangelical morality it is necessary to first understand the ethical operation of the individual believer in the community of the faithful.

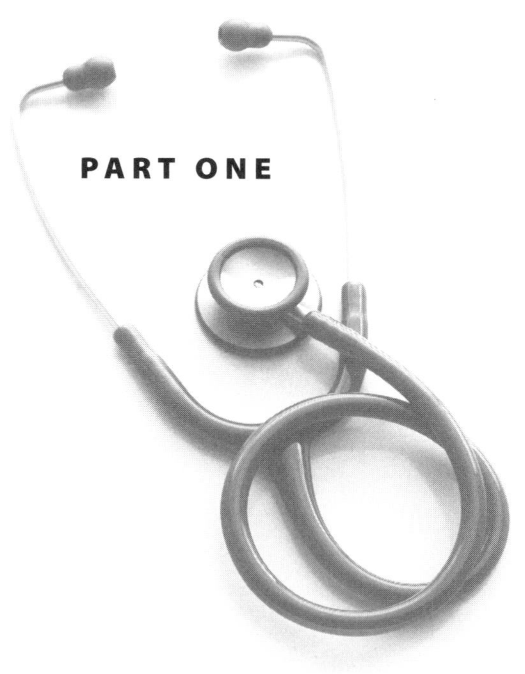

PART ONE

The Theological and Ethical Nature of Evangelical Faith

1

Evangelicals in the World

Evangelicals must function in societies that may be more or less tolerant of their beliefs. In the late modern West there is an increasing effort to silence religion in public discourse. Evangelicals should reject this call, even while agreeing that there should be strong separation of church and state. This means that evangelicals must develop their own ethical understandings of social concerns and have their own standards for the behavior of believers. They, then, must have the capacity to make their positions understandable for others engaged in social discourse.

Human life is good—flawed, but good.

Human life is good in at least three senses. First, it is good to experience living. Of course, suicides, both self-inflicted active euthanasia, and those not specifically associated with the deterioration of physical health, indicate that not everyone experiences this sensation of goodness. Still, the struggle of almost all living things, including humans, to continue earthly existence seems to warrant the claim that being biologically alive is generally perceived positively.

Second, people can be morally good. Though, as Jesus clearly pointed out, in the absolute sense "no one is good—except God alone" (Mk 10:18; Lk 18:19), individuals (and their communities) can be more or less relatively good. To some, such language is difficult as it asserts there is some standard of evaluation and that persons can move toward that standard. Yet, with the exception of true nihilists all persons act as if some choices and some behaviors are ethically preferable to others.

Third, and perhaps most importantly, individual humans are not morally neutral entities. Rather, each can and should be recognized as a being of value. Some sociopolitical groups can clearly be defined as oriented toward evil, and some individuals seem bent toward injuring others and themselves. Still, though all people fail to be good at some times or even most times, every one of them has worth. Human life matters. It matters to other people because individuals are, for others, means to ends. Also, they are ends in themselves. This is the claim of Christians, and to a greater or lesser degree is the claim of most societies at the end of modernity.[1] For Christians, finally, this claim is made because humans matter to God.

Generally, then, efforts to improve the spiritual and physical condition of persons, including the effort called health care, are morally desirable for the sake of all three types of the "goodness" of humans. This does not mean that any actual practice of health care might not be flawed, even while health care generally is a moral good. Nor does it mean that those who render care are inevitably virtuous. Nor does it mean that individuals who seek the services of those giving such care are doing so for morally appropriate reasons. Still, care-giving and care-receiving are moral goods; sometimes demanded by justice, sometimes as expressions of the merciful character of the individual or community, sometimes as an expression of personal purity, and sometimes all three.

According to evangelicals, the right and good are genuinely possible for believers, by God's grace. This means that right and good are sufficiently, even if not entirely, knowable to those who stand in need of knowing them for the purpose of moral action. A favorite verse of evangelicals is 1 Corinthians 10:13: "No temptation has seized you except what is common to man. And God is faithful; he will not let you be tempted beyond what you can bear. But when you are tempted, he will also provide a way out so that you can stand up under it." The ethical implication is that Christians can understand well enough what God expects so that they can, relying on his strength, act accordingly. Not surprisingly, then, the vast majority of moral analysis within the evangelical community occurs not in the classroom or in scholarly papers, but in the congregation listening to a sermon, in the small-group fellowship, and between individual believers.

Still, though Christian morality is always first of all *Christian*, it does over-

---

[1]Of course, not all who might enter into the American discourse on bioethics would share the belief that humans are moral goods. For instance, various supporters of strong animal rights (e.g., PETA, advocates of "deep ecology" and Singerian utilitarians), reductionists (i.e., those who assert that humans have no existential worth since no meaning can be posited given the purely naturalistic essence of human beings), and strong elitists (i.e., those who hold to Nietschean-like or social Darwinist arguments) might disagree. On the other hand, some have argued for the human as moral good, but only as a pooled group, thus offering a sort of optimist view of humanity, but not of all persons (e.g., some crass utilitarians and Marxists). Interestingly, evangelical Christians share with many so-called secular humanists and some socialists the belief that individual humans are moral goods. Evangelicals, however, do not agree that humans are intrinsically morally good: "All have sinned and fall short of the glory of God" (Rom 3:23). The "means-end" language is Kantian.

lap at points with the morality of the world. To use an example from daily life, the believer makes the moral choice to obey traffic laws. Of course, some might assert such is simply adherence to the requirement for such obedience in Romans 13. Yet, Christians do not blindly obey, they agree with these laws. In doing so, the follower of Christ is declaring that the state is to be obeyed (unless such obedience is fundamentally contrary to the gospel). The believer is also declaring that human life has value, for while traffic laws exist to minimize aggravation and to help with economic development, they exist first and foremost because human life has been deemed *of value.* This is a moral claim and it is a claim expressed by believers and nonbelievers alike when they cooperatively develop and then obey traffic laws. Of course, most immediately, such obedience may arise from a desire to avoid a traffic citation or higher insurance rates, but these too are based finally on some valuing of human life. These are agreed to by Christians and those of the world on the basis of different fundamental claims, but shared assertions, that human life matters and that the State should be obeyed unless there is a good reason not to do so.

Obedience to traffic laws does not require much thought on the part of believers. Still, it is a specific moral cooperation with those of the world that is not in its particulars required by Scripture. Indeed, it would be absurd to suggest that the Scripture provides specific instructions on following traffic laws. No Scriptures refer to octagonal, red signs requiring *stop* nor yellow flashing lights encouraging *caution.* Likewise, some other moral interactions with the world, far more complicated ones, lack specific scriptural instruction. Nowhere is this more evident than in the arenas of the applied biological sciences. As Christians live within the world and interact with those who are not of the faith and do not want to be, they must at times work with nonbelievers toward common proximate moral ends.

Sometimes Christians in health care will cooperate with those of the world, sometimes actively oppose them, and sometimes simply tolerate actions. Not surprisingly, abortion, euthanasia and eugenic genetic engineering are points of significant conflict. Yet, that does not mean understanding and even some cooperation on health-care concerns are impossible. Regardless of the specific foundational variation, in the West at the end of modernity, most people seem to think that humans as individuals have worth. To use language common to social ethics, the assertion that humans have worth is a middle axiom.[2] In

[2]The term is now in common usage; it appears in works by William Temple, J. H. Oldham and

other words, regardless of the foundational reason, the basic moral principle is shared. This is particularly significant for bioethics. In fact, though it may not always be readily acknowledged, the concept of health care only makes sense if it assumes that the individual person is a *good,* that individual life matters. For Christians this should be obvious, but it is also a point of agreement with most other people.

Some evangelicals, if the term is used broadly, would assert that this minimal commonality does not mean the church and committed believers should participate in the world's politics (in both the informal and formal sense of that word). Aversion to the institutional politics surrounding health-care organizations on matters like abortion, euthanasia and the use of generic pharmaceuticals should be respected as it can be morally legitimated using both the history of the early church and the Text, and it remains the basic position of conservative Anabaptists and some in stricter Holiness churches.

If the faith community, though, makes the choice to engage the broader society, it is not enough to simply understand its own positions on moral issues. It must attempt to understand the moral positions of those in the world. In order to participate in discussions in the civil arenas (from hospital hallway decisions in secular medical centers to political debate), Christians must understand the secular language. Further, it facilitates cooperation (when such is possible) for Christians to "engage" using secular ethical terms and reasoning. This means, as a matter of practice, evangelical Christians should defend the idea that public forums ought to be available to those holding any moral perspective (at least any that is not genuinely, immediately and violently destructive to the social foundations). Such is desirable for the church in protecting itself from persecution and in providing freedom to those of the world to accept or reject Christ. This does not mean Christians believe that all moral positions are equally valid or should be tolerated to equal degrees.[3]

John Bennett. Their use of the term is not as expansive as here, especially the above use that asserts these can be drawn on the basis of various philosophies.

[3]The dominant interpretive model is "inclusive/exclusive/pluralistic," developed by Alan Race, *Christians and Religious Pluralism: Patterns in Christian Theology of Religions* (Maryknoll, N.Y.: Orbis Books, 1983). These distinctions can be applied to a single evangelical approach that is exclusive on central doctrine and basic ethics, while pluralistic on some issues (e.g., baptism) and inclusive on others (e.g., worship styles). See also Terry Muck, "Instrumentality, Complexity and Reason: A Christian Apporach to Religions," *Buddhist-Christian Studies* 22 (2002): 115-21; Lesslie Newbigin, *The Gospel in a Pluralistic Society* (Grand Rapids: Eerdmans, 1989); and Bernard T. Adeney, *Strange Virtues: Ethics in a Multicultural World* (Downers Grove, Ill.: InterVarsity Press, 1995).

The faithful cannot give up any core moral belief in the name of expediency. For evangelicals, as for all social groups, moral issues have frequently and appropriately been boundary shaping. Sometimes this leads to some degree of intolerance for those of the world and sometimes even disfellowship of Christians who align themselves too much with the morality of the unbelieving culture. In at least some situations this intolerance is not only morally understandable, but strongly preferable. Two examples are the abolition of slavery and prolife/antiabortion advocacy.

Learning from and cooperating with those of the world is limited by the foundational claims of the gospel, yet this is not as great a restriction as some believers may think. Taking the moral life seriously means taking living in the world seriously. While there may be times and places that require believers to come out from and be totally separate from those who do not follow the Lord, this is not the pattern established for the normal Christian life.

People tend to analyze, especially their opponents, in nominal terms—yes/no, good/bad, on/off. Either one is or is not an ally, with being an ally requiring full agreement simply because there is no "in between." Jesus, after all, said, "He who is not with me is against me, and he who does not gather with me scatters" (Mt 12:30). Being a Christian, being in the vital relationship with God through Christ, is either-or; one either is a Christian or one is not.

Yet, the Christ also said, "No one who does a miracle in my name can in the next moment say anything bad about me, for whoever is not against us is for us. I tell you the truth, anyone who gives you a cup of water in my name because you belong to Christ will certainly not lose his reward" (Mk 9:39-41). A similar verse is found in Luke: "'Do not stop him,' Jesus said, 'for whoever is not against you is for you'" (Lk 9:50). The Matthean passage and a parallel verse in Luke are different: "He who is not with me is against me, and he who does not gather with me, scatters" (Lk 11:23; see also Mt 12:30).

In other words, some issues and some relationships are more complex than is revealed by the use of nominal terms. For example, analysis by the dominant media and by the spokespersons of the American political system, especially during the height of the presidential election cycle, is so simplistic in its use of nominal analysis that it becomes deceptive. Sadly, evangelicals have not always been known for their subtle analysis of moral variation, and often criticisms are well founded. It is important that those of the faith discern what is and what is not "either-or," and then properly distinguish appropriate degrees of tolerance for those matters that are more complex.

"[T]olerance is not the same thing as affirmation."[4] To the contrary, one tolerates that which one considers wrong, but chooses to not act coercively because of a greater good. Toleration is not affirming whatever someone does on the basis of moral subjectivity. Tolerance is not a sort of utilitarianism either. Tolerance is moral rejection of an act or attitude without acting to prevent another from acting or holding that attitude, except possibly through persuasion.

The issue of tolerance is further complicated as it must be applied differently within the church and outside, for instance with alcohol intoxication and homosexual behavior. The person acting in a particular way as one in the body of believers or as one outside calls the Christian to different types of toleration with two different epistemological approaches and two types of moral analysis. Toward those of the world, there should be high tolerance. Christians should be willing to accept much of the immorality of those in the world, though tolerance should never become approval of the moral behavior. Christians can even advocate for social standards that ostracize and shame the grossly immoral, but should not support the deprivation of liberty by the state for such, unless there is genuine and significant danger. In other words, to use social contract language, people have the right to be immoral—unless that immorality injures another.[5]

While patient and understanding with the spiritually immature, believers have stricter moral requirements for those of the faith, and there should be little tolerance for those in the community of Christ who selfishly attack others by their wantonness, harshness or indulgence, thereby damaging the body of believers. The church should operate with a strong communitarian ethic and with high expectations of accountability for itself and its members. Paul summed up these dual levels of tolerance:

> And you are proud! Shouldn't you rather have been filled with grief and have put out of your fellowship the man who did this? Even though I am not physically present, I am with you in spirit. And I have already passed judgment on the one who did this, just as if I were present. When you are assembled in the

[4]Daniel Taylor, "Are You Tolerant? (Should You Be?): Deconstructing the Gospel of Tolerance," *Christianity Today,* January 11, 1999, pp. 42-52. See also Daniel Taylor, *Is God Tolerant? Christian Thinking About the Call for Tolerance* (Wheaton, Ill.: Tyndale House, 2003).

[5]This is actually a point of disagreement among some evangelicals. Those with more of a libertarian orientation would be more tolerant; those leaning toward "Christianization" would be less. Historically, evangelicals have held a position between two extremes, but have moved in one or the other direction depending on the times and the issues.

> name of our Lord Jesus and I am with you in spirit, and the power of our Lord Jesus is present, hand this man over to Satan, so that the sinful nature may be destroyed and his spirit saved on the day of the Lord. Your boasting is not good. Don't you know that a little yeast works through the whole batch of dough? Get rid of the old yeast that you may be a new batch without yeast—as you really are. For Christ, our Passover lamb, has been sacrificed. Therefore let us keep the Festival, not with the old yeast, the yeast of malice and wickedness, but with bread without yeast, the bread of sincerity and truth. I have written you in my letter not to associate with sexually immoral people—not at all meaning the people of this world who are immoral, or the greedy and swindlers, or idolaters. In that case you would have to leave this world. But now I am writing you that you must not associate with anyone who calls himself a brother but is sexually immoral or greedy, an idolater or a slanderer, a drunkard or a swindler. With such a man do not even eat. What business is it of mine to judge those outside the church? Are you not to judge those inside? God will judge those outside. "Expel the wicked man from among you." (1 Cor 5:2-13)

Tolerance can be understood as functioning to greater or lesser degrees. Toleration always requires, contrary to the way those of the world sometimes portray it, an initial and ongoing objection to a specific immorality. Then without accepting it as morally desirable, the one who is tolerant withholds coercive power.

Tolerance requires[6]

- initial objection;
- withheld coercive power;
- a limit to the tolerance (no moral person can tolerate everything, by definition);
- a recognition that it is an inadequate basis for deeply developed human relations (though not "neighborliness").

A scale or spectrum can be described using seven categories of response to the behavior of others:

1. Affirmation and Active Participation: Morally desirable behavior for an ordered society and for the well-being of the church and believers. This behavior is to be encouraged by believers in the body of believers and, if in the secular sphere, both among the faithful and the worldly. This includes basic requirements of citizenship, or at least supporting basic human rights for all.

---

[6]Modified from Taylor, *Is God Intolerant?*

2. Full Affirmation and Encouragement: Morally desirable behavior for a faithful witness within and outside of the church. This behavior is required of believers, but not for those of the world. This includes matters of "civility."
3. Partial Affirmation and Minimal Support: Morally preferable over other options, but incomplete or morally "tarnished" behaviors. To act on such creates what is often called "the problem of dirty hands." Dirty hands may be acceptable, but not if they lead to spiritual staining.
4. Neutrality: Morally neutral behavior. This includes so-called matters of taste and is not toleration as there is no opposition or affirmation of the act.
5. Weak Tolerance: Morally questionable behavior that does not impede the civil freedom of the believers to act in a Christian manner nor destroy the foundations of the society that provides that freedom; an example would be nonmarital sexual intercourse between two unmarried 40-year-olds in a private situation. Weak tolerance requires the believers to distance themselves from the action but not necessarily from the persons who act in the immoral way.
6. Strong Tolerance: Morally repugnant behavior that is destructive to the individuals involved and that may weaken the society, though is not directly injurious to the faithful or socially vulnerable. This must be tolerated, but with strong public protest; also, those participating in such behaviors would be excluded from the community of faith, an exclusion the world must "tolerate."
7. Rejection: Socially destructive behavior. Christians may protect themselves and the society against an immediate threat.

Toleration of non-Christians operates differently than for those who disagree within the faith. On the one hand, the believer seeks the conversion of the nonbeliever. The faithful seek not, first and foremost, to defeat earthly enemies, but to make them family members, workers in the spiritual guild, part of the new ethnicity. There should be a high toleration of the moral failings of those in the world, and believers should work with those of the world to accomplish common moral tasks. On the other hand, on most matters of morality, the faithful ones have (or should have) a much lower tolerance of moral failure among those of the body of Christ, while at the same time seeking to restore the fallen Christian.

Believers' moral toleration of the world has historically varied for at least four reasons:

1. how much cooperation from the worldly can serve a common proximate end;
2. how much the believer feels his or her other moral obligations would be threatened;
3. how important the issue at hand might be;
4. an erroneous assumption that the cultural values shared by Christians are actually Christian values, even when those values are not required of the faithful.

If evangelicals are to enter into civil discourse, they should be tolerant of others and others should be of them. Sadly, Christians may have to learn to tolerate the intolerance of others, especially when it is immersed in the self-deception of the worldly who define toleration as agreeing with them. However, how Christians act is more significant spiritually and is something that they can always control. Drawing from both Mouw and Taylor (though with significant modification), believers should[7]

- see themselves as called to be agents of God's righteousness within the church (a primary scriptural image portraying God's relationship to the individual believer and to the church is as the bridegroom to the bride—the primary moral task of the church, then, is to "be the church," the obedient servant, the good child, the pure bride);[8]
- recognize God cares about public righteousness (the creation, including the social existence of humans, is a good);
- see themselves as called to be agents of God's righteousness within the world and, therefore, try to bring God's standards to bear on public life (sometimes only by individual and ecclesial community example; sometimes also with words in public discourse);
- acknowledge that Christians are sometimes selective in their moral outrage;

---

[7]Modified from material by Taylor, *Is God Intolerant?* p. 46; and Richard Mouw, "Tolerance Without Compromise: Christian Engagement in an Era of Political Rancor," *Christianity Today,* July 15, 1996, <http://ctlibrary.com/ct/1996/july15/6t8033.html>. See also Richard J. Mouw, *The God Who Commands* (Notre Dame, Ind.: University of Notre Dame Press, 1990).

[8]Stanley Hauerwas, *The Peaceable Kingdom* (Notre Dame, Ind.: University of Notre Dame Press, 1983), p. 99.

- acknowledge that Christians need to act tolerantly toward those of the world unless life or liberty are truly threatened;
- engage modestly (being faithful to where God has placed the believer, given the resources God has provided, and in light of the necessity for tolerating moral differences that are not a direct threat to the proclamation of the gospel or the immediate well-being of persons);
- evangelize with the understanding that the first apologetic is living an exemplar Christian life.

The faithful should ignore matters of taste as a concern only of the individual. Matters of civility should be discussed publicly as manners, but must be recognized as culturally specific. Matters of citizenship should be addressed as part of the long-term protection of the social order which, in turn, protects individuals and their rights. Immediate threats to the social order and to individuals must be addressed, if necessary, using the force of the state. Obviously, this leaves one significant category of particular difficulty: what to do when the state itself oppresses or persecutes groups or individuals within the society or in other nations for reasons inconsistent with the fundamental purpose of the state to protect its members' life and liberty. This includes, most significantly for those in the evangelical tradition, when the state impedes the proclamation of the good news. It also includes the state endorsing the killing or significant marginalizing of the vulnerable.

If Christians are to interact with the world, then it is necessary, to the extent possible, to explain their moral activity to those of the world in language that makes sense to them. Such an exposition of Christian moral positions cannot be done using the Scripture, even though for themselves Christians must make appeal to the Text as the authoritative report of the good news. Those of the world will not find the Scripture compelling. Believers should translate. After all, Christianity is not a hidden religion. There is no secret knowledge *(gnosis)*. Believers should tell the world how decisions are made, which virtues are promoted within the community of faith, and how they are led to hold specific moral positions in agreement with the broader civil society. There are worldly persons of good will who honestly want to understand why Christians claim certain moral positions, and Christians should be willing to explain.

If others can understand the general moral reasoning of Christians, it may facilitate cooperation. At one level, the world is the opposite of the community of the faithful. Certainly, circumstances arise when the world must be seen as the spiritual enemy of those following Christ. However, in an earthly sense, unless these circumstances include persecution, Christians are better served by seeing the world not as opposed to the body of Christ as much as juxtaposed—the saved and those who might yet be saved. Though Christians will often believe that the moral position they hold is definitive, it might be that certain occasions within secular settings call for believers to represent their moral arguments as one set next to many competing responses to a need or a dilemma.

The faithful should not be misled into believing that such openness of options exists for the moral discourse within the church. High tolerance of error in the world cannot be matched by a similar level of tolerance within the community of faith for at least two reasons. First, Christians do not believe that their moral understanding is one among many equally legitimate competitors, but is one that stands distinct from all others when honest and pure. The willingness to not assert such preferability in discussions with the world is for evangelistic and pragmatic moral reasons. Christians should not appear arrogant. There is nothing they have to boast about except that they were lost and found, undeserving and have been loved anyway. Second, in the West, Christians have as much of a right to be heard on the public square as any other social group, but believers should not mistakenly allow an emphasis on rights language to lead to an acceptance of subjectivity within the community of faith. When this strong sense of uniqueness is combined with the Western notion of individual rights, the believer can appropriately claim a *right* to engage in civil discourse as an equal participant. Under a genuinely secular state (not a secular society, for there is no such thing), in which the religious have as much of a right to speak, hold office and make moral claims as any others, believers can and should engage the broader society rather than withdraw from or despise it. The same right does not exist in the church.

Confusion over this distinction of expectations for society and higher expectations for believers leads some of the world to become anxious, even fearful, about participation of evangelicals in the public forum. They fear that evangelicals will seek to establish a theocracy. This is historically unfounded—especially when considering evangelicalism as a movement initiated in the revivalism of the late eighteenth century rather than characterizing it as a contemporary expression of sixteenth century Reform Protestant theocracy, or inquisitional Counter-Reformation Catholicism. Indeed, the oppression of people and the slaughter of innocents over the past century by those claiming to be "secular" has vastly exceeded all those killed under commands by the various immoral leaders of Christendom since Constantine. Though some evangelical Christians do favor theocracy, they seem far less common (or at least less published) than their equivalents among atheists (the Maoists, Leninists and radical secularists) who advocate social control of religion. Theocrats are few and far between, serving more as "straw-persons" for opponents than prophets for the faithful. Even so, tit-for-tat comparisons are not useful in bioethics discussions, though they may have a place in apologetics or broader political discourse.

There are many evangelicals who combine conservative religious doctrine with conservative social morality and politics within a democratic framework. These do not seek a theocracy (a fact demonstrated by alliances with conservative Jews and with Mormons). They desire a social order that is noticeably less libertarian and/or libertine.

Even more evangelicals, however, are politically moderate, though as a group more socially conservative than the nonchurch attendees. Some evangelicals are *politically* liberal, for instance, Evangelicals for Social Action and Sojourners, though these do not seem to make up a large proportion of American evangelicals. These groups are roughly paralleled in Catholicism by the Catholic Workers movement. Still other groups among evangelicals claim that they are excluded from many public and major religious forums because they do not readily fit into the American political spectrum. These may vary in political orientation from libertarian Christians (not *libertine*—an evangelical libertine is an oxymoron) to African American evangelicals.

Since the ethical starting point for the believer is the trust relationship with Jesus Christ as understood through the Text, the faith community and the intervention of the Holy Spirit, the faithful should not expect those of the world to readily accept or even understand at a deep level this moral order. Nonetheless, communication is required for the shared proximate moral needs of believers and nonbelievers. Therefore, Christians should be able to "translate" their morality into that of the world. These translations cannot be into metaethical "Esperanto"—the philosophical language of the academy and ethics committees that do not actually function in clinical care or in the community at large—but to the language generally understood in the United States, specifically social contractarian deontology.

Christians living in the West at the end of modernity must simultaneously be believers with a faithful *orthopraxis* (or correct moral practice), and able to translate their ethics into non-Christian, that is secular, moral language in order to function with that faithful worldview in a non-Christian world. Minimally, Christians should endorse a thin notion of the social contract. The contract for safety and liberty assumes that the individual is not a rights holder by reason of being a contract maker, but is a contract maker by virtue of biological existence within the state and intrinsic rights that exist prior to the state. These concepts fit well with evangelicalism. The social contract as generally understood in the United States allows a high degree of liberty, which serves the church, but is not so thin as to allow liberty to trump all other values.

CONCLUSION

Numerous historical factors have worked together to lead evangelicals to assert that they are holders of a peculiar truth. Outsiders may well be uncomfortable with such exclusivity, but they should "tolerate" it just as evangelicals should tolerate, whenever possible, those with whom they disagree. From within the community of faith, though, this exclusivity is considered a manifestation of the blessing of God, legitimated among the faithful by appeal to the Scripture.

This exclusivity is not the position of one Scriptural author or another, but is a dominant theme of the Text. For instance, Peter states:

> But you are a chosen people, a royal priesthood, a holy nation, a people belonging to God, that you may declare the praises of him who called you out of darkness into his wonderful light. Once you were not a people, but now you are the people of God; once you had not received mercy, but now you have received mercy. Dear friends, I urge you, as aliens and strangers in the world. (1 Pet 2:9-11)

Paul declares:

> Therefore, my dear friends, as you have always obeyed—not only in my presence, but now much more in my absence—continue to work out your salvation with fear and trembling, for it is God who works in you to will and to act according to his good purpose. Do everything without complaining or arguing,

> so that you may become blameless and pure, children of God without fault in a crooked and depraved generation, in which you shine like stars in the universe as you hold out the word of life. (Phil 2:12-16)

And Jesus is reported as saying:[9]

> Whatever town or village you enter, search for some worthy person there and stay at his house until you leave. As you enter the home, give it your greeting. If the home is deserving, let your peace rest on it; if it is not, let your peace return to you. If anyone will not welcome you or listen to your words, shake the dust off your feet when you leave that home or town. I tell you the truth, it will be more bearable for Sodom and Gomorrah on the day of judgment than for that town. I am sending you out like sheep among wolves. Therefore be as shrewd as snakes and as innocent as doves. (Mt 10:11-16)

The first-century Christian called *Mathetes* (perhaps a person of that name or a pseudonym; the word means disciple or follower) wrote "Letter (Epistle) to Diognetus" (ca. A.D. 130):

> For the Christians are distinguished from other men neither by country, nor language, nor the customs they observe. For they neither inhabit cities of their own, nor employ a peculiar form of speech, nor lead a life which is marked out by any singularity. . . . They dwell in their own countries, but simply as sojourners. As citizens, they share in all things with others, and yet endure all things as foreigners. Every foreign land is to them as their native country, and every land of their birth as a land of strangers.[10]

Yet, being "other" to the world and the world "other" to believers does not eliminate the need or opportunity for common endeavors. From the Christian perspective, the possibility of working together arises out of the three notions of goodness listed at the beginning of this chapter. The individual, almost without exception, experiences his or her own life as a good, and this provides a common basis for discourse. There are some, albeit significantly limited, points of shared morality that allow the valuing of certain moral goods. And

---

[9]Some New Testament scholars argue that this specific text cannot be attributed to Jesus. Many evangelicals find such arguments pointless. The text, that is the whole canon, is inspired by the Holy Spirit and is presented to the body of believers as the written Word of God that always points to the living Word of God (Jesus; see Jn 1). For more on moral epistemology, see chapter 3.

[10]Miroslav Volf, *Exclusion and Embrace: A Theological Exploration of Identity, Otherness and Reconciliation* (Nashville: Abingdon, 1996), p. 27, uses this quote as the basis for a discussion on Christian engagement with enemies.

humans experience at least some other people as relatively good, which means there is a possibility of real cooperation if Christians and those of the world recognize one another as ends in themselves.

The greater moral burden, from the Christian perspective, is on believers. Yes, it is true that sometimes power imbalance prevents Christian engagement, but that is generally not the case in the West. Given that evangelicals simultaneously claim to understand true virtue better and that, by the Spirit, they have greater strength to act upon it—with all other things being equal—it is incumbent on believers to kindly and politely initiate discourse. To not do so is to take up the mantel of Jonah in his bitterness.

Further, any dialogue with those of the world is meaningless if Christians do not first demonstrate their own willingness to live by the moral standards they proclaim. For believers to offer tolerance or, even more, to demand rights is a dreadful witness if the Christian moral life is not lived within the community and among believers. In spite of some pitiful failures, Christians must continue to declare that theirs is a religion that requires the actual expression of faith in behavior and to expect such of one another.

The reason for this is simple: Christianity is not a religion of "faith" as an intellectual endeavor, though there are right beliefs. Rather, Christianity is a religion in which *faith* refers to a trusting relationship. A relationship is not simply thoughts about that relationship; such is no more than fantasy or daydreaming or wishfulness. Rather, as a relationship, Christianity is to be lived now in light of the Eternal One. This living today has, according to Christianity, everlasting implications.

Those of the world and believers must recognize that tolerance is not the same thing as affirmation. Evangelicals who engage the world are not to endorse the central value of the world. Taylor correctly notes that toleration is an inadequate basis for substantial human relations, but that the lack of deeply developed relationships is sometimes acceptable. There is, after all, a distinction "between healthy tolerance and a diseased moral passivity or indifference."[11] To use the language of Catholic ethicist Wildes, sometimes we must acknowledge that people can be moral "acquaintances" rather than moral friends or enemies.[12] Still, this never elim-

---

[11]Taylor, "Are You Tolerant?" p. 42.

[12]Kevin Wm. Wildes, *Moral Acquaintances: Methodology in Bioethics* (Notre Dame, Ind.: University of Notre Dame Press, 2000); James R. Thobaben, "Pleased to Make Your Acquaintance: A review of Kevin Wm. Wildes' Moral Acquaintances: Methodology in Bioethics," *Christian Bioethics* 7, no. 3 (2001): 425-39.

inates the Christian's obligation for neighborliness or, in the health-care setting, collegiality, but it does give the highest priority in human relationships to the community of the faithful. Practically, Christians should operate with two levels of explanation and two degrees of tolerance—one for the world and one for the church.

2

Evangelicalism as a Historical Movement

Evangelicalism is a social movement that arose out of pietism and revivalism. It is marked by four dynamics: (1) particularism and universalism, (2) primitivism and progressivism, (3) purity and graciousness, and (4) spiritual knowledge as universal and the limit on obtaining that knowledge. Currently, evangelicalism as a movement allows for the sociopolitical participation of Christians, but with some suspicion of the corrupting influence of the world. Evangelicalism is highly engaged on some bioethical issues.

The Christian faith has many forms, and in spite of some significant disagreements, there are striking similarities among them. Almost all adhere to trinitarian monotheism and indeed those who do not would generally be viewed as outside the faith. All recognize that the mercy of God is necessary to have an ongoing relationship with him. All assert that conversion should be accompanied by changes in moral behavior. All have some form of ritual behavior that reiterates the salvation story.

Evangelicals as a subset affirm those beliefs and practices, but emphasize certain interpretations of doctrine and expectations for behavior. All evangelicals accept that salvation—specifically salvation from hell, though that term may not be used as frequently as in the past—is possible only through Jesus Christ. Though with varying degrees of fervor, evangelicals claim that this is good news for all people and, therefore, it is necessary to evangelize. Since the first days of the gospel, there has been a tension among Christians (and among outsiders) between a claim to exclusivity and a sense of call to influence the society.

Further, though there are some significant differences on matters of authority, church polity and epistemology, there is far more agreement on moral positions than might be expected. This is particularly notable given the vast social and cultural differences within the earth's largest and most widespread Protestant movement.[1] To a large degree, evangelical culture transcends eth-

[1]Consider participants in Lausanne Movement and World Evangelical Fellowship, and see

nic and national boundaries. Across the world, along with basic orthodox doctrine, evangelicals assert that

- the new birth prior to biological death initiates a new life and relationship with God that moves a person toward holiness by God's Spirit;
- the Text (Christian Scriptures) sufficiently describes the means to enter into this trust relationship with God;
- the interpretation of the Text and holiness occurs within the community of faith and through accountability.[2]

Though the dating of historical movements is always contestable, the beginning of modern evangelicalism can be reasonably traced to the Wesleyan revivals in Great Britain and the Great Awakening in the United States.

The Wesleys and early Methodists did attempt to directly influence social policy, notably toward the abolition of slavery, and the limitation of distilled alcoholic beverages. They also developed educational facilities to evangelize students, to prepare individuals for ministry, and to provide skills for success in the marketplace. The Wesleys' greatest social influence was through the sectarian oriented small groups that included high membership expectations (including service to the poor and otherwise marginalized, as well as strict personal behaviors, which transformed the lives of many at the bottom of the social order). Responsibility and accountably applied to one's health and the health of others. Not surprisingly, the early Methodists established clinics, and John Wesley's bestselling book during his lifetime was likely a self-treatment book called *The Primitive Physick*.

The Great Awakening, which occurred at about the same time in the United States was essentially a series of evangelistic meetings (the theoretical underpinnings were provided by Jonathan Edwards; the lead preacher was George Whitefield, John and Charles Wesley's sometime compatriot). Though some claim that these provided a basis for the "democratization" of religion and, consequently, the political change of broader society, that was not the intention of the preachers. Still, the social impact was real, as evidenced by the negative response of the social, political and religious elite toward revivals held among the agrarian and emerging working classes and the petty shop owners. As with John Wesley, Edwards was

---

"Bioethics: Obstacle or Opportunity for the Gospel?" Lausanne Committee for World Evangelization 2004 Forum <www.lausanne.org/documents/2004forum/LOP58_IG29.pdf>.
[2]Ibid.

favorably inclined toward new medical technologies and science in general as a means to improve society. (Ironically, Edwards died following an inoculation he had taken to demonstrate the safety of that new public health technique).

The wilderness revival camp meetings, half a century after the Great Awakening, at the beginning of the nineteenth century, began the displacement of the previously dominant denominations with the Baptists, Methodists, the Disciples and other smaller groups. These groups tended to place a strong emphasis on individual moral improvement (often referred to as "holiness") with the main limit on their immediate broader social and political influence being their concentration in relatively low population areas.

When the next period of revival came a quarter century later, this desire for moral improvement combined with American optimism and economically improved social location. Especially northern evangelicals began to assert a political agenda. Abolition and prohibition became the central social moral concerns of the evangelicals. Several notable examples of this expression of evangelicalism were the Tappan brothers, Charles Finney and Sojourner Truth.[3]

Following the Civil War, evangelicals continued to express interest in social issues, but emphasis was then placed on improving the self in order to improve society. This was manifest in the conservative side of the feminist movement and a deeper concern for prohibition. Both were combined into moral arguments about the family as it faced modernization and urbanization. The best examples were the Women's Christian Temperance Union (WCTU) in the United States and the Salvation Army in England (and later the United States). The WCTU's watchwords were "Agitate—Educate—Legislate."[4] The Salvation Army established a defiant presence serving the poor in spite of harassment from the political right and political left. However, a shift toward privatizing religion had begun.

Eventually, as Methodists in the South and North, Baptists in the South, and smaller evangelical groups throughout the country were accepted by the middle and even the upper strata of society, the ability to hold social justice and personal purity together diminished. The response of these groups—who had once loudly and simultaneously proclaimed the need for

---

[3]Sojourner Truth's Christology was ambiguous. On the one hand, she sometimes sounded like a Finneyite evangelical, and at others she sounded like a Hicksite Quaker. See Margaret Washington, ed., *Narrative of Sojourner Truth* (New York: Vintage Classics, 1993).

[4]WCTU History website <http://www.wctu.org/earlyhistory.html>.

individual salvation and social transformation—to economic and social responsibility was to separate individual salvation from social transformation. By the end of the nineteenth century, some members and denominational agencies started focusing on what was known as the Social Gospel. Others emphasized what was called personal holiness. Most who continued to self-define as evangelicals (including those remaining institutionally located in denominations like Methodist and Presbyterian) belonged in this latter category.

As Pentecostalism developed in the early twentieth century, that movement and others asserting a pretribulation rapture seemed to become even less concerned with social change, thinking it mere window-dressing.[5] The evangelical sense of being outsiders was exacerbated when doctrinally orthodox and morally conservative Christians were increasingly branded as fundamentalists, and fundamentalists as bigoted. Without denying the bigotry that may well have existed among evangelicals, it was no less present among their opponents—both secular and religious. Indicative of this tendency was the cultural annihilation of the working class hero, William Jennings Bryan, using media caricatures drawn by the cynical and the powerful during the Scopes trial, eventually culminating in misrepresentations on stage and in film in the mid-twentieth century. Still, significant portions of the evangelical movement brought this on themselves, with only a few groups, like the Salvation Army, attempting to hold evangelism for eternal salvation and insistence on earthly justice together as worthy ends.

The early twentieth century, with the possible exception of the rescue missions, was a time of withdrawal from civil discourse by evangelicals. Evangelical Christians rejected the radical politics that were finding some acceptance in the cities (e.g., anarchism and most forms of socialism). The rural populists, with whom they often aligned, fell apart as a movement. The watershed event was the Scopes trial. The leftist populist William Jennings Bryan won the trial, but lost the media. Evangelicals were

---

[5]The *Scofield Reference Bible*, a very popular work among evangelicals of various stripes, but especially fundamentalists, during the first half of the twentieth century, described the return of Christ in such a way that the continued decay of the world should be expected and any effort to impede it was a fool's errand. Dake's Bible rose to prominence among Pentecostals in the mid-twentieth century. It asserted the same.

A good primary reference on Pentecostals and healing is Oral Roberts, *The Oral Roberts Reader* (New York: Zenith Books, 1958), especially chapter three, "What Is Healing By Faith?"

branded as backward bigots impeded by their own anti-intellectualism, and many withdrew into what became fundamentalism or strict forms of Holiness Methodism. The new form of evangelicalism, Pentecostalism, started to capture the minds and hearts of white and black members of the American working and impoverished classes in both urban and rural areas, but there was little political involvement—except occasional local efforts by persons such as Four-Square Gospel Church founder, Amie Semple McPherson, for moral purity, and all but ignored radio sermons by anticommunist preachers.

The idea of social improvement at that point belonged almost exclusively to theological liberalism. Consequently, the rise of Christian religious hospitals in the early twentieth century, that replicated a nineteenth century pattern of religious schools and orphanages, was institutionally based within the mainline denominations, along with Catholic orders and diocese. The exceptions were evangelical participation with clinics that were part of rescue missions, overseas medical missions and the founding of a few colleges as substitutes given what was considered the failed higher education of the mainline denominations.

Though a strong social presence, evangelicals were generally overlooked by politicians and demeaned by scholars as a remnant of a dying age, and they usually stayed on the sociocultural margins for the first half of the twentieth century. When African American evangelicals became involved with social change through the civil rights movement, nonblack northern evangelicals generally remained uninvolved. Northern evangelicals were simply disengaged, held back by intimidation, embarrassment, cultural inertia or a general disdain for the corruptions of the world. Southern evangelicals, in line with a general social conservatism not originally associated with the evangelical movement, often stood in opposition to the civil rights movement—overtly or tacitly. In the meantime, mainline/oldline denominations did address the issues of civil rights. Their bureaucracies and organizational leaders expanded their portfolio to include a variety of social issues.

Evangelicalism remained off to the side of civil discourse until several European and American theologians (most notably Dietrich Bonhoeffer, Karl Barth, C. S. Lewis and Reinhold Niebuhr) began to question the idea of inevitable social progress and, even more, the liberal belief that evil was mere illusion or ignorance. Preachers appropriated portions of their thought. Other leaders gaining voice through yet another revival movement, this one spearheaded by Billy Graham, brought evangelicalism out of the "backwaters" of American social thought in the 1950s. In the late 1960s and early 1970s, a youth-based revival occurred, taking forms such as the Jesus People and the One Way program. The former was an informal development often including persons from the drug/hippie culture with a few converts from political radicalism. This movement was open to anti-Vietnam War and other leftist political positions. The latter developed into a formal effort by Billy Graham and Bill Bright of Campus Crusade, along with parallel efforts from Youth with a Mission. An intellectual movement grew up alongside, exemplified by L'Abri, led by Francis Schaeffer and his wife, Edith.

By the late 1970s, certain leaders among fundamentalists and Pentecostals began to assert the need for renewed "Christian" participation in the political sphere. Sometimes this was closely linked to specific political parties or candidates, such as with Jimmy Carter's presidential campaign and the Moral Majority. The decade of the 1980s was a period of increased social approval of evangelicals, with the beginning of the megachurches and the aging of the baby boomers. Political and social engagement tended to be defined either as an activity for individual Christians to be supported by other believers or as an integral part of the life of the church, with specific issues woven into ongoing ministries. Either way, the marginalization of evangelicals seemed to have ended. Increasingly, by the 1990s, more subtle sociopolitical analyses arose from evangelicals, with more leaders asserting their *right* to participate in public debate without demanding they dictate final conclusions. By 2000, evangelicals were considered a powerful political force and in 2008 were the object of active courting by both major parties.

With the beginning of the twenty-first century, evangelicalism in the United States is marked by two opposite ecclesiological trends: the continuing growth of megachurches with multiple cell groups and the rise of the house church. Also, the evangelical movement seems to be taking seriously its global nature, with various Pentecostal, Anglican and neoevangelical expressions. Inevitably, this includes consideration of justice and mercy issues without inevitably forcing responses into neat categories along the American political spectrum.

An associated trend is toward denominational realignment and changes in local church affiliation without strong regard for old-line designations.[6] When evangelicals define themselves as *Christians*, it is not in the sense of the weak ecumenicalism of old-line churches, but with the sense that being a follower truly redefines who one is, and to what communities one belongs.

As Robert Wuthnow noted over two decades ago:

> On the whole, denominational differences by no means drop out of the picture, even when the differences between religious liberals and conservatives are taken into account. But the gap separating liberals and conservatives generally tends to be wider than that separating any of these denominations.[7]

In other words, evangelicals have more in common with other evangelicals than they do with others within their own historical traditions and, in some cases, ecclesial organizations. This is particularly noticeable in the conflicts that have arisen in old-line denominations. Still, evangelicals are not all identical.

There are six "types" of evangelicals, though the distinctions are only analytical and only tendencies. In practice, persons of several types worship together in the same church and, certainly, work together on issues of justice, mercy or purity.

- Fundamentalists: Usually independent, Southern Baptist or conservative Presbyterian; strong tendency toward Calvinist Baptist or Calvinist theology.
- Holiness: Strong tendency toward Wesleyan/Arminian theology.
- Neo-Evangelicals: In mainline and independent congregations; part of renewal movements.
- Pentecostals: Usually independent or in a distinctly Pentecostal denomination; emphasis on mystical experience (usually requiring the gift of tongues and often belief in healing).
- Charismatics: Located in mainline or independent congregations; accept legitimacy of "gifts" but do not require specific expressions as proof of the full indwelling of the Spirit; emphasis on contemporary worship styles.

---

[6]Barry A. Kosmin and Ariela Keysar, American Religious Identification Survey 2008 <www.americanreligionsurvey-aris.org>.

[7]Robert Wuthnow, *The Restructuring of American Religion: Society and Faith Since World War II* (Princeton, N.J.: Princeton University Press, 1988), p. 220.

- Anabaptists: Similar theology to, and influenced by, but not derived from eighteenth-century revivalist-evangelicals.

Evangelicalism operates, as do most social movements, within a range created by a set of values. Within this range, though differences can be significant, the consistency on moral choices among evangelicals across cultures is dramatic. This dynamic does impact how evangelicals talk about and, depending on the issue, how believers respond to moral concerns. These values shape how evangelicals engage within their own communities and interact with those of the world.

For evangelicalism, these tendencies can be described using four sets of polarities. Each of the six types of evangelicals expresses agreement with these values to some extent.

- Particularism and universality
- Primitivism and progressivism
- Moral purity and the acceptance of grace
- Knowledge as universally accessible fact and knowledge as personal spiritual experience

PARTICULARISM AND UNIVERSALITY

There is no doubt that Christians, perhaps especially evangelicals, believe they are part of a special group. This "peculiar people" (1 Pet 2:9 KJV) has often sought to have a moral impact on the societies in which it finds itself, even while holding a group understanding that the believers are "other than" those societies and so must never fully and noncritically participate in the general culture (Deut 14:12; Tit 2:14). The particularism arises from the theological assertions evangelicals make about Jesus the Nazarene. For believers the Savior is not a vague "Christ-Spirit," but Jesus who was and is and will forever be the Christ. Jesus was, as he walked upon this earth, simultaneously fully human and fully God. To use technical language, evangelicalism is a theocentric religion, but only when theocentrism is understood as Christocentrism and only when that, in turn, is defined by the claim that Jesus of Nazareth is the God/Human. This aspect of the particularism of evangelicalism is certainly that which most irritates those of the world. For evangelicals, to borrow a phrase from the Jesus People Revival of the late 1960s and early 1970s, Jesus is the "One Way." At least in theory, this claim of particularity should lead to graciousness on the part of believers—after all, if evangelicals are right, then their salvation is an undeserved gift from God through Jesus Christ, even while they declare with confidence the uniqueness of salvation through Jesus Christ. Admittedly, this humility does not always find expression.

The universality of evangelicalism actually rests in the depths of its particularism. Everyone needs Jesus because everyone has the same needs, if not in the specifics, at least in that all are separated from God by the brokenness of sin (sin being both violation of God's will and acting in a manner contrary to one's own most fundamental well-being). It is said that death is the great leveler, and so it is, but from the evangelical perspective so is sin. The universal condition that "all have sinned and fall short of the glory of God" (Rom 3:23) does not for evangelicals lead to pessimism. Instead, for most, though certainly not all believers, the human condition when coupled with the potential for individual redemption pushes the typical evangelical toward a pragmatic optimism. Anyone is redeemable. It pushes evangelicals toward a valuing of all individuals, regardless of ethnicity, age, gender and so forth. Of all the theological doctrines accepted by evangelicalism, the valuing of the individual may have the single greatest impact on how bioethical concerns are considered.

In terms of social ethics, where a given group of evangelicals finds equilibrium in this tension varies. Some will focus on the morality of the "peculiar people" arguing that those of the world are not their concern, except evangelistically. Others will claim that they collectively must not only encourage the restraining of evil, but must demonstrate the positive good throughout the society, including in the political and other social spheres. Some who find themselves between these two positions will declare that the community of the faithful must focus on serving the believers and bringing others to a salvific relationship with the Christ, but the transformed individual must, as an individual, fully engage the social order.

The universality of Christian claims means that often evangelicals will have moral opinions about social concerns. These opinions may find expression in the standards of the fellowship. The particularity of the moral life means that only some of those opinions will rise to the level of needing to be expressed and acted upon in the broader culture. For example, while evangelical Christians may not favor in vitro fertilization being used for unmarried heterosexual couples, it will not often become so significant an issue as to elicit public activity. Abortion, since its legitimacy centers on denying human status and the associated rights necessary for societal functioning, will elicit advocacy activity. Advocacy for the unborn is viewed as both a basic civil restraint of evil directed against the legally innocent individual and a necessary spiritual intervention that more might have the opportunity to hear the gospel and live their lives by God's mercy. Some moral standards apply only to believers, while others should apply to society at large.

PRIMITIVISM AND PROGRESSIVISM

Arising out of the belief in universal truth about Jesus Christ, evangelicals tend to question the legitimacy of any explanation of meaning (metanarrative) that is counter to their own. The universality of that message is both spatial and temporal. In other words, evangelicals consider cultural moral fads to be a form of temporal provincialism. Words like *popular*, *new* or *evolved* have little theological currency. Great favor, rather, is given to what is the earliest (or what they claim is the earliest) form of Christianity. This desire to remain true to that which has once been given can be seen in favorite Scriptures and in some of the music that has served evangelicals until recently.[8] *Old-time religion* and *pure religion* are extolled.[9] Sometimes this is simply reluctance to adapt to changing circumstances, or a misunderstanding of what is fundamental to the faith, or sheer bigotry. More often this desire for pure, old-time religion is an expression of primitivism, the belief that something significantly true from the past must be maintained against a series of continuing threats.

Though the terms can be defined in a variety of ways, for the purpose of understanding contemporary evangelicalism, *primitivism* is the assertion that the simplest theological doctrine and the most basic organizational structures of the early church are the best. Frequently in past decades, primitivism was strongly associated with *restorationism*, which is the effort to return to a bygone day in which the organizational structures and philosophy/theology were supposedly purer or, at least, more accurate. Increasingly, evangelicals mark primitivism as simple disregard for organizational structures that have grown over the past two centuries. Historically, it would be

[8]Among the Bible passages to which evangelicals turn on this are 1 Corinthians 1:18-23; 2 Corinthians 11:4; Galatians 1:8; and 1 Timothy 6:3.

[9]See the spiritual "Give Me That Old-Time Religion," edited by G. D. Pike, 1873, and further adapted by Charles D. Tillman, 1891; and the recording by Gary Davis, "Pure Religion," *Pure Religion and Bad Company* (Washington, D.C.: Smithsonian Folkways, 1957).

difficult to identify where the desire for primitive church organization and doctrine leaves off and a general suspicion of centralized organizational authority begins.

The progressivism of evangelicalism is often an expression of pragmatism in meeting the standards of what is believed to be the primitive truth of the gospel. Since its beginnings, with Wesley and Whitefield/Edwards, evangelicalism has been extremely open to the newest communication, organization and leadership techniques. Sometimes this has also meant being tied to other progressive aspects of the culture, as in the nineteenth-century membership overlap between evangelicalism and the progressive sociopolitical groups. That, however, for various reasons, including the tendency to personalize religion (both from the influence of American Romanticism and the rise of premillenialism), along with the political marginalization associated with the fundamentalist/modernist controversy, did not continue with evangelicals in the early twentieth century.[10]

Evangelical progressivism, starting in the 1940s and genuinely advancing in the 1960s and 1970s, centered not on progressive politics but on using and developing the most current communication technologies and organizational theories. For example, in the 1970s, evangelicals mastered the use of mass mailings and broadcast television while old-line denominations were still depending on monthly newspapers. In the 1980s and 1990s, parachurch groups, megachurches and house churches began using organizational theories such as continuous quality improvement and management by presence while the old-line denominations were still clinging to grossly inefficient and highly centralized bureaucracies.

At the turn of the twenty-first century, evangelicals have developed electronic forms of education and computer-assisted worship forms to a far greater extent than the old-lines. Evangelicals, while often suspicious of cultural progressivism when that means doctrinal and moral change, are more than willing to use business and political organizational models, music styles and instruments, and various communication technologies if they think they are useful. The evangelical movement, after all, is the one from which Wesley

---

[10]See George M. Marsden, *Fundamentalism and American Culture: The Shaping of Twentieth-Century Evangelicalism 1870-1925* (New York: Oxford University Press, 1980); Timothy L. Smith, *Revivalism and Social Reform: American Protestantism on the Eve of the Civil War* (Baltimore: Johns Hopkins University Press, 1980); and Donald W. Dayton, *Discovering an Evangelical Heritage* (Peabody, Mass.: Hendrickson, 1976).

and the Methodist class system, Whitefield's field preaching, Finney's altar calls, camp meeting mass gatherings, and the military structure of the Salvation Army arose—all of which were considered organizationally revolutionary in their time.

These polarities—progressivism in organization and technology and primitivism in doctrine—can create tension among contemporary evangelicals. For instance, over the past three decades, denominational designations have become less significant. Evangelicals have been prone to cross denominational lines for local revivals, for social issues and, lately, parachurch organizations like Campus Crusade and Promise Keepers. Still, evangelical ecumenicalism always is limited by the movement's general distrust of bureaucracies (now exacerbated by a broader so-called postmodern suspicion of centralized "voices") and sometimes by suspicion of the doctrinal integrity of others.

In social ethics the biggest point of conflict among evangelicalism arising from the tension of primitivism and progressivism is over materialism—how "successful" should churches and believers be? Those strongly favoring numerical growth, almost of necessity must use organizational methods similar to those of large corporations and communication technologies that are often like intrusive marketing. Others declare that the "remnant is few" and there is no need to "polish"—which to them really means to obscure—the presentation of the primitive gospel message. In its worst form, those in the first camp will claim that God is specially "blessing" the church with numbers and prosperity.[11] In its worst form, those in the latter will sink into bitter, self-righteous legalism about what they think are primitive church positions, but which actually developed in the past two centuries in the United States.

MORAL PURITY AND THE ACCEPTANCE OF GRACE

Historically, the distinctives of evangelicalism began to coalesce with the Wesleys, Whitefield and Edwards, taking clear shape with the wilderness revivals and then the urban revivals of antebellum America. Having said this, evangelicalism is also very much the grandchild of the Reformation. Salvation, as both the early reformers and the later evangelicals have asserted, is by grace through faith.

Grace is the unmerited favor of God, or to use the word in its original

---

[11]See C. Leonard Allen, "Roger Williams and 'the Restauration of Zion,'" in *The American Quest for the Primitive Church*, ed. Richard T. Hughes (Urbana: University of Illinois Press, 1988).

sense, the indulgence of God. It is an offering from a greater to a lesser, from one in a position of dominance in a relationship who condescends to lift the weaker. Evangelicals often cite Paul's letters to the churches at Rome and at Ephesus to explain grace; respectively, they say:

> For while we were still helpless, at the right time Christ died for the ungodly. For one will hardly die for a righteous man; though perhaps for the good man someone would dare even to die. But God demonstrates His own love toward us, in that while we were yet sinners, Christ died for us. (Rom 5:6-8 NASV)

> For by grace you have been saved through faith; and that not of yourselves, it is the gift of God; not as a result of works, that no one should boast. For we are His workmanship. (Eph 2:8-10 NASV)

The "acceptance of the Lord" is passive in that it is the removal of active barriers against his love, rather than any action that would satisfy the infinite debt created by the individual's transgressions. All sins, even those directed against other human beings, like murder or adultery, are ultimately sins against God. Having said this, conversion is often associated with internal struggles, including active defiance of God. In the past, these moments were sometimes called "running from the Lord" or "wrestling like Jacob." Now these moments are more likely to be framed in psychological and/or Kierkegaardian-like existentialist language of emotional *baggage* (the former) or *crisis* (the latter).

Though altar calls may be going the way of the camp meeting, the revivalist theology of those gatherings remains an underlying assumption of both the seeker-sensitive megachurches and the strict, rural congregations in clapboard buildings with hand-painted signs. Evangelicals, with few exceptions, argue strongly that a person must choose to receive the grace of God. This was, and remains, one of the biggest distinguishing characteristics of evangelicalism from one of its immediate predecessors, colonial New England Calvinism. The emotions associated with this acceptance of Jesus as Lord, though taking a variety of forms, are another distinguishing characteristic. As much as a decision of the intellect or commitment of the will, this is also a reorientation of the affections.

The dominant model of conversion for evangelicals is that of Saul of Tarsus on the road to Damascus, though—in fact—many conversions are of those reared in the church or moving from lukewarm congregations to evangelical churches. Still, almost all conversions, be they dramatic, or developed over time, begin with some form of tension. This tension may be due to a family, financial, and/or health crisis. Frequently conversions are associated with the transitions into adulthood. Especially outside the United States, class-associated deprivation and political turmoil may raise questions about the social order that are addressed religiously. Less frequently, but importantly as such are more common with intellectuals, persons may experience philosophical or theological inconsistencies they seek to address with a new religious commitment.

The best word to use for this tension is *anomie*.[12] The converted Christian has usually faced some kind of existential crisis or tension that results in a sense of meaninglessness, and then entered the Christian community finding that the relationship with Jesus Christ (as reinforced by the community) provides a foundation for living, regardless of the problems one might have. In a sense, evangelicals claim that every conversion is a "foxhole" or "jailhouse" or "crutch" conversion, for everyone is "under attack" or "imprisoned" or "diseased" until she or he is with Christ.

Though there are numerous ways to describe the conversion experience, one from sociology of religion can provide an operating model.[13]

1. Tension: usually between one's self-understanding/emotions and the subculture of which one is part, perhaps triggered by a traumatic event or developmental transition.
2. Anxious curiosity: often specifically directed toward religion or other alternatives, though it may take the form of exploration of "alternatives."
3. Recognition of anomie/dismay: the awareness of the inadequacy of one's social identification and, generally, the assumption that the current operational interpretation of the world does not work (need for reidentification asserted); the process is seemingly driven by exasperation with the status quo.

---

[12]See Emile Durkheim, *Suicide: A Study in Sociology,* trans. John A. Spaulding and George Simpson (New York: Free Press, 1951), pp. 241-76; and Peter L. Berger, *The Sacred Canopy: Elements of a Sociological Theory of Religion* (Garden City, N.Y.: Doubleday, 1967), pp. 49-50. For an explicitly Christian understanding, going beyond human social dislocation to existential or spiritual dislocation, see Søren Kierkegaard, *Sickness Unto Death.*

[13]The model is significantly modified from John Lofland and Rodney Stark, "Becoming a World-Saver: A Theory of Conversion to a Deviant Perspective," *American Sociological Review* 30, no. 6 (1965): 862-75; John Lofland, "'Becoming a World-Saver' Revisited," *American Behavioral Scientist* 20, no. 6 (1977): 805-18; John Lofland and Norman Skonovd, "Conversion Motifs," *Journal for the Scientific Study of Religion* 20, no. 4 (1981): 373-85.

4. Seeking: formal intellectual exploration, often following affective bonds, interest-group affiliations and so forth.
5. Evaluation of options: weighing options on the basis of coherence with other aspects of life; work toward equilibration through reinterpretation of other relationships and new self-indentification.
6. New affective bonds and modification of prior affective bonds: depending on how friends and family are associated with the new worldview, relations may strengthen, or may weaken.
7. Commitment activities: participation, both individually and corporately, in commitment mechanisms.[14]
8. Experience of acceptance: life is "perceived" or interpreted as balanced.
9. New tension: all worldviews and self-identifications are dissonant with some portions of the societies and broader cultures of which they are a part; to no small degree this is because those societies and cultures are not consistent; the new worldview (in this case, evangelical Christianity) may then create or exacerbate inconsistencies.

This process sounds like a philosophical or psychological self-structuring, and perhaps it is. The aspect of "choice" is rarely emphasized in traditional sociological models, but it should be. In evangelical language, this means that the Holy Spirit coaxes or woos with gracious love until the individual accepts or dies. Rejecting God is not final in most evangelical theology formulations until one has ceased to be in the physical realm. Evangelicals understand the process in terms of biblical examples and passages. These selections from Romans can serve as an example.

Tension:

> For although they knew God, they neither glorified him as God nor gave thanks to him, but their thinking became futile and their foolish hearts were darkened. Although they claimed to be wise, they became fools and exchanged the glory of the immortal God for images made to look like mortal man and birds and animals and reptiles. (Rom 1:21-23)
>
> All have sinned and fall short of the glory of God. (Rom 3:23)

Anxious curiosity:

> To those who by persistence in doing good seek glory, honor and immortality,

[14]Rosabeth Moss Kanter, *Commitment and Community: Communes and Utopias in Sociological Perspective* (Cambridge, Mass.: Harvard University Press, 1972).

> he will give eternal life. But for those who are self-seeking and who reject the truth and follow evil, there will be wrath and anger. (Rom 2:7-8)

Anomie/dismay:

> What a wretched man I am! Who will rescue me from this body of death? Thanks be to God—through Jesus Christ our Lord! (Rom 7:24-25)

Seeking:

> Brothers, my heart's desire and prayer to God for the Israelites is that they may be saved. For I can testify about them that they are zealous for God, but their zeal is not based on knowledge. Since they did not know the righteousness that comes from God and sought to establish their own, they did not submit to God's righteousness. Christ is the end of the law so that there may be righteousness for everyone who believes. (Rom 10:1-4)

Evaluation of options:

> Therefore, brothers, we have an obligation—but it is not to the sinful nature, to live according to it. For if you live according to the sinful nature, you will die; but if by the Spirit you put to death the misdeeds of the body, you will live, because those who are led by the Spirit of God are sons of God. For you did not receive a spirit that makes you a slave again to fear, but you received the Spirit of sonship. And by him we cry, "Abba, Father." (Rom 8:12-15)

New affective bonds and modification of prior affective bonds:

> I urge you, brothers, to watch out for those who cause divisions and put obstacles in your way that are contrary to the teaching you have learned. Keep away from them. For such people are not serving our Lord Christ, but their own appetites. By smooth talk and flattery they deceive the minds of naive people. Everyone has heard about your obedience, so I am full of joy over you; but I want you to be wise about what is good, and innocent about what is evil. (Rom 16:17-19)

Commitment activities:

> Therefore, I urge you, brothers, in view of God's mercy, to offer your bodies as living sacrifices, holy and pleasing to God—this is your spiritual act of worship. Do not conform any longer to the pattern of this world, but be transformed by the renewing of your mind. Then you will be able to test and approve what God's will is—his good, pleasing and perfect will. (Rom 12:1-2)

Experience of acceptance:

> Who will bring any charge against those whom God has chosen? It is God who justifies. No, in all these things we are more than conquerors through him who

> loved us. For I am convinced that neither death nor life, neither angels nor demons, neither the present nor the future, nor any powers, neither height nor depth, nor anything else in all creation, will be able to separate us from the love of God that is in Christ Jesus our Lord. (Rom 8:33, 37-39)

New tension:

> Who shall separate us from the love of Christ? Shall trouble or hardship or persecution or famine or nakedness or danger or sword? As it is written:
>
> "For your sake we face death all day long;
> we are considered as sheep to be slaughtered."
>
> No, in all these things we are more than conquerors through him who loved us. (Rom 8:35-37)

The character of a complete evangelical conversion, then, is simultaneously passive and active. The former is manifest in the soteriological claim that Jesus came to us while we were still sinners, that he died for the ungodly and that it was not we who first loved God, but he who first loved us (Rom 5:6-8; 1 Jn 4:10, 19). The latter, the activity of salvation, is expressed in evangelism and ethics. If one has been so graciously, so undeservedly saved, then a response is necessary. At one level, these are simply expressions of good manners—Jesus saved the believer from hell, so the least the believer can do is respond with a "thank-you note" of Christian service. More deeply, the believer who has fully experienced conversion of the intellect, will and emotions has an extraordinary sense of gratitude. The believer responds with evangelism and a changed morality expressing gratefulness. For some groups, especially those that might be designated *traditional* evangelicals, the standards for behavior following conversion can be strict. Fundamentalist and holiness subsets of evangelicalism, as well as the related Anabaptist groups, have high expectations for the behavior of the individual believer—including in the arena of bioethics.

Evangelicals generally would assert that while God seeks a loving relationship prior to justification, it is only after one chooses to affirmatively respond that morality can be properly called Christian. To say yes to the moral good, we must first say yes to the divine Jesus Christ (2 Cor 1:18-20). To use traditional theological language, truly virtuous morality is a component of sanctification, the ongoing love relationship between God and creature, and his creatures among themselves, made possible by the renewing influence and indwelling presence of the Holy Spirit.

While in *evangelical* Protestantism the decision to enter into a relationship with Christ is radically individual, the changed and changing life of the one in a relationship with God through Jesus Christ is not. The convert is initially part of the communities of the world. In a moment of complete isolation before God, the individual decides whether to identify with the body of Christ or those of the world. Generally, evangelicals assert that everyone has this awful and awesome opportunity to come before the living God and make a choice. The moment of individual re-forming immediately becomes the moment of reidentification with the community of faithful believers and entry in the body of Christ, the church.

At different times over the past two hundred years, evangelicals have combined their belief in an active response to salvation with a commitment to progressivism, and a confidence in their particular version of what ought to be universally accepted in such a way as to become a genuine political force. Currently, this is not the case. Still, most evangelicals want to be heard. They do want to promote values that can be shared under the limits of the social contract, and the majority would assert that some of those potentially shared and potentially helpful values are currently being ignored.

Contrary to some popular media representations, evangelicals are actually significantly less involved in the political sphere than in rendering direct service. Christians generally have been disproportionately present in serving and funding others in serving the hungry, building houses for the working poor, assisting with disaster cleanup and in overseas outreach. They do not necessarily become active with advocacy groups on such issues. It is almost as if they sense a Christian duty to provide mercy, but are uncertain about the possible contamination of being involved in the politics of the state, even over matters of injustice. This may be a remnant of early twentieth-century reticence or hesitation due to popular media disdain. Also, believers disagree on the question of civil participation as Christians per se.

Evangelicalism is one voice among many in the public square and individual believers are likely to use their faith to make social ethical, including bioethical, decisions. When they think that innocent individuals are being hurt or their own religious well-being threatened by compelled acceptance of non-Christian morality, they may participate in advocacy. For instance, abortion is much more significant to contemporary evangelicals as a religious concern than euthanasia. On the former there is functional unanimity on the prohibition but for an exception to save the life of the mother, though political toleration of exceptions for cases of rape and incest may grudgingly be given. Indeed, opposition to abortion is often an ethical litmus test for evangelicals. Euthanasia, on the other hand, is discussed with more distinctions and categories.

KNOWLEDGE AS UNIVERSALLY ACCESSIBLE FACT AND KNOWLEDGE AS PERSONAL EXPERIENCE

Evangelical epistemology (or theory of the nature of knowledge) is discussed below, but it is important to rehearse some of the differences of opinion that have arisen over the past two centuries among evangelicals and how those might impact a discussion of bioethics. Essentially, there is a debate in Christianity over whether or not basic, true morality is accessible to non-Christians. Generally speaking, in the eighteenth century among the fathers of evangelicalism—specifically John Wesley and Jonathan Edwards—it was claimed that those not in a relationship with Jesus Christ could not truly know or act upon the good. They could not be truly virtuous. This did not mean that nonbelievers could not be positively engaged to cooperate on social concerns, only that they would never fully recognize the good that can be achieved through an intentional response to God's grace. This position was juxtaposed with some Reformed views of general revelation and to Roman Catholic natural law theory.

A shift occurred in the early nineteenth century. The strongly progressive evangelicals elevated the possibility of all members of society knowing the good and acting upon it, even to the point of directing the government in what they considered a Christ-like way. So, Finney asserted that the opposition to slavery demanded by Christ was intrinsic to good social order and that everyone should readily see it. Further, and this is the distinction, the government should be used to provide "moral suasion" to compel the changing of minds.[15] His was not a social contract argument to end slavery, but a Christian one calling for moral conversion.

Theological liberals picked up the idea of a generally accessible, pure moral truth by the early twentieth century, as the evangelicals began their social retreat. The rise of the Nazis and later revelations about Stalinism

[15]Charles G. Finney used both natural-law like arguments and a "moral suasion" argument (similar to other "true virtue" arguments with a strong emphasis on perfection/sanctification). See "Lecture XL: Regneration," *Lectures on Systematic Theology* (1846). Interestingly, John Wesley, fifty years earlier in a manner quite atypical for him, used some natural-law reasoning along with assertions about Christian virtue in an abolitionist tract, "Thoughts Upon Slavery."

divided old-line Christians, with some asserting that the moral good was generally "knowable" and should be taught in the church and society (*education*—variously defined—was seen as the solution to all social ills) and others claiming that the moral good would not be chosen by most even if knowable (this latter position was rooted in the thought of the neo-orthodox movement).[16]

Those of the world broke along similar lines. Some said humans could "be good," claiming society was progressing, or could with proper leadership and education. This in the most extreme form, ironically, became a liberalized version of social Darwinism, promoting eugenics and state-controlled education. A touch of Darwinism was blended with just a bit of nineteenth-century evangelicalism's desire to "establish the kingdom of God," but now without God. Others of the world dismissed the idea of "good" people, accepting the logic of reductionism, advocating a civil nihilism, or in some cases a not-so-civil version.

CONCLUSION

Though somewhat simplistic, the movement of evangelicalism from Edwards, the Wesleys and Whitefield through the current era can be described as a series of stages. The earliest is represented by the Wesleys' expectation that members in the Methodist bands would maintain personal purity and serve the socially marginalized. Charles Finney and his use of vigorous opposition to slavery as a primary indicator of one's personal sanctity best represent the next era, roughly from 1820–1860. Following the American Civil War, groups that had held views similar to Finney's switched their emphasis, using abstinence from alcohol in particular as the great social project, but framing it in terms of the pure individual and the pious family. The turn of the twentieth century marked solidified social acceptance of the mainstream Baptists in the South and Methodists throughout the nation and the beginnings of splits within those movements typified by the fundamentalist/modernist controversies. From the 1920s to the early 1960s, the mainline came to include several former evangelical denominations; in these groups social action was left to bureaucrats and congregations focused on the domestic needs of families,

[16]See Karl Barth, Dietrich Bonhoeffer and Jacques Ellul. See especially Reinhold Niebuhr, *Moral Man and Immoral Society: A Study of Ethics and Politics* (New York: Charles Scribner's Sons, 1937).

especially after the birth of the baby boom children.

Eventually, the reduction of Christianity to, first, a vague "Judeo-Christian" religion and, eventually, to one acceptable choice among many equally acceptable choices, led to the marginalization of the mainline, now old-line, denominations. At the same time, evangelicals—some within these same denominations, some acting in other denominational groups and some acting in independent congregations—began to draw larger numbers from the middle and upper-middle classes. The evangelical presence among the working and poor classes was already secure. Simultaneously, evangelicalism exploded in the non-Western world. Evangelicalism has now displaced the former mainlines as the dominant form of Protestantism worldwide.

And, once again, there is an effort to yoke together social action and service with personal moral purity, but with the recognition that Christianity is not to be the "assumed" religion anywhere. Ethically, this means that evangelicals will assert their values on the public square, but recognize that there are competing "voices" that may or may not speak of compatible positions on specific social issues yet *have the right* to be heard just as they do.

Since the initiation of the evangelical movement (Wesleyan revival in England and the Awakenings in America), the primary reason for interacting with other people has been to convert them. At the end of modernity in the West, and even with the acceptance by most evangelicals of the need for civility in public discourse and the general tolerance of them by those of the world, there remains a belief among evangelicals of the uniqueness of Jesus Christ and the community he initiated. This means the following:

1. There is a belief that society needs at least some of the values evangelicals promote for its own well-being. "Assisting" society is, then, a matter of prudence.
2. Specific protection for the marginalized is morally required. Protecting the vulnerable, especially when ignored by the state that has the specific duty to defend them under the social contract, is a demand of justice.
3. Evangelicals have a fear that their increased social acceptance will lead to compromised faith and compromised morality within their own community. The pattern has appeared repeatedly in the history of Christianity. This fact, if no other, calls for personal virtuosity and community consistency.

Through most of its history as a movement, evangelicalism has included a yoking of specific positions on particular moral issues with rebirth in Christ. This is certainly true today when it comes to issues in bioethics. Aside from evangelistic efforts, evangelicals at this time generally consider engagement with those of the world on sociopolitical concerns, including bioethical ones, appropriate, but it must be done acceptably.

3

Knowing Ethically

AN EVANGELICAL CHRISTIAN MORAL EPISTEMOLOGY

E*pistemology* is the analysis of how one knows what one knows. Evangelical epistemology tends to include two distinctions: (1) between salvific and moral knowledge, and (2) between knowledge accessible to all persons and knowledge accessible only to those in a saving relationship with God through Jesus Christ and guided by the Spirit. Moral guidance of believers on matters not propositionally considered in the Text can often be understood analogically. Christians must then "translate" those analogical understandings for those of the world in order to cooperate morally.

> The disciples came to him and asked, "Why do you speak to the people in parables?"
>
> He replied, "The knowledge of the secrets of the kingdom of heaven has been given to you, but not to them. Whoever has will be given more, and he will have an abundance. Whoever does not have, even what he has will be taken from him. This is why I speak to them in parables:
>
> "Though seeing, they do not see;
> though hearing, they do not hear or understand.
>
> In them is fulfilled the prophecy of Isaiah:
> "'You will be ever hearing but never understanding;
> you will be ever seeing but never perceiving.
> For this people's heart has become calloused;
> they hardly hear with their ears,
> and they have closed their eyes.
> Otherwise they might see with their eyes,
> hear with their ears,
> understand with their hearts
> and turn, and I would heal them.'
>
> But blessed are your eyes because they see, and your ears because they hear.

> For I tell you the truth, many prophets and righteous men longed to see what you see but did not see it, and to hear what you hear but did not hear it. (Mt 13:10-17, quoting Is 6:9-10)
>
> Jesus spoke all these things to the crowd in parables; he did not say anything to them without using a parable. So was fulfilled what was spoken through the prophet:
>
> I will open my mouth in parables,
> I will utter things hidden since the creation of the world." (Mt 13:34-35, quoting Ps 78:2)

EPISTEMOLOGICAL CLAIMS, PART ONE: THE TEXT AS THE TRUE STORY

Jesus spoke in parables. Though childlike in innocence, they were not and are not childish in naiveté. For even though they were readily accessible to those without highly developed academic skills, they were not presentations of simplistic truisms, but declarations meant to fundamentally alter the hearer. Yet, that only begs the question: why, then, would the Messiah speak in veiled language? Why would he create analogies that were difficult for some to understand?

The intention of the parables was to inform. Still, it is clear that his use of them often created confusion, or at least ambiguity. Certainly, Jesus' reference to the Isaiah passage in Matthew 13 is, in part, a messianic claim—as he further asserts by referring to Psalm 78. Is there a "messianic secret"? What is the point of eternal truths that cannot be cognitively grasped and, subsequently, incorporated into one's understanding?

Matthew, in his presentation of the stories, seems to indicate something is concealed, not through obfuscation, but by the hardness of the hearts of hearers. It is not the Speaker who fails to communicate, but those who should be hearing. Communication requires participation from both parties. If there is a "messianic secret," it is not a secret accessible only to those who advance through stages to some complex of Gnostic-like knowledge. Nor is it a secret that only the scholarly or even the morally precise can know. God does not, on a whim, deliver only a select few from ignorance. The revelation of eternal truth is not arbitrary or capricious.

The Text makes clear the standard is set by God, not God subject to some outside standard:

> As the heavens are higher than the earth,
> so are my ways higher than your ways and my thoughts than your thoughts. (Is 55:9).

The revelations of God vary in expression according to his unvarying love. God presents Truth (both for salvific and moral purposes) in accordance not with the human expectation of right and wrong or good and bad but with the divine expression of love.

Assuming, then, that God's actions do not need to be justified for human beings, what is the instrumental purpose of parable secrecy? Why does Jesus use these brief vignettes and stories? Most evangelicals believe that the failure to understand God's true knowledge is due to humans stubbornly refusing to relinquish their own prideful self-understanding. The knowledge necessary to enter into a saving relationship with God is available to anyone, regardless of intellectual capacity, who in humility turns to the Divine. The use of simple narratives (parables) to convey truth to the faithful and to those willing to become faithful allows access to information for any who would choose to continue growing in the faith.

Jesus cites Isaiah, which is also echoed in Jeremiah.

> And I said, "Here am I. Send me!"
> He said, "Go and tell this people:
> "'Be ever hearing, but never understanding;
> be ever seeing, but never perceiving.'
> Make the heart of this people calloused;
> make their ears dull
> and close their eyes.
> Otherwise they might see with their eyes,
> hear with their ears,
> understand with their hearts,
> and turn and be healed." (Is 6:8-10)

The passage that Jesus takes from Isaiah follows the call of the prophet. He is told that the people are unfit to hear the Truth, even though it ought to be obvious to them. They are unfit because they are not in a proper relationship with God. Similarly, in the parallel Jeremiah passage, it is the fear of the Lord that conditions the capacity to know. *Fear* is understood as proper awe and respect, though terror at the majesty of God without the protection of his grace is not inappropriate. Without such recognition, the absolute Truth is not a truth knowable by the hearers.

Hear this, you foolish and senseless people,
who have eyes but do not see,
who have ears but do not hear:
Should you not fear me?" declares the LORD.
"Should you not tremble in my presence?
I made the sand a boundary for the sea,
an everlasting barrier it cannot cross.
The waves may roll, but they cannot prevail;
they may roar, but they cannot cross it.
But these people have stubborn and rebellious hearts;
they have turned aside and gone away.
They do not say to themselves,
'Let us fear the LORD our God.'" (Jer 5: 21-24)

EPISTEMOLOGICAL CLAIMS, PART TWO: THE SALVIFIC USE OF THE TRUE STORY

Jesus, in explaining why he uses parables, seems to be assuming his hearers understand, at some level, the declarations made in the casting out from Eden and the scattering of Babel. Individuals are fallen and their institutions are morally shattered. Even so, the stories in the parables indicate that God in the story of Jesus Christ provides the means for restoration and even more. The parables are told to convey that truth, though in particularized ways. They are told to make divine truths concrete. In this, they parallel the life, death and resurrection of Jesus, which is the offer of access to the universal but particularized to the life of the individual. This means, and Christ demonstrates by his parabolic teaching, that knowledge does not have intrinsic good. Knowledge, all knowledge, is in some way or another instrumental. It is always a penultimate good that points to the ultimate good of a relationship with God through Jesus.

Most evangelicals claim that any reasonable person can discern fundamental facts about the reality of God from a careful analysis of that which God has created, though most evangelicals would clearly assert that such is not salvific. These forms of knowledge merely *convince* one of the general need for a god. Generally evangelicals doubt that such natural proofs will *convict*—or draw one into a relationship—without self-examination and the recognition of personal need as guided by the Spirit. Further, virtually all evangelicals would assert that the character of God can be genuinely known only through a direct experience of Christ, simultaneous with or subsequent to that recognition of personal need.

In other words, evangelical epistemology is two-layered. Christians claim that God can be known in the sense of a mathematical fact. One does not, after all, *only* know a friend as a friend, but also as a human being with a particular color of hair, a specific accent, and a particular social and historical location. Yet most evangelicals would claim that the deep characteristics of God cannot be truly known, only philosophized about, prior to a salvific relationship with him. The human need for God can be knowable as "fact" before conversion, but the reality of God can only be known after. As the great hymn of fear, awe, and humility at the edge of humiliation declares: "I once was blind, but now I see."

Simply put, if "God is love," then one cannot *know* love until being in love and being loved (1 Jn 4:8). For example, humans know their friends in at least two ways. On the one hand, a friend is known as, say, a human woman with brown eyes who is thirty years old. In addition, a friend is known as *friend*, as one with whom one has a distinguishing relationship—a relationship that differentiates that individual from other individuals who are female, thirty and with brown eyes by virtue of how she relates. To know a friend in this sense is different from knowing that a triangle has 180 degrees within the constraints of Euclidean geometry. All Christians claim that one can know God in the same sense as knowing a friend. Christianity is a religion of relationships, and those relationships cannot be reduced. Christianity can be understood intellectually by study, but can be understood existentially only by those who *know* God as friend.

"Objective" knowledge about God, even if available, is of no value eternally without being accompanied by trust (faith of relationship).[1] The practical claim, then, of most evangelicals is that Christianity is a religion of relationship, and only in the relationship can one "know" how to live a good or right life. The individual enters into a community with God through Jesus Christ, and God assumes a place within the individual through the Holy Spirit. Though it is considered offensive by some outside the faith, the New Testament implies strongly that only those in that relationship have God as Father, for only they are "born again" or "adopted" into the holy family. Only the child can honestly recognize the reality of the parent. As Billy Graham, one of the preeminent leaders of evangelicalism put it, "I accept the revelation of himself by faith."[2]

[1]"You believe that there is one God. Good! Even the demons believe that—and shudder" (Jas 2:19).

[2]Billy Graham, Los Angeles Revival, 2005.

This is not the same as knowing an impersonal, philosophical fact.

One can understand a deer tick or a bald eagle as individuals and as parts of systems and, indeed, that knowledge can be useful morally. One can understand carbon as an atom having six protons and an atomic mass of approximately twelve, and as a significant component of organic systems, and understand far more complex aspects of biochemistry which will serve well the health-care professional. The capacity to know in this way does not significantly assist in obtaining existential (that is, in the Kierkegaardian sense of the eternal expressed in the temporal moment) knowledge and can, indeed, become an impediment if the knower becomes arrogant about his or her capacity to proximately *know*, mistaking it for eternal *understanding*.

Persons may use reason or sociocultural conditions or psychologically threatening experiences or other ways of knowing their own spiritual condition to discern the need for God, but one can only know God through meeting him. In other words, even the Bible is not proof of God to the unbeliever, since accepting its authority presumes conversion. Yet, afterward, it is authoritative for the faithful, though it cannot be read and understood in isolation, but requires interpretive boundaries established within the body of Christ.

One scholar, David Lawton, considering how the Text is used within the community of the faithful, states that "[w]hat readers read in the Bible are words; only the interpretation will make them Word."[3] More precisely, for evangelicals, what readers read in the Bible are words fully and uniquely divinely inspired, but only by the grace of the Holy Spirit in one's life, through direct inspiration and the community of the faithful, can one interpret them so as to make them "the Word heard." This does not mean that the Scripture is not the Word from the moment it is spoken by God, for it is according to evangelical theology, but it is not fully accessible without grace. As Lawton continues, "the Holy Spirit must read, as well as write, the Bible."[4] And this is accomplished within the accountability of the community of faith.

The description of that proper relationship and how one enters into it is sufficiently found in the scriptural canon. Yet, it is the relationship through which God saves, not the Scripture; indeed, one might never read a verse and still be saved as are many young children and persons incapable of reading. This does not diminish the significance of the Scripture as the given Word of

---

[3]David Lawton, *Faith, Text and History: The Bible in English* (Charlottesville: University Press of Virginia, 1990), p. 33.
[4]Ibid.

God. It does mean that the Scripture is never to be worshiped, for it is only instrumental. God alone, a Being and not a book, is to be adored. Further, though sufficient for salvation and guidance in virtue, the Scripture sometimes does not provide specific procedural or propositional guidance about particular moral concerns. As John said, all that Jesus did could not be contained in books, so all that Jesus wants Christians to do morally is not either. Still, the pattern of the Text provides important guidance even when specific propositions are not evident. And, importantly, new moral analysis should never contradict the consistent message of Scripture.

EPISTEMOLOGICAL CLAIMS, PART THREE: THE MORAL USE OF THE TRUE STORY

Knowing in the parables of Jesus is never abstract. What is true of the parables is true of all Christian knowledge; it is purposeful. One of the *ends* of the Scripture story is moral, specifically guiding Christians in living day to day. This is not the only nor even the most important end, but it is an aspect of the divine intention in telling the good news in the Text.

A genuine moral life is possible *after* one enters into a relationship with Jesus Christ. Evangelicals draw on the arguments of Paul, specifically in Romans and 1 Corinthians, to make such an assertion.

> In the same way, the Spirit helps us in our weakness. We do not know what we ought to pray for, but the Spirit himself intercedes for us with groans that words cannot express. And he who searches our hearts knows the mind of the Spirit, because the Spirit intercedes for the saints in accordance with God's will. (Rom 8:26-27)

> Therefore, I urge you, brothers, in view of God's mercy, to offer your bodies as living sacrifices, holy and pleasing to God—this is your spiritual act of worship. Do not conform any longer to the pattern of this world, but be transformed by the renewing of your mind. Then you will be able to test and approve what God's will is—his good, pleasing and perfect will. (Rom 12:1-2)

> The Spirit searches all things, even the deep things of God. For who among men knows the thoughts of a man except the man's spirit within him? In the same way no one knows the thoughts of God except the Spirit of God. We have not received the spirit of the world but the Spirit who is from God, that we may understand what God has freely given us. This is what we speak, not in words taught us by human wisdom but in words taught by the Spirit, expressing spiritual truths in spiritual words. The man without the Spirit does not accept the

> things that come from the Spirit of God, for they are foolishness to him, and he cannot understand them, because they are spiritually discerned. The spiritual man makes judgments about all things, but he himself is not subject to any man's judgment: "For who has known the mind of the Lord that he may instruct him?" But we have the mind of Christ. (1 Cor 2:10-16)

Note the reference to "we." Conversion by grace through a faithful relationship with God is subjective and personal, but the subsequent moral knowledge of God is not. The conversion of the individual takes one from the "community" of the world into the "community" of the saved. The transition from *against God* to *with God* is highly individual, according to evangelicals, but the continuing transformation of the individual following spiritual rebirth occurs only in community. In the community of those who have experienced a true relationship with God, the Christian comes to understand that the true story of Jesus Christ has moral meaning.

The Bible, then, gains moral epistemological priority after individuals have committed themselves to relationships with God through Jesus Christ and entered into the community of the faithful. This does not mean the Scripture was not morally "correct" before conversion but that it was not truly accessible without the indwelling of the Holy Spirit. The knowledge of the Bible is available in a special way to those who have had a religious conversion.

The conversion experience is necessary for true moral understanding. More broadly, what is known must be experienced, either directly through the "senses," including the spiritual "sense," or can be learned secondarily through authoritative voices of those who have themselves "sensed" the love of God directly. This assertion may come as a surprise to those who erroneously assume that scriptural reductionism is the dominant evangelical epistemological claim. Yes, "the Bible says it, I believe it, that settles it" appears on the bumpers of some, but even such presumes the transformation of one's understanding through *knowing* God personally.

As ethicist Tristram Engelhardt says:

> [T]o put matters another way, the collapse of Christian bioethics into secular bioethics is only avoided when one recalls that the epistemological claims of Christian bioethics are rooted in a real experience of a transcendent God.[5]

Not surprisingly, the senses—including the spiritual sense—can be de-

[5]H. Tristram Engelhardt Jr., *The Foundations of Christian Bioethics* (Lisse, Netherlands: Swets and Zeitlinger, 2000), p. 168.

ceived. Even if not *deceptive*, sensory input is processed into "information" that is mediated through cultural location and psychosocial capacity, and that can lead to mistakes. Therefore, sensory input requires verification. Everyone needs secondary sources by which to "test" sensory input and interpretive knowing. The Scripture, besides providing direct moral guidance for the believer on some issues, also provides a check on the spiritual sense.

It is not an accident that persons, when seeing something for which they do not have previous experience, will say to another, "Did you see that?" Simultaneously this question indicates the initiation of interpretation of sensory input into knowledge and a request for verification that the input was satisfactorily accurate. Evangelicals turn to the Text for that verification. The two disciples meeting Jesus on the Road to Emmaus is one example. "They said to one another, 'Were not our hearts burning within us while He was speaking to us on the road, while He was explaining the Scriptures to us?'" (Lk 24:32 NASV).

So, for instance, if a "still small voice" (1 Kings 19:12 KJV) speaks to a believer and gives a command similar to that received by Elijah, that person had better verify with the teachings of the whole Text and the counsel of mature believers that she or he is really supposed to consecrate a national leader and kill the priests of other religions (by the way, it will not be confirmed). Likewise, though "to obey is better than sacrifice" (1 Sam 15:22), the slaughter of the disobedient is now not consistent with the whole Text and the teaching of Jesus, who fulfilled—and thereby transformed—that which had been written before. Indeed, for evangelicals, the whole Bible, even the Old Testament (Hebrew Scriptures) can only be read from the perspective of belief in Jesus; the New Testament is the standard for interpretation of the Old.

A problem arises that can go on *ad infinitum*. The authenticating process too can be wrong. Evangelicals using the Bible respond with the assertion that, because they have the certainty of a relationship with Christ, they can recognize or sense the Scripture is authoritative. This apparently tautological statement rests on the assertion that different people wrote the Text, but the grace of God inspired and assembled it. In other words, God guided those who wrote *and* those who canonized the Text and guides those who read it with a trusting heart. The Bible is a whole made up of parts, which has full meaning only within the community of faithful believers, and for that community is the check on morality.

This does not mean that the Text addresses every moral concern with all pertinent particulars. Certainly this is not the case with bioethics. Still, the general rules and patterns are sufficiently revealed for living a holy life following rebirth. To put this in negative language, there are degrees of ignorance. Evangelicals clearly believe that they can *know* enough to act morally in accordance with the purpose of God, even if they do not understand everything about every variation on the moral concern. Just because there is a line of gray it does not mean there are not black and white, right and wrong.

That does not solve the problem of how to explain Christian morality to those of the world. And, certainly, it does not provide a basis for moral cooperation when such is deemed ethically desirable. Some evangelicals claim that Christian moral arguments should be made in the public arena using scriptural propositional statements. On occasion, Christians will declare that the Scripture should be universally respected and universally accepted as a moral authority. They will say, for instance, that the Scripture expresses a general opposition to abortion and that is sufficient for public debates. A far more effective approach is to recognize the expectations for believers and to distill Christian moral positions to specific propositions (sometimes called middle axioms), and then apply them to social moral problems in a way that makes sense to nonbelievers.

In spite of the interpretative task of the community and even given that some moral problems are not directly considered in the Bible, evangelicals do not consider scriptural truth conditional. Its accuracy is not based on the individual reading it being "saved," though to a great degree the capacity to understand that truth is. Any variation should be within a range of interpretations if one is to remain doctrinally orthodox and express that in orthopraxis.

EPISTEMOLOGICAL CLAIMS, PART FOUR: THE USE OF THE TRUE STORY ANALOGICALLY

Unfortunately, and contrary to what some suggest, direct biblical instruction is simply not available for many contemporary ethically complex situations. This should be expected because the Bible is not primarily a philosophical text or even a moral guide. It is not primarily a discourse. It is essentially a narrative that tells the story of God's gracious love and that, by the Spirit who wrote it, invites the reader to fully participate in that story. The moral discourse in the Scripture is almost always a secondary reflection on the activity of God in his people, and their loving response. Still, though it is not the primary purpose of the Text, moral instruction is an inextricable expression of that primary purpose. To put it another way, being in a relationship with the Lord inevitably elicits a moral response. The Scripture offers patterns that guide, foundational truths upon which to build and allegories that instruct, but no direct commands on many matters of bioethics. When possible, evangelicals can rely on direct and specific biblical moral instruction, but should not expect it for many issues in bioethics.

Evangelicals assume that direct commands present in the Text are to be followed. Usually, those that are problematic (ones that seemingly conflict with other direct commands or violate broader scriptural principles) are prioritized or reinterpreted by common assent or tradition on the basis of broader scriptural themes. When uncertain about whether a particular command is morally compelling in a given moment, evangelicals tend to seek confirmation by prayer and/or by the discernment of the community. Some believers would challenge this and say they "simply" read the Book and follow the commands. However, there are commands that should be obeyed without variance and commands that are to be usually disregarded, or claimed to be specific because they refer to exceptional cases (usually commands peculiar to the situations in which they were first received). In other words, the degree of moral obligation depends on the moral whole of the biblical text. Any conclusions must be framed by the larger story from which they are drawn. This is not a decision for the individual, but is to be verified by accountability within the community.

Prooftexting is considered legitimate if it occurs within the confines of the broader narrative. Of course, the community of faith has sometimes inadequately evaluated such uses of the Scripture, though no more so than "scholars" who have attempted to justify their own philosophies or to find something "new" in their quest for peer approval by pulling out isolated phrases to construct sweeping arguments. Still, the follower who uses prooftexts is best served using Paul's approach rather than attempting to justify his or her own political or cultural values (otherwise, the reasoning will be truly tautological; the value is "assumed" and then texts are "selected" to justify the value). The story is a whole but expressed in the particulars. Thus prooftexts make sense when they express the whole, but are spurious or even destructive when not. Practically speaking, the text should be read and used dialectically; from the whole to the specific, from the specific to the whole. The gospel is not a vague myth about love or niceness or even the golden rule, but a story about real events that continue to be expressed specifically in the lives of believers and the church.

The Bible has sufficient information for a saving relationship, including all general guidance for following Christ, but it does not include all the particulars in the form of injunctions on how to live the Christian life in a specific time in a specific place. The moral epistemological question for evangelicals, then, is how to use the Bible when the Text does not directly inform the moral issue at hand. This is particularly true in bioethics. While it is pointless to try to excuse adultery as morally legitimate, given the clear commandments against the act and the clear affirmations of marital integrity, this is not true about abortion, euthanasia and genetic engineering. Still, the Text can provide the believer with guidance through the presentation of patterns and examples even when direct propositional instruction is not available. These can be applied in bioethics analogically.

Practically speaking, evangelicals tend to approach the Text using five methods of moral reasoning. First, they read the stories that are part of the true story of Christ and recognize in them specific constructs according to which their lives should be shaped. This moral reasoning is *virtue reasoning*. Second, they seek direct instruction. This can be further divided into direct command and direct example. Sometimes these are accumulated so that principles can be established. This moral reasoning is *deontological*. Next, they make calculations about benefit and loss, considering spiritual benefits and detriments in the calculation. When making such calculations in regard to a group, like a church or family, the third method of moral reasoning, *utilitarianism*, is used. When calculating the plusses and minuses only in regard to themselves as individuals, the moral reasoning is *hedonism*, which is fourth. Except in the narrowest sense, such as preferring to enjoy God over experiencing hell, hedonism is not a method that evangelicalism endorses. Utilitarianism is acceptable as a method secondary to deontology or virtue.

When utilitarianism is unacceptable, analogy may be used. The fifth reasoning method, and the method most important for addressing concerns over new technology and forms of organization, is *analogical*.[6] It is similar to virtue reasoning, but is based on structural rather than content similarity. It is ethically useful because it allows a basis for considering, at least initially, morally complex, seemingly novel, concerns. As a moral method, analogical reasoning

[6]For a consideration of analogy in ethics from a Catholic perspective, see William C. Spohn, *Go and Do Likewise: Jesus and Ethics* (New York: Continuum, 2000).

is quite vulnerable to interpretive error, which can lead to false or imperfect conclusions. The source analogue and target analogue may be mismatched, or salient commonalities ignored in favor of less significant matters. Such interpretive errors, in turn, cause moral error. Still, analogy is necessary with brand new technologies and organizational forms.

The stories that serve as analogues for Christian ethical analysis do not appear in isolation, but are told over and over again. Children raised in the community are taught the stories from a young age. So, most children raised in English-speaking evangelical churches know that "Zacheus was a wee little man" and they know that David killed Goliath. Much of the preaching and the Sunday-school education in evangelical churches involve learning these stories and how they should shape the individual believer's life. That is, evangelicals are told the stories and then asked to conform their lives to the pattern found in the stories. In fact, they are taught that the stories of these "heroes of the faith" are part of the same story to which they belong, the story of God's saving love. Evangelicals not only use direct commands and preponderance of evidence, they look for structural patterns in Scripture that reveal moral truth.

Preaching is the primary form of evangelical moral discourse. The preacher will read a passage of Scripture and expound, usually beginning with some exegesis, and then provide an application to current circumstances, often accompanied by extrabiblical illustrations. Usually these are stories analogous to the story read from Scripture. The congregation responds to the preaching discursively. In some congregations this occurs with a verbal encouragement or warning during the preaching itself. In others, it comes afterward in formal or informal discussion of "what the preacher said." The evangelical approach to ethics is that of the pulpit filled with a "Bible preacher."

The use of specific references is governed by the whole story. In fact, the beginning point for Christians struggling with moral concerns should never be specific verses, but the story into which, by God's grace, the believer has woven his or her own story (what Hayes calls the symbolic world; what now is popularly called the metanarrative).[7] Of course, this is actually just a manifestation of the internal logic of the faith. One is saved, then becomes moral. One hears the story, accepts the story, becomes part of the story and then starts to apply specific passages.

[7]Richard B. Hayes, *The Moral Vision of the New Testament* (San Francisco: HarperSanFrancisco, 1996).

Let it also be noted that there may be epistemological disagreements between evangelicals and others who are Christians. For instance, Roman Catholics tend to use strong tradition arguments and, if tied to conservative academic circles, may specifically make appeal to Aquinas or the church fathers. Evangelicals are unlikely to do anything similar. Even though they may refer to Wesley in the broad Methodist tradition, or Edwards or Calvin in the broad Calvinist tradition, it is not definitive even if it may be instructional. Old-line Protestants may appeal to the social sciences or to higher critical exegetical analyses of the Scripture, perhaps prone to use such as morally authoritative. Evangelicals, again, may refer to such, but as a means to understand the Scripture and their own experiences of the Spirit. Indeed, exegesis as an approach to the Scripture remains valuable but secondary to the informing of the Text by the Spirit. Evangelicals tend to weave the hermeneutical task into the descriptive.

In looking at bioethics and how it should be understood among evangelicals, it is best to use the primary means of evangelical moral analysis, which looks a lot more like a Sunday morning sermon based on a key Scripture from the life of Christ than deductive philosophy, social science or biblical critical approaches based in nineteenth-century notions of objectivity.

The emphasis should be on the discursive presentation of the whole story, and how any direct moral guidance fits into the broader report of God's reaching out in love. Evangelicals "love to tell the story" and, in doing so, set parameters that define the limits of moral response. To use an evangelical phrase, "the Bible interprets the Bible." So, the best way to understand this aspect of typical evangelical moral reasoning is to see the Bible as the primary epistemological source for the person who has a true experience of God, but with specific commands and analogies understood as part of the larger salvation story. The connection between the specific commands and analogies are either taught by the current community of faith or verified by its historical authorities. This means that evangelical ethics is "peculiar"—both in the sense of being distinct and, to some outside observers, in the sense of being bizarre.[8]

One of the best descriptions of the Protestant appeal to the Text as the source of moral instruction is from Richard Hayes.[9] He refers to the four-

[8]Stanley Hauerwas and William H. Willimon, *Resident Aliens: Life in the Christian Colony* (Nashville: Abingdon, 1989); and Rodney Clapp, *A Peculiar People: The Church as Culture in a Post-Christian Society* (Downers Grove, Ill.: InterVarsity Press, 1996).

[9]Hayes, *Moral Vision of the New Testament Community*, pp. 3-7. Hayes would probably not agree

fold task to be taken up by those seeking New Testament guidance for contemporary moral concerns. The descriptive task is *exegetical,* that is, a consideration of what the Text meant to the writer and within its original setting as it was written. Hayes correctly points out that this should include consideration of both *didache* (specific teachings) and *ethos* (the community character shaped by stories, symbols, social structures and practices).[10] Second is the *synthetic* task, which is the effort to find canonical consistency. Of course, evangelicals assume such consistency is intrinsic since the text is not only written by inspiration, but also the books of the Bible were canonized as a whole by the inspiration of the Holy Spirit.[11] The *hermeneutical* task, third, is the crossing of the cultural and temporal gap between the writers of the text and circumstances of today. Finally, the fourth task is the *pragmatic,* that is, the "embodying [of the] Scripture's imperatives in the life of the Christian community."[12] These final two tasks he refers to as "application" of the text.[13]

Another way of talking about analogues is with the language of *types,* as used by David Lawton.[14] The Scripture is full of examples of typological identifications; for instance, Paul's reference to the Second Adam (1 Cor 15), Peter's use of the term the "Holy Nation" (1 Pet 2:9-10), and the author of Hebrews referring to the order of Melchezedek (Heb 5). The analogy contains the reality of the type represented. This is not unlike the reality of Christ's suffering within the sacrament of Communion, even though evan-

---

with the shorthand descriptions of the fourfold task given here, especially exegesis, but they are sufficient for this setting.

[10]Ibid., p. 4.

[11]Hayes claims that this process is assisted by three textual foci: community, cross and new creation (ibid., p. 5). The first two are certainly central. The third is important, but perhaps no more so than other themes. Still, this does not diminish from the excellent analysis by Hayes nor his arguments about the use of the text today.

[12]Ibid., p. 7. Hayes uses the word *imperative* and seems slightly more oriented toward discerning the command implications of the text. In this, his emphasis appears to be more deontologically oriented than my own. The difference may be only a slight difference in emphasis. The application of his method to abortion (chapter 18) comes the closest to the use of the Text in this work.

[13]See also Sondra Wheeler's and Allen Verhey's uses of Scripture in bioethics: Sondra Wheeler, *Stewards of Life: Bioethics and Pastoral Care* (Nashville: Abingdon, 1996); and Allen Verhey, *Reading the Bible in the Strange World of Medicine* (Grand Rapids: Eerdmans, 2003). For Southern Baptist perspectives, see the various works of Richard Land, Albert Mohler, David Gushee and Ben Mitchell.

[14]For the use of types within Scripture (esp. Jesus as New Adam, New Joshua, New Melchezidek, etc.) see Lawton, *Faith, Test, and History.* Lawton argues that "[t]ypology is the central link from the Old Testament to the New Testament" (p. 19).

gelicals do not consider the consecrated elements to be transubstantiated, as would Catholics.

In cases of moral analysis, common typological characteristics are discerned, and the claim is made that these commonalties allow extension to the current moral concern or characteristic. "[S]ome of the content of a source analog is transferred to a target analog."[15] In one sense, this might be called a precise kind of deontological thought, or it might be called a form of casuistry. Most appropriately, analogical thinking is to be understood as the community seeking consistency in a given decision specifically, and behavior generally. It arises from the desire to be virtuous, with this virtuosity being understood as consistency with the character of Christ.

The power of analogy for evangelicals lies in the claim that the moral concern of the Christian today is of like kind with those reported in the Text. The believers' moral issues are like those that Jesus experienced; though not in specifics, they are of like types. This is not simply a moral assertion; it is a soteriological (salvation doctrine) claim. The early church declared, and evangelicals continue to believe, that Jesus was tempted (including facing morally ambiguous situations) in every way that we are (Heb 4:15-16). This, the salvific impact of the Incarnation (including the temptation, betrayal, and crucifixion), is the source of the typological connection between the Bible and the life of the believer.

When direct instruction is available, it is used. When strong precedents accumulate to create a pattern, they are followed. To supplement these or to provide guidance in their absence, the community uses analogy. The congregation shares, reads, acknowledges and analogically extends the validity of the Scripture. The application, if it is true to the analogue, appropriates spiritual validity in that it arises from the Text. This is more than a metaphorical or allegorical reading.[16] The capacity to use analogies within the community of faith is contingent upon the following: (1) faithfulness in allowing the Spirit to be active (or Christian humility), (2) understanding of the specific texts (e.g., parables) as part of the Text and (3) testing of the

---

[15]Paul Thagard, *How Scientists Explain Disease* (Princeton, N.J.: Princeton University Press, 1999), p.14. This is a reference to understanding diseases analogically. Thagard is referring to "analogical mapping" according to Richard Hadden.

[16]For a metaethical or philosophical explanation of metaphor and analogy that includes historical references to Aristotle and Aquinas as well as more recent philosophers and which includes consideration of scientific and theological uses of analogy, see David Burrell, *Analogy and Philosophical Language* (New Haven, Conn.: Yale University Press, 1973).

analogies for consistency and internal logic. These cannot be successfully accomplished without the community of faith. In other words, the ability to use moral analogies in Christianity assumes, namely, the person using them has been altered toward wisdom by the Holy Spirit and is morally embedded in a community of faith.[17]

Analogy is similar to metaphor, but—for purposes of this study—will be differentiated to the extent that the similarities with an analog are similarities of type, rather than superficial similarities that can be used for heuristic purposes. Metaphors may sometimes represent similarities that are of the same type (they may be analogical), but they also may simply serve as reminders of characteristics that are, in fact, not genuinely shared between the two situations or decisions. Importantly for evangelicals, the nature of a moral similarity must be analogical. The internal order must be the same and represented in the analogous situations and decisions. While certainly the language can be debated, for the purposes of this analysis, *metaphor* is a broader category than analogy. A metaphor is figurative, likened to another, but not necessarily a literal comparison.[18] The analogy is literal in the sense that the analogue is the same in moral structure or proportion.

Also, analogy is not the same as allegory. Allegorical readings of the Bible have their place, but generally not in ethics, because their use disregards the historical reality of the events in the Text. Certainly some passages of Scripture are meant to be allegorical or symbolic; fiction designed for truthful pedagogical purposes. However, allegorizing events intended to be understood as real in the modern historical/scientific sense, such as the life of Jesus himself, would be problematic to evangelicals.

An example of analogical reasoning in mathematics can be applied *analogically* to ethical reasoning.

> The use of analogy and similar relational comparisons . . . promote[s] flexible

---

[17]See also Duns Scotus's various responses to Aquinas. One of the clearest descriptions of Christian analogy appears in the work of Thomas Aquinas. Analogy in Aquinas, as developed out of Aristotle, is understood as coming in two basic and related forms: analogy of attribution and analogy of proportionality. If an analogy is an intrinsic attribution it bears similar characteristics, because it has a similar existing purpose or common origin. If it is an extrinsic attribution, the similarity may be in instrumental purpose. Of the second kind, analogy of proportion can be real, in which the relational or structural similarities of the analogues is a reflection of the essential nature of each, or can be metaphorical, in which case the relationships and structures are relatively similar.

[18]Modified from *Merriam Webster's Collegiate Dictionary*, 10th ed. (Springfield, Mass.: Merriam-Webster, 1995).

> conceptual learning and problem-solving. Analogy allows [the learner] to use commonalities between mathematical representations to help understand new problems or concepts, thereby contributing to integral components of mathematical proficiency.[19]

This analogy on the use of analogy makes sense for understanding morality. The common use of analogy within moral reasoning extends to moral reasoning itself. Among the favorite analogues for morality are the law, etiquette, language, the enjoyment of beauty and mathematics.[20] In other words, morality is like

- the law in providing rules with sanctions;
- etiquette in that it provides a way for interacting;
- language because the patterns are learned within communities;
- the enjoyment of beauty because fairness is a symmetry;
- mathematics because the "parts" fit together and unknowns can be determined from knowns.

Evangelicals use analogies to understand the new and complex, and it makes sense best within the community of believers, because of the prior univocal presentation of God through his Spirit to each believer and to the body as a whole. Subsequently, evangelicals may need to translate these analogies and the moral conclusions they reach in order to enter into discourse with the world, because the analogies and conclusions are based on that spiritual presence unique to the faithful. But this should not be difficult, if explicitly done. In bioethics particularly, both believers and those of the world use analogy extensively for argumentation. Sometimes this is explicit.[21] Sometimes it is simply an unconsidered component of discourse. Regardless, it is understandable.

Analogy is particularly useful in ethics because it allows the individual to

---

[19]Lindsey E. Richland, Osnat Zur and Keith J. Holyoak, "Cognitive Supports for Analogies in the Mathematics Classroom," *Science,* May 25, 2007, 1128-29.

[20]Morality analogized with law (traditional; e.g., Kant), etiquette (e.g., Philippa Foot), language (e.g., Rawls), biological life (e.g., developmentalists, sociobiologists), enjoying beauty ("sentimentalists" such as Shaftesbury, Hutcheson and Hume; in J. Edwards symmetry of beauty is found in morality; in Kant the analogy is used with the source and target analogs reversed), mathematics ("rationalists"). On the last two, see Michael B. Gill, "Moral Rationalism vs. Moral Sentimentalism: Is Morality More Like Math or Beauty?" *Philosophy Compass* (November 2006).

[21]Eric Wiland, "Unconscious Violinists and the Use of Analogies in Moral Argument," *The Journal of Medical Ethics* 26 (2000): 466-68.

not only "understand" cognitively but also sympathetically, to use the traditional language of Adam Smith.[22] The novelty of new technologies for the culture, or the survival of persons with disabilities who might well have died in the past, or simply the experience of severe illness in a culture that distances itself from suffering and illness, are either disordering or unordered. This means that reliance on unambiguous precedents or directives, including those in Scripture, may not—indeed, often are not—available for making sense of a morally confusing situation.

The distinction between sympathy and empathy is difficult to make. Generally, sympathy is an affective response to another which draws forth concern, ranging from momentary worry for another to compassion that elicits advocacy or action. Empathy is a matter of recognizing structural similarities, but without concern for the other. Some might argue that sympathy is a category contained within the broader category of empathy as emotional knowledge of another's circumstances, while others prefer to think of empathy as self-oriented and distinct from sympathy, which is described as other or communally oriented. Using the first understanding, empathy is affective knowledge while sympathy is affective knowledge with favorable identification expressed as concern.[23]

---

[22]There is a significant popular disagreement on when to use which term. To a great extent the selection of *sympathy* as the more invested term is arbitrary. In their fine article, "Empathy and Analogy" <http://cogsci.uwaterloo.ca/Articles/Pages/Empathy.html>, Allison Barnes and Paul Thagard seem to favor *empathy* over *sympathy* as a term to explain how analogy is used in novel situations. For moral decision making, though, analogy is usually used to not only understand but "identify with" for the purposes of assuming a position of affirmation or advocacy or, at least, genuine concern (even if very weak).

[23]Adam Smith, in *A Theory of Moral Sentiments,* argues for sympathy as the basis for community interactions with persons who would otherwise be strangers. This sympathy, though, can wear thin. At which point (though Smith does not use the language) it could be called an empathy of disdain. Such a process can be observed in those who are concerned for someone who is hurt in an accident, but who is eventually redefined as a malingerer. Others would suggest that interactions with moral strangers are interpreted through rational decision. For more on the Christian engagement with strangers, acquaintances and friends, see the following: Engelhardt, *Foundations of Christian Bioethics*, especially pp. 168-79; Kevin Wm. Wildes, *Moral Acquaintances: Methodology in Bioethics* (Notre Dame, Ind.: University of Notre Dame Press, 2000); James R. Thobaben, "Pleased to Make Your Acquaintance: A Review of Kevin Wm. Wildes' *Moral Acquaintances: Methodology in Bioethics*," *Christian Bioethics* 7, no. 3: 425-39. Engelhardt, Wildes and Thobaben—an Eastern Orthodox, a Roman Catholic and an evangelical, respectively—would disagree on the mechanism or knowing process, but agree on the human condition of having two broad categories of moral knowledge: that knowable by those of the world and that knowable by those who follow the Christ. Wildes and Thobaben would also agree, and Engelhardt seems to imply, that there is a category of acquaintance between stranger and friend, or that there is a continuum of stranger and acquaintance that allows varying degrees of understanding.

Analogy for moral purposes requires empathy. It is needed to make sense of new situations, using old situations as the basis for interpretation. For Christians there is often a sympathetic component to analogy. After all, the words used to construct most of the primary moral analogies call for concern and action. Applying the stories of the true gospel story calls for purity in oneself and justice and mercy for others. Inevitably, justice and mercy require more than abstracted empathy; emotions require sympathetic identification with the aggrieved or the sufferer.

The three primary weaknesses in the use of analogies are these: (1) analogues may be only superficially related;[24] (2) even if they are fundamentally related, the specific selected characteristic may not correspond and, therefore, the analogy may be inapplicable; and (3) circumstances not revealed by the use of the analogy may call for a different response even if there are fundamental similarities between analogue and the subject/issue of concern. A fourth weakness, not for those within the community of faith but from the perspective of those outside, is that the analogue from Scripture may itself be dismissed as having no validity because the Scripture has no validity. Those of the world do not agree with the moral epistemological significance of the Bible and this is one reason why the Scripture cannot be used authoritatively in secular settings.

One way of addressing these weaknesses from within the faith community is simply to recognize that for evangelicals the Gospel story is *the* analogue. It is the pattern for the moral life. Consequently, while there may be debates as to which portions of the story to use in a specific situation or how to place an emphasis, there is no disagreement about the priority of the good news as the analogue for all moral choice and all moral virtue. This, however, is not persuasive to those of the world. Still, an appeal to justice and mercy, and sympathy for the sufferer and the aggrieved may be starting points for the use of analogy, which in turn may help clarify real needs and real solutions. Believers do not doubt that other persons can "know," but in making a claim for a greater access to the Truth, Christians are claiming that the moral knowledge of others is sometimes fundamentally deficient and inadequate. This does not, by the nature of the gospel, allow arrogance or intolerance. Rather, it means cooperation is possible, but limited.

---

[24]Thagard, *How Scientists Explain Disease*, p. 141.

CONCLUSION: THE STORY, CHRISTIAN BIOETHICS AND THE WORLD

To this point, it has been emphasized that the story of Jesus Christ, from Genesis through Revelation and as expressed in the life of individual believers and the community of faith, is the means of knowing morally for evangelicals who have previously experienced God's grace. This might lead to the conclusion that only the Scripture can be used. That conclusion would not be accurate. By temporal calculation, the church existed before the New Testament. The church is the interpretive community for the Scripture. Of course, one could claim that ontologically the Text is in the mind of God from before time. But, finally, this distinction should make no practical difference since there is no other Holy Text and there is no believer who exists outside of the church. This is a two-edged sword, to modify the Pauline image. It means that believers must turn to the Bible for their moral instruction and that believers cannot use it as the *primary* means for moral reasoning with those outside the community, since it can only be genuinely understood within the church. Some might claim that evangelicals are part of an overlapping moral-linguistic community—one with a moral order that in some ways transcends the faith. While having much in common with non-Christians, believers do make moral claims that are distinct in content or in explanation.

Believers may make appeals to some level of general moral knowledge among all humans. Depending on the theological tradition from which the particular evangelical group sprang, this may be understood as natural law (e.g., evangelicals, including charismatics, in Anglican/Episcopal churches or Catholic congregations), general revelation (most Calvinist traditions) and/or prevenient grace (e.g., Wesleyan traditions). The claim may be that forms of ethical structure and even some moral "knowing" are intrinsic to the human condition because of neurophysiologic processes, or social structures, or the created *telos* of each individual, even while allowing that particular expressions get worked out differently in different times and different places. Another argument for points of agreement can be made using "middle axioms" in which there is no fundamental agreement on why a moral value should help or a principle be affirmed, but the fact that it is commonly held or affirmed will allow cooperation on policies that may spring from that value or principle.

Furthermore, Christian moral knowledge dictates that Christians not act in immoral ways toward unbelievers. Some degree of cooperation is necessary, though the level of that cooperation is certainly a contested point. At the least, Christians can agree that God has established an order beyond the church that operates to prevent humans from destroying one another, and Christians should cooperate with that order. When those of the world seek to promote, in a morally acceptable manner, values that are compatible with the Christian notion of the Good, then believers should cooperate with that as well.

This is not a philosophical argument for which evangelicals, generally speaking, care all that much. While the parables and the entire gospel story may have been concealing for some, for believers they are to be revealing, and that tends to be accepted as sufficient for their own moral needs. The Text as interpreted in the community provides guidance in living the Christian life. Metaethical debates about neuroethics and sociobiology, about culture and psychosocial development are interesting, but the real question that concerns evangelicals is how to practically know the good and right, and how to do them—to the extent demanded for the church, or to the extent possible for those of the world. In other words, the evangelical use of analogy for moral knowing involves two broad moves: first, finding analogies that make "sense" of a new moral situation for the believer and, then, the believer using the structural similarities discerned to help nonbelievers understand a Christian moral position allowing cooperation with nonbelievers when possible.

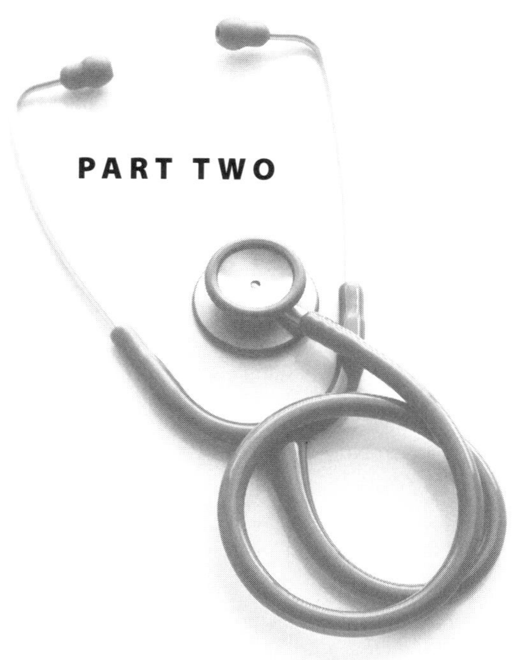

PART TWO

Characteristics of Humanity and Bioethical Debates

4

Theodicy and Healing

HUMANS AS DISORDERED

Humans suffer. The experience of physical suffering can disorder one's life if there is not a sufficient explanation. When illness or injury occur, if one defines one's purpose by roles that are lost or one's worldview requires that only the bad or otherwise inadequate have significant problems, then anomy may arise to which one can only respond with desperation or some kind of faith. Evangelicals claim that Christianity is the single sufficient explanation for suffering that provides true hope for continued living.

> As he went along, he saw a man blind from birth. His disciples asked him, "Rabbi, who sinned, this man or his parents, that he was born blind?" "Neither this man nor his parents sinned," said Jesus, "but this happened so that the work of God might be displayed in his life. As long as it is day, we must do the work of him who sent me. Night is coming, when no one can work. While I am in the world, I am the light of the world."
>
> Having said this, he spit on the ground, made some mud with the saliva, and put it on the man's eyes. "Go," he told him, "wash in the Pool of Siloam" (this word means Sent). So the man went and washed, and came home seeing.
>
> His neighbors and those who had formerly seen him begging asked, "Isn't this the same man who used to sit and beg?" Some claimed that he was. Others said, "No, he only looks like him." But he himself insisted, "I am the man." "How then were your eyes opened?" they demanded. He replied, "The man they call Jesus made some mud and put it on my eyes. He told me to go to Siloam and wash. So I went and washed, and then I could see." "Where is this man?" they asked him. "I don't know," he said.
>
> They brought to the Pharisees the man who had been blind. Now the day on which Jesus had made the mud and opened the man's eyes was a Sabbath. Therefore the Pharisees also asked him how he had received his sight. "He put mud on my eyes," the man replied, "and I washed, and now I see." Some of the Pharisees said, "This man is not from God, for he does not keep the Sabbath."

> But others asked, "How can a sinner do such miraculous signs?" So they were divided. Finally they turned again to the blind man, "What have you to say about him? It was your eyes he opened." The man replied, "He is a prophet."
>
> The Jews still did not believe that he had been blind and had received his sight until they sent for the man's parents. "Is this your son?" they asked. "Is this the one you say was born blind? How is it that now he can see?" "We know he is our son," the parents answered, "and we know he was born blind. But how he can see now, or who opened his eyes, we don't know. Ask him. He is of age; he will speak for himself." His parents said this because they were afraid of the Jews, for already the Jews had decided that anyone who acknowledged that Jesus was the Christ would be put out of the synagogue. That was why his parents said, "He is of age; ask him." . . .
>
> Jesus heard that they had thrown him out, and when he found him, he said, "Do you believe in the Son of Man?" "Who is he, sir?" the man asked. "Tell me so that I may believe in him." Jesus said, "You have now seen him; in fact, he is the one speaking with you." Then the man said, "Lord, I believe," and he worshiped him. Jesus said, "For judgment I have come into this world, so that the blind will see and those who see will become blind." Some Pharisees who were with him heard him say this and asked, "What? Are we blind too?" Jesus said, "If you were blind, you would not be guilty of sin; but now that you claim you can see, your guilt remains. (Jn 9:1-23, 35-41)

PART ONE: THE TEXT

A pool is the center of activity—this time Siloam rather than Bethesda. Contrary to the Bethesda pool healing earlier in the Gospel, at Siloam Jesus directs the person who is diseased to wash per his instructions. The diseased man is to follow the prescription of the healer. Jesus, as he had with poverty and oppression, is challenging the accepted understanding of disease as moral disorder. He also demonstrates a willingness to use the healing "technology" of the day. Certainly, John writes of the pool in a matter-of-fact way. Whether or not the healings were considered miraculous, as those of Bethesda, is immaterial. Jesus does not contraindicate the use of the waters but rather combines his activity with an accepted, common healing mechanism.

The Pool of Siloam—unlike the Bethesda pool—though apparently used as site for healing, was more notable to the residents of Jerusalem as the only permanent water source within the city during the first century, being substantially fed from a spring apparently diverted to the site during the reign of Hezekiah in the eighth century B.C. in order to prevent access to any invading force that might take up siege against Jerusalem. The water was likely that used for temple services. The name means "sent." While there are speculations as to the symbolic significance of these two pools, Siloam and Bethesda, it is generally assumed that the pools are mentioned simply because they are the sites of the miracles.

Jesus' offer of healing at both pools appears to be based on the assumption that the disorders go far beyond physiological or anatomical failures. Though they are that, they are something more. Perhaps the man at the Bethesda Pool relishes the pity, or the excuses disease provides for a failed life. Perhaps the man who washes in the Siloam Pool is passive in his illness. Possibly the culture has deemed all these individuals impure or inadequate or somehow deserving of sickness. One way or another, both Jesus and the men recognize that the society or the men themselves or both have declared the paralytic and the blind man invalid beings.[1] When Jesus asks the question of the first—"Do you want to be healed?"—and when he gives the command to the other—"Go wash in the pool"—he is challenging the operating interpretations of the culture—and of all cultures.

The healing of the blind man with spittle and washing is preceded and followed by religious leaders questioning Jesus' sanity. Like political leaders that simply cannot, or will not, conceive of anyone disagreeing with their interpretations of reality, they challenge Jesus for challenging them. Perhaps the best contemporary parallel would be the medicalizing of anti-Marxist political positions in the former Soviet Union. Anyone who rejected the worldview could do so only as an enemy of the state or out of insanity. To a lesser degree of severity, but nonetheless similar, is the medicalizing of moral positions—both for and against—on the legitimacy of homosexual behavior. Regardless of whether the behavior is or is not natural, opposition or support is not a matter of sanity or phobia but of morality.

People have been defined by their disorders as long as history has been recorded and, though there is variation with different diseases and disabilities, the same remains true today. In part, these miracles are Jesus' rejection not of the category of blind or leper or paralytic but of the defining of a person's

---

[1]The following note important structural flaws in the cultural understanding of illness. This does not mean that their solutions are necessarily preferable: Ivan Ilych, *Medical Nemesis: The Expropriation of Health* (New York: Pantheon Books, 1976); Hans-Georg Gadamer, *The Enigma of Health,* trans. Jason Gaiger and Nicholas Walker (Stanford, Calif.: Stanford University Press, 1996); and Thomas Szasz, *The Theology of Medicine: The Political-Philosophical Foundations of Medical Ethics* (Syracuse, N.Y.: Syracuse University Press, 1988).

significance before God—and therefore before others—by such categorization. For this and other challenges to the social order, he was deemed a rebel, a heretic and a mad man.

Both by the specific words and by the location of the miracle in the Text, it appears that Jesus is rejecting the cultural explanation about disease and disability specifically and the claims made about suffering and marginalization more generally. In doing so, Jesus corrects an error. Those who think that physical existence has no connection to the spiritual are wrong, as well as those who believe that there is a direct, one-to-one correspondence between physical and spiritual "disorder." Rather, all of existence—physical, spiritual or any other kind of existing—is subordinate to the Divine. The distinction that needs to be made, whether enduring suffering or enjoying bounty, is not between corporeal and ethereal but between following God's divine purpose and not. In this passage, there is no mistaking that Jesus wants all to recognize that the severity of spiritual blindness is far greater than physical, but without minimizing the significance of the latter.

Given the other healing miracles of Jesus (and it is important to note how weighted the Gospels are toward presenting these as significant events of his earthly ministry), it seems quite clear that the physical body matters to the Christ, but that it matters penultimately—that it gains its value by the relationship to the ultimate, which is the relationship with God. While Jesus sometimes differentiates the body, soul, mind, strength, heart and spirit, he apparently does not understand them as radically separable. The individual does not "possess" a soul, for that implies an individual prior to the soul itself. The individual is the soul and the soul is the individual, at least in some sense. Some of the terms Jesus uses mean different things and some may be almost synonymous. He gives priority to the soul, but that seems to be something more akin to what is now meant by the word *person* rather than animating spirit.

When Jesus heals the man at Siloam, he is declaring that (1) the world is fallen, but that he can restore it, (2) individuals can be restored as well, (3) all of life (including the experience of illness) is simultaneously a social and an individual experience, (4) human physical existence and spiritual existence are inextricably linked, and (5) life and wholeness in the "now" are linked to the eternity of the Divine.

PART TWO: CHRISTIAN BIOETHICS

From a Christian perspective, any form of suffering, including that which is primarily physical, is in one way or another an expression of the falleness of humanity and the brokenness of nature. For the follower of the suffering God, it is—or should be—coincident with hope.[2] What is hope?[3] Hope is a fourfold understanding of the future: (1) desire (pointed toward a *telos* or goal), (2) yoked with a willingness to act, (3) believing that one's actions and other factors can lead to change, (4) all while having the capacity and willingness to change oneself for that *telos*. Hope is not merely an attitude or belief—it is an activity. Christian hope is always finally directed toward God, always directed toward the wholeness of the divine order for which every individual was created.

Hope for the sick person might legitimately be for physical healing. Or for the one who is dying, there may be hope to die well as a ministry for the living, and the sure and true belief in the resurrection to come. In the end, hope in the midst of illness and death, for the evangelical believer, must hinge on the relationship with God. Anything else is mere wishfulness.

Real hope does not deny real suffering. The difficulties associated with illness can be significant, but these burdens—and burdens they may be—remain secondary to the spiritual reality of the whole person and the communities to which that person does and can belong. Evangelicals readily acknowledge that disease is usually a biological phenomenon, but one that may in turn have roots in spiritual reality.[4] No one is reducible to his or her physiological processes, even while those processes are part of the complex biological, cultural and social interaction of a spiritual being. Paul, at one point, declares that the body is but an "earthen vessel" and elsewhere compares it to the seed that dies in order that the plant will arise (2 Cor 4:7; 1 Cor 15). Perhaps the greatest distinguishing characteristic of the biological body is that, in its physicality, it bears more of the obvious marks of finitude. For this reason, it serves as a reminder of human weakness.

Still, the temporal characteristic is not, in and of itself, sinful. The creation

---

[2]This is not a reference to patripassionism, but to the suffering of the Christ. Having said that, patripassionism should not be considered one of the fundamental heresies of the church, though it is an error that demonstrates an inadequate theology of the Trinity.

[3]These thoughts were spurred on by Janet R. Nelson's paper presented at the 2003 Society for Christian Ethics in Pittsburgh, "Mental Illness Is Missing—and Why This Matters to Bioethics."

[4]An excellent description of the ways in which the scientific world tends to understand disease is found in Paul Thagard, *How Scientists Explain Disease* (Princeton, N.J.: Princeton University Press, 1999). The author looks in particular at the very recent change in descriptions of the etiology of ulcers.

from dust means vulnerability, but it does not necessarily mean evil. Sin comes into the world after creation of the physical existence. God declares the physical, along with the spiritual, as good (Gen 1). The full human, including the finite and damageable biological body, is believed to be worthy of Christian concern. The body, soul, spirit, mind, heart and strength (however they may individually be defined) exist only as an inextricably linked unity as long as one exists here.[5] The person created in the image of God bears that image with the dust of the earth. Somehow the individual, with all his or her component parts (including the physical body) is a bearer of the divine image, though not deity.

To use theological language, the components of the whole person might be thought of in the same sense as the Trinity. Christians are monotheists, yet they claim that God has manifest himself and exists within himself as three *hypostases* of one *ousia* (consubstantiality). In an analogous way, Christians can understand the whole human as a whole who exists only as a whole, even while being able to distinguish differentiating characteristics among the component parts. Though only an analogy (and though, perhaps, only for this life), if this is even partially applicable, then the spiritual reality amplifies the value of the physical rather than diminishes it.

Apparently Jesus thought the earthly body of an individual has real value. He chose to heal the sick not as an expression of Gnostic pity for their spiritual weakness but because, all other things being equal, it is good to be physically healthy. The miraculous healings of the Lord are the most frequently recorded activity in the Gospels. And, as is apparent from the healing miracles of Jesus, physical well-being is not to be separated from the well-being of the whole person.

Any extreme separation of the physical body from the rest of what constitutes the individual is not historically appropriate. Though there is a variety of opinions on the concept of heaven, there is a belief among all evangelicals that the individual will be recognizable and will have limits after death. According to Paul (1 Cor 15), the raised shall have identifiable bodies, but spiritual bodies rather than physical bodies in the earthly sense. Further, in some sense the heavenly body is an expression of the reality of the physical body. Though

[5]There is a tendency to use the categories of body, soul and sprit as if these were comprehensive. This is based on a Pauline passage in 1 Thessalonians 5 and should be compared to other patterns, for instance that of the Lord Jesus in Matthew 10:28; Mark 12:30; Luke 10:27, and Old Testament passages such as Deuteronomy 6:5; 2 Kings 23:25; Psalm 31:9; 63:1; and Micah 6:7.

there is not unanimity among evangelical Christians on what is meant by the terms *body, soul* and *spirit* and what of the individual will be raised at the end of time, some evangelical Christians see radical differentiation of the soul and body as a reflection of pre-Christian Greek thought, or that of early modernity as typified by Cartesians, not the gospel.[6] All evangelicals do agree that in some way the body is simultaneously a piece of pottery, a temple of the Holy Spirit and shall be raised transformed to live through eternity.

The complexity of the Christian understanding of physical well-being arises in part through confusion over the concept of body. The "body" in Christianity sometimes refers to the earthly, physical body and sometimes refers to the expression of the individual through eternity. In the case of the latter, the body is eternal and not finally subject to disease. In the case of the former, the body can be disordered by injury or illness. Adding to the confusion over the word *body* is the fact that numerous, related terms are used in Scripture to refer to the individual human being and its various components.

Most notably, Paul's use of the term "flesh" (usually *soma* for body, but *sarkinos* for flesh) sometimes leads to misrepresentations of the significance of the physical body. While in the Gospels *flesh* is understood more or less positively or neutrally as the created physical component of the human that

---

[6]See, for instance, Joel Green, "Eschatology and the Nature of Humans: A Reconsideration of Pertinent Biblical Evidence," *Science and Christian Belief* 14, no. 1 (April 2002): 33-51. It may be that the best term to describe this unified whole is *individual*. The problem with that language is that in the West it also implies a sharp distinction from being part of the social entities. See also John A. T. Robinson, *The Body: A Study in Pauline Theology* (Philadelphia: Westminster Press, 1952). Robinson provides some clarity on the distinction of flesh and body and on the necessity for Christians to understand their resurrection *body* in social terms which include the individual (social as in the *body* of Christ or the *bride* of Christ). On the other hand, some of the final conclusions, which seem to go far beyond the prior work on the texts, are not going to be found acceptable to most evangelicals. See too J. Keir Howard, *Disease and Healing in the New Testament: An Analysis and Interpretation* (Lanham, Md.: University Press of America, 2001). The book provides a solid accounting of the scholarship on sickness in the New Testament and good presentation on the different approaches of the various New Testament authors. However, I must take issue with two points, both fairly minor, though with broad implications: (1) Howard states that, for the church today, miracles should not be understood as mechanisms of healing, but as an "interpretive term" (p. 297); while it is indeed interpretive, to suggest that this is not part of the mechanism of healing or that God cannot directly intervene would be problematic both for postmodern understandings of sickness and health and for evangelicals; (2) there seems to be a slight tendency, in the end, to return to a Cartesian-like mind (spirit)-body dualism. Still, he does correctly challenge those who would use only such an understanding. As will be argued in this chapter, these are not mutually exclusive categories and their simultaneous (or coincident) use does not exclude the legitimacy of the other. Also see Hector Avalos, *Health Care and the Rise of Christianity* (Peabody, Mass.: Hendrickson, 1999); and John J. Pilch, *Healing in the New Testament: Insights from Mediterranean and Medical Anthropology* (Minneapolis: Fortress, 2000).

is united in marriage and is the food symbolized in the sacrament, for Paul the term is sometimes negative. For instance, Paul speaks of the flesh in Romans 7:5 and Romans 7:25. The New International Version translates this as the "sinful nature," which may be preferable in that it distinguishes the flesh as a word for evil from flesh as the physical, which God created as good. Yet Paul also uses flesh to describe human temporal existence that becomes an opportunity for sinful desires when combined with the sinfulness of pride before the Infinite.

God became incarnate. No one can be a Christian who does not accept that God took upon himself human form, including the frailties of temporal existence. If such is not the case, then there is no significance to the crucifixion, nor does the resurrection have any meaning, for it is simply a magic trick of a mocking deity. Indeed, one is simply not a Christian if there is not acceptance of the resurrection. The same God-human who performed healing miracles for others was himself raised and, in so doing, declared both the opportunity to enter eternity and the significance of the temporal before that time.

Extreme differentiation of the physical and spiritual minimizes the significance of Jesus' sacrifice. It also creates a risk to which evangelicalism has been vulnerable in the past and may still be, namely the subsequent minimizing of ethical responsibilities for the physical well-being of persons. Though the heritage of evangelicalism is marked by strong efforts to unite concern for the earthly well-being of individuals and the state of their souls, since the beginning of the twentieth century the broad movement has not been as demonstratively concerned as it should be. This body, soul and spirit, as a unity, are the individual and all of that individual is a moral concern for believers. The Scripture demonstrates that (1) the categories of mind, body, soul and spirit are not to be understood in a rigid, exclusive manner, and (2) the ultimate concern is relationship, not philosophical constructs.

Regardless of the philosophical questions, two assertions about the body/soul do matter for Christian ethics, specifically bioethics. First, there is a functional holism in the New Testament.[7] Second, though the specifics do not matter on any major issue in bioethics (as to whether there is an immediate resurrection, an intermediate state, or any other specific form of eternal life), it is imperative that Christian ethics accounts for the fact that the person sur-

[7]As J. P. Moreland and Scott B. Rae correctly note in *Body and Soul: Human Nature and the Crisis in Ethics* (Downers Grove, Ill.: InterVarsity Press, 2000). They would emphasize inextricably linked dualism, rather than heterogenous unity of the human.

vives death, somehow, in some way. Eternal survival provides teleological value back upon this life.

The reality of the eternal impingement upon the temporal can sometimes lead to incorrect assertions about the causes of suffering. Claiming that any given experience of disease or injury is a direct consequence of specific sinful activities is problematic. Even when a physical casual relationship exists between an immoral act and illness or injury, it is almost always also associated with other causal factors that were beyond the control of the sick or injured individual. To claim otherwise moves one quite close to the religious arrogance of Job's comforters, something some evangelicals did when AIDS exploded in the West.

Another risk is putting all the moral responsibility on coping with sickness or injury on the one who is directly suffering. When evangelicals choose to focus exclusively on how God can "use" illness and injury to spiritually better the life of the sufferer, they risk denying the goodness God intended for this creation. They also commend endurance and patience while not recognizing that their own failures to manifest those virtues in serving the sick or injured may be more egregious. Further, they do not see that, regardless of the causes of the other's suffering, their own spiritual needs must be met through service to individuals and such must always be marked by kindness and gentleness. It is true that God can and will use anything for his end in our lives, especially as we consent to his Spirit, but focusing on the sufferer's response instead of the necessity of ministering to that suffering person can result in a docetic minimizing of physical need and a blaming of the sufferer as if his or her sins were worse than the comforter's. God can transform all things into a means of grace, even illness and injury, but this does not mean that physical suffering is a good. To the contrary, it is always in some way an expression of evil. If the wellness of the body is considered a penultimate good, then disease and injury must be considered bad.

Yet, any bad can be transformed to God's end. For, as the good of the physical body is penultimate, so is the evil of disease. In other words, being physically sick or injured is not the worst thing that can happen to someone. Hence, if something grander is occurring, then the physical suffering can be transformed by that grander thing. Sickness and injury can be transformed from an evil into something from which good springs. Since the body is inexorably woven together with the spirit and soul, both physical disorder and health-care treatment can affect the spirit/soul, just as the disorder and healing of the spirit and soul can be contributing causes in illness and in the effectiveness of care. The inverse, though, is also true: the spirit and the soul can transform the meaning and experience of physical suffering.

Based on traditional interpretations of the first three chapters of Genesis, evangelicals claim that persons are simultaneously dust (finite), the image of God, and fallen sinners in need of grace. This means suffering and sin are inevitable and God is correcting the causes of suffering and the consequences of sin.

When thinking of suffering and its causes, evangelicals do not tend to specifically use Aristotelian language *(material cause, formal cause, efficient cause, final cause)* or that of any other philosophical school, but the arguments are not entirely dissimilar from traditional philosophy either.[8] Typical of their pragmatic spirituality and belief in an engaging God, they speak of:

Ultimate cause: the perfect and final will of God, which is both the first and final good of all activity, and which for love allows freedom.

Penultimate cause: aspects of being (when these are properly directed it is "rightly ordered love"[9]), which orient freedom.

- human falleness (the reorientation of the human heart away from the Good (original sin);
- the "dustiness" of human existence (finitude);
- "evil" as a reality distinct from humans and the Divine which is oriented toward human destruction and the dishonoring of God (usually, though not always, personified as Satan).

Proximate cause: willfulness (be that conscious or not) or freedom enacted leading to action; includes both individual and structural "willfulness."

- the human being who is hurt;
- another human agent;
- societal structures;
- God;
- nonmaterial "evil force or being";

[8]Perhaps the most important work on the subject of God's will and suffering for evangelicals is Leslie Wetherhead, *The Will of God* (Nashville: Abingdon, 1972). The only other book that approaches its influence would be C. S. Lewis, *The Problem of Pain* (New York: HarperCollins, 1996).

[9]Augustine of Hippo, *The City of God,* book 15, chap. 22.

- usually, nonhuman animals are understood as *not* willfully causing suffering; though this is debated for certain higher animals.

Immediate causes: the immediate cause that precedes material or substantive change.

In clinical settings, then, theologically grounded evangelicals will acknowledge their "part" in their own suffering and that of others, without denying that at different levels other "causes" may be acting. These different levels of causation operate simultaneously, or coincidentally. In other words, a believer may say all of the following when facing suffering:

- "We are all under the will of God" (ultimate purpose of God will not be defeated).
- "That drunken person driving that car was doing an evil thing. I don't care if he's an alcoholic. He chose to drink. He chose to not get enough help. He chose to act in a way that hurt me" (individual sin as penultimate and/or proximate causal factor).
- "There is too much excessive drinking going on in this society and the government should at least do something about how many people drive impaired" (structural sin as proximate causal factor).
- "But the Lord can use this to accomplish his purpose in my life" (proximate cause of suffering retroactively transformed by divine grace at the penultimate level).
- "That car came at me and there was nothing I could do to avoid it. It was metal on metal" (immediate material cause).

Evangelicals generally agree that all or most of these levels of causation are operative, but they will not necessarily agree on emphasis. An example may help explain some of the differences among evangelicals. Almost without exception, evangelicals understand that all suffering has, at its root, the general broken state of human nature. This, for some, is understood to be expressed almost exclusively in individual decisions for evil. So, some extremely conservative evangelicals might assert that the immediate cause of AIDS in a practicing homosexual was HIV, but that it was proximately caused by God as a warning or opportunity to repent, with the penultimate causes being the punishment to the sinner and the ultimate cause the glory of God. However, most evangelicals would not constitute the argument that way. Most would probably claim the proximate cause was a human choice to act in risky manner and that there is a structural sin in society that encourages such promiscuity, even while allowing that God permits consequences for sinful action in response to the corporate and individual rejection of him.

The immediate causes (material or substantive mechanisms) of physical disorder are (1) physical factors, (2) psychological factors, (3) social factors and (4) spiritual. The latter can be distinguished into the positive directly miraculous (divine testing or punishment) and negatively miraculous (evil). Those who are not Christian might prefer to refer to these as *luck* or the chaotic (in the sense of completely unpredictable); regardless, they are causes that are beyond the natural or, at least, beyond the measurable. These various categories are not mutually exclusive.

Physical factors that immediately cause physical disorder are infectious organisms (with that term understood broadly to include viruses and prions), injuries, nutritional deficits, molecular-genetic malformation and so forth. Psychological factors can include conditioning that leads immediately to destructive behaviors or an inability to respond in constructive ways to situations requiring decisions. Psychological factors also include physiological or anatomical failures in the brain that, in conjunction with other inadequacies in coping with social existence, can result in serious psychological malfunction. Society can help or hurt the physical well-being of individuals through the presence or absence of good public health services and reasonable legal protections (e.g., clean water, pure foods, etc.). Persons without such social care will, as a group, be sicker than those in the general population. Evangelical Christians also believe that God sometimes directly acts, miraculously healing or punishing. Some, probably most, evangelicals also believe that evil (usually understood as the personal being, the devil) can do the same, though at a far lower level than God (in Christian theology, the evil one is not the opposite of God as in Manichean or Zoroastrian religion, but is a created, fallen being who presumes to claim the prerogatives of the Divine).

All suffering, according to orthodox theological ethics, is eventually related to the falleness of humans, usually in combination with the finitude of human creation. So, in one sense, evangelical Christians do assert that disease and injury are consequences of sin. However, that is a universally shared penultimate cause and consequence. Ethical analysis tends to be focused on causality at the proximate and, sometimes, immediate levels, while consideration of larger religious questions occurs at the penultimate and ultimate levels.

Morality tends to center on which human being or beings are responsible for and could willfully change a given outcome most directly.

Three arguments about causes of suffering warrant specific mention. First, some evangelicals emphasize the presence of "evil" and demonic negative miracles. In response they may use some form of exorcism. This is not as generally portrayed by the popular media, but rather is "laying on of hands" and extensive prayer, sometimes quite demonstratively and sometimes quite calmly.

Most evangelicals do use the laying on of hands in some circumstances. While perhaps not attributing the immediate cause of the disease or injury to Satan, they do see the suffering as transformable by God and consider laying on of hands a mechanism of prayer. It is a divine opportunity to manifest spiritual power through the faithful action of the believers.

Second, some groups view suffering as a mark of inadequate faith rather than of specific sins. Thus, the lack of a curative miracle is deemed a sign of weak trust. Though often portrayed in the media as a common attitude within the evangelical cohort, it actually is rare. Extremes are sometimes falsely generalized to the entire movement by those who prefer to stereotype. The representation of evangelicals is no different, though it may also be due to the fact that a disproportionate number in popular media and teaching in secular institutions simply do not know, due to self-imposed avoidance, many evangelicals or understand evangelical thought.

Third, evangelicals assert that though God is immutable, he is effectible, specifically through prayer. This is usually understood as the individual's and the church's cooperation with the Holy Spirit. So, the cooperation is actually bringing the well-being (spiritual well-being always, physical sometimes) of the object of prayers into alignment with the will of God.

To use popular language, then, virtually all evangelicals believe in miracles. God does intervene in human affairs, yet without depriving humans of their individual and corporate capacity to choose—to cooperate with or act against the divine purpose. These interventions, or *miracles*, can be good or bad. There is significant difference among evangelicals on how and how often such miracles occur. Some evangelicals assert that God is directly intervening on virtually every occasion in a material way, so miracles (defined as direct proximate and immediate causation by God) occur all the time. Others claim that freedom of the will is operative and the proximate cause of suffering and, to a lesser extent, healing is almost always the choice of some individuals, though God sometimes acts directly. A few aver that the *dispensation* of direct material miracles is past, so the only specific miracles that occur are those within human souls. Another group claims that God's will establishes and specifically predestines the entire order of time, thus God is the direct proximate and immediate cause of all events. And these positions exist in a variety of combinations. It should be noted that the phenomenal growth of evangelicalism in the developing world is often of a form that emphasizes the tangibly miraculous.

Regardless of the position on miracles, evangelicals realize that a spiritual aligning with God's love may or may not lead to physical healing in a specific case, but will also claim that such is always better for the whole person. Sometimes the body gets sick even while the individual may be thriving in every spiritually significant sense (relationally with family, friends and God). Christians must claim this, regardless of one's spiritual worthiness, since the physical body dies.

The following list clarifies how moral culpability is assigned by noting the proximate cause of suffering. Obviously, it is not a list of disease etiologies, as they tend to be descriptions of immediate causes. Also, contrary to popular thinking in the modern West, evangelical Christians do assert that communities can suffer since they can be the seat of sin or the object of the wickedness of others. Ethical precision, then, requires that these categories of moral causation of disease and injury be refined. Blame or culpability for suffering varies.

Natural consequence of immoral behavior
Natural consequence of erroneous behavior[10]
The sinful action of others
Consequence of natural order
Divine punishment for sin
Testing/training by God
Forces of evil

These are not mutually exclusive categories and, further, there can be change over time. For instance, someone might be paralyzed due to another's intoxicated driving, which then becomes an opportunity for training by God or instructing others. This, however, is not something that anyone should ever impose on another (and certainly not in the ICU). It may be, after all, that

[10]Some might assert that individuals and communities are culpable for ignorance, and sometimes they are or should be. For reasons of clarity, and given that such culpability might not always exist, the category is kept distinct.

God does not want the *training* or *growth* of the suffering individual as much as justice against the perpetrator.

Still, it is more than just a truism that living according to the flesh (sinful desires) does tend to hurt one physically, even though other factors always enter in. Sinful behaviors, as commonly defined among evangelicals, generally increase the risk for disease and injury, though there is not a one-to-one correspondence. For instance, alcohol abuse increases the probability of liver disease and motor vehicle accident injuries. This does not mean that all persons who behave in a particular way will become diseased, only that the probability increases. Further, and more importantly, this does not mean that all persons with certain diseases or disabilities have participated in particular sins or are worse sinners than anyone else. From Job through the teaching of Jesus, it is clear that such an absolute correspondence cannot be asserted and to do so is itself sin. Some previous attributions of self-exacerbated disease have proved correct (e.g., the use of tobacco and cancer), but some incorrect (e.g., stomach ulcers and self-inflicted stress), and some remain uncertain (e.g., anorexia), and all are almost inevitably partial. One way to describe this is using the BEING model: behavior, environment (natural and social), acquired immunities, nutrition and other inputs, and genetics all influence whether or not one gets ill.[11]

Even when persons contract sexual diseases through their own promiscuity, believers should avoid—for moral and evangelistic reasons—the claim that this is the direct punishment of God. From a Christian perspective, any suffering might be attributed to the direct activity of God, but the definitive assertion of such in a given case would require certainty and that is inevitably lacking without direct prophetic inspiration. No believer should assume that direct, divine condemnation is falling on another in a particular way unless that believer is willing to accept the condemnation that she or he deserves before the Righteous One for his or her own particular sins. Should the infected person make such a connection, then so be it—but that is something for the mature in the faith to do for himself or herself.

This is not to say that general understandings of injury and illness, of risk factors that are immoral behaviors according to the faith, of population trends, of the sick role and disability, and of other health related matters are not useful. It is to say, however, that the general is useful only when it is applicable,

[11]Yale University, Public Health (division of Medical School, now a distinct college) used the BEING model of disease etiology in the 1980s.

and the applicability in individual cases should always be done with great caution—for both medical and spiritual reasons. The individual's body, when sick or injured, becomes a site for the intersection of the complexity of health care and the complexity of morality.

At the deepest level, in specific cases of the disordering of health, the evangelical response to questions of culpability should be "it is not our place to ask"—at least not at first. The patience of Job—which he did not demonstrate until late in the story—is realizing some things just happen, and that includes on many occasions unfairness in a broken world. The entire conclusion of the book of Job, even taking into account the prose section at the end in which Job receives compensatory earthly blessings, is that the Divine can always challenge an earthly challenge of him. In other words, when all is said and done, who are we to even ask the question? When Job does demonstrate patience, it is as endurance and a continued relationship with God in spite of never being provided a sufficient etiology of his suffering.

Evangelicals believe they can ask theodicy questions, but they must exhibit humility and accept that an answer about proximate causes may not be given. Rather, the problem of theodicy should become an opportunity to enter into dialogue with God and to cling to assurance of a merciful relationship with the Father. From within such a relationship we may ask about suffering, but simply so we can go on in following the Lord. Knowing why suffering occurs, albeit always to a limited extent, helps the redeemed Christian respond to the circumstances of the world. The faithful community can then understand whether or not the preferred response to a given situation is advocacy for justice or the offering of mercy or both.

Regardless of what one believes about the exact relationship of body/soul, and regardless of whether one knows the proximate causes of specific experiences of suffering, the believer remains obligated to care for the broken individual in this life, not just wait for something good to happen in the life to come. The New Testament does not clearly resolve some of the esoteric questions about the relation of body and soul and human suffering. At the opposite extreme, the questions of whether or not one should accept Jesus as Lord or assist the poor are clear and unambiguous.

Perhaps Christian scholars should engage philosophy and perhaps the clergy should be educated so as to respond apologetically to philosophical schools, but Christians would be making a grievous mistake to think therein lie sufficient responses to moral uncertainty. They would be far better served, in the case of bioethics, entering into service to the poor and the sick from which they could gain a better understanding of the human condition and the humanity of those who physically suffer.

The value of the physical body resides in the relationship the whole person has to God, posited in the creative act and upheld by God's continuing grace. The body, in some form, will continue—though for the redeemed, without the disorder that marks all flesh in this life. Yet even prior to that final redemption the physical body matters and can be temporally redeemed—as was the blind man's who had not sinned anymore than anyone else, nor had his parents.

The blind man whom Jesus healed had hope that in spite of the proximate and immediate causes of his impairment, his life had order within the will and affections of God. The man, perhaps triggered by desperation or simply having been overwhelmed by the cultural branding of those with blindness, listened to the Christ, had hope in his words, believed that God cares about physical well-being. The reality of the physical body, according to evangelical theology, continues through this world and, albeit transformed, into the life to come. The significance of biological existence, then, arises from the ultimate relationship of the whole person to the Divine. The full human, including the damageable and disorderable biological body, is worthy of Christian concern because it is one of God's concerns.

PART THREE: CHRISTIAN BIOETHICS AND THE WORLD

Debates about exactly how the soul (or person) relates to the body and how that affects the understanding of suffering can be traced back as far as written language. Philosophers, including Christian philosophers, have engaged in an ongoing argument about the relationship of the body and the soul or mind for millennia. Too often this has apologetic significance but is not immediately pertinent to ethics, except as after-the-fact justifications for predetermined choices. Still, to understand how suffering is interpreted in the secular world it is helpful to describe how the mind/body or soul/body relationship is interpreted. The range of positions on mind/body or soul/body constructs can be understood as a scale imposed on a triangle (see diagram on p. 108). Expanding the scale to include non-Western philosophies and religions certainly should be done when considering bioethics in other settings, but is not necessary when considering dominant themes in the so-called West.

There is a variety of positions on the continuity, or lack thereof, of individual identity. For heuristic purposes, the arguments of theologians and philosophers about identification, personhood, etc. can be put into categories of monism, dualism, plurism and "noneism."[12] The categories should be imagined on a continuum. All the arguments address, one way or another, the body/soul or body/mind problem. That is to say, they are attempts to claim or deny that the whole is more than the sum of the parts. Each position or argument is part of a long tradition, either in the church or in secular philosophy or both. Of course, there is variation among and within these different argument categories, sometimes overlapping with neighboring positions.

Monism. Monism is the claim that the identity of the individual is somehow a unified whole, or perhaps more properly, the individual is a unit. It can be differentiated into three major subcategories (though other forms can and certainly do operate): physicalist monism, idealist monism and heterogeneous monism.

The *physicalist monist* asserts that all mental (or spiritual) activities can be reduced to physical processes (a sort of biological equivalent of double predestination, except with no heaven). The physicalist monists are best represented by scientism reductionists who claim that individuals are no more and no less than their genetics worked out phenotypically. Contrary to what many atheistic philosophers and bioethicists claim for themselves, few actually fit into this category when making day-to-day decisions. The theodicy is highly rational but somewhat cynical. The cultured elites can know that all of existence is reducible to physical processes temporarily conspiring to form the individual. The masses, they imply, are generally better off not understanding that existence is utterly meaningless in any eternal sense. Most physical monists would deny there is an ultimate cause but would assert that nontheistic evolution or some other physical process is purposely working itself out from the penultimate to proximate to immediate levels of causation. More precisely, all events are immediately caused by prior physical events and, so, there are only immediate causes. In practice, no society can be maintained with this worldview, hence the advantage of the illusion.

Idealist monists deny the reality of the physical. Their arguments can be traced to Eastern religions and to a few Western philosophers. The monism of body/soul or body/mind is often a reflection of an ontological monism, that is, a monism of all of reality. As examples one can look to Hinduism and

[12]The word *pluralism* might be preferable grammatically, but its use would create too much confusion given its use for other purposes.

New Age religions that emphasize the transmigration of the soul, and to some degree Christian Science with its denial of the reality of physical suffering. In Western philosophy, one can see this tendency, though in a different way, in Leibniz. This is not a common approach in Western bioethics. Their theodicy is highly rational. Assuming the starting assumption of ontological monism is accepted, the claim is made that all suffering is ultimately an illusion. Even so, in the illusory world, the experience of suffering arises from the proximate cause of previous errors (in the case of Eastern-based philosophies) or intellectual fault (in the case of Western neo-gnostic movements, like Christian Science). The victim, finally, is to blame for the experience of suffering. This does not eliminate the need for the more enlightened to render compassionate care.

Heterogeneous monism is one of the two classical positions of orthodox Christianity and of humanist philosophers who assert there is something unique to humans. A unity of the ideal or spirit or soul is assumed to exist with the physical or the body. Christians who argue for this may emphasize that the soul is a component of the whole, but that on earth and in heaven it is always yoked with a body (physical body on earth; spiritual body in heaven). Or, they may claim that *soul* is a term better used to describe the whole, with the physical body and mental capacities subsets of or perspectives on that; the body in a general sense, then, refers to the delimited soul that exists here and through eternity. Christian heterogeneous monism can also be called strongly unified dualism.

Humanists offer other versions of heterogeneous monism. These may be of an atheistic or deistic existentialist orientation with the claim that somehow the individual constructs his or her personal identity. Or, they may favor a notion of evolution in which humane values and human character emerge when a threshold of biological development is crossed. They run into some of the same theodicy problems that arise with physicalist monism. If reality is reducible, then from what springs purpose? The argument is made that as water has characteristics that are completely different from oxygen and hydrogen, so can humans have more significance than their components; the whole can be more than the parts. But this does not satisfactory address injustice when the entity maltreated or when the "loser" of the so-called natural lottery simply suffers to no end but oblivion. The theodicy appears irrational as it is an attempt to create a *telos* to give meaning while denying there is a *telos*. The closest parallel in world religions may be Jainism, but Jainism is rational in that it includes the concept of karma and samsara to explain the suffering of apparently just or innocent individuals.

Dualism. Dualism seems to operate in two dominant forms in contemporary debates about identity: nontheistic and theistic. Philosophers or bioethicists interested in elevating one or more "personhood" characteristics usually argue the former, sometimes using arguments that would allow the assignment of personhood to some nonhumans and almost always the denial of personhood to some humans. Though usually not a Cartesian form, nontheistic bioethical arguments are frequently dualistic with the distinction being drawn between biological human and person. The human and the person may or may not coincide at any given moment in any given being. Personhood becomes the secular equivalent of the soul—the part of the individual that is deemed morally significant.[13] This leads to highly irrational theodicy claims that depend on the defining of suffering and the justice of that suffering entirely by the individual—whether the one who is sick or injured, or one observing such a person. The consequence is that sick and injured can be deemed if not worthy of suffering, at least not worthy of care since the defining is an autonomous act of the person and, not surprisingly, the person with the most power gets to decide who counts and what form of suffering has meaning.

Persons of Western religions who assert some form of strict body/soul (spirit) dualism, often with the possibility of "disembodied existence,"[14] typify theistic dualism. Christian, Jewish and Islamic versions of dualism generate highly rational theodicies. Any unfair suffering is addressable in the afterlife. The biggest risk is that physical suffering will be dismissed as nothing in comparison with the benefits of heaven. To use the language once pejoratively directed at evangelicals, it is "pie in the sky, by and by." The response for evangelicals is that the comparison with heaven is not the only comparison that can be made. This life can also be compared to the creative intention of God. Injustice can be despised, suffering should be alleviated, compassion is required not in spite of eternity but because the Eternal God has decreed it is so.

Another form of secular dualism draws on classical utilitarianism and is typified by the substitution of continuing interest for a divinely created moral identity. At first glance, one might assign such theorists to the physi-

---

[13]Gilbert Meilaender, "Terra es Animata: On Having a Life," *Hasting Center Report* 23 (July-August 1993): 25-32.

[14]Moreland and Rae, *Body and Soul,* p. 57.

calist monist category, but the role of interests outside of primary physical characteristics make it more appropriate to define them as nontheistic dualists. This reasoning, to say the least, becomes problematic for persons with disabilities or anyone else whose interests might not measure up to the combined interests of the broader society.

Plurism. Plurism is the claim that identities, and subsequently moral identifications, come and go. Theorists holding such a position assert that any given human can be at any one time or through time, identifiably different persons. Social constructionists represent the plurism category, especially with individuals who are defined as having changing ethnic identities or gender identities, which the individual assembles into himself or herself. It is functionally quite similar to noneism. There is no coherent theodicy because there is no coherent person to experience suffering, though an effort is often made to assert that evil is attributable to the social order without providing a basis for defining either evil or good.

Noneism. Some philosophers claim there is no such thing as meaningful identity or the possibility of actual identification or, if there are such, they have no final moral significance. Some even go so far as to assert that there is no such thing as self or person and that the notion of human is meaningless. This is interesting philosophically but almost pointless politically unless one favors anarchy. The most extreme noneism starts with social constructionist or psychological self-constructionist arguments that are then deconstructed resulting in nihilism. In bioethics, this position is sometimes used to disempower the vulnerable; for instance, significantly disabled traumatic brain injury survivors are sometimes defined as nonexistent.

The noneists generally follow Hume's arguments or some version of westernized Eastern philosophy. Their theodicy tends to be an expression of skepticism because, after all, there is no one to suffer, at least no one who can be demonstrated to actually exist. Noneism denies the reality of ongoing identity of any given individual in this life or the next; it is a sort of hyperdeconstruction.

Practically speaking—and that is the real concern of ethics—just about everyone acts in daily life as if there is a person, soul, mind or whatever one chooses to call "it." Further, given the impact of illness and injury on well-being—both for good and ill, both in creating suffering and in building character—this reality is generally understood as either inextricably woven together with the body or as a unity of the self that is heterogeneous. The

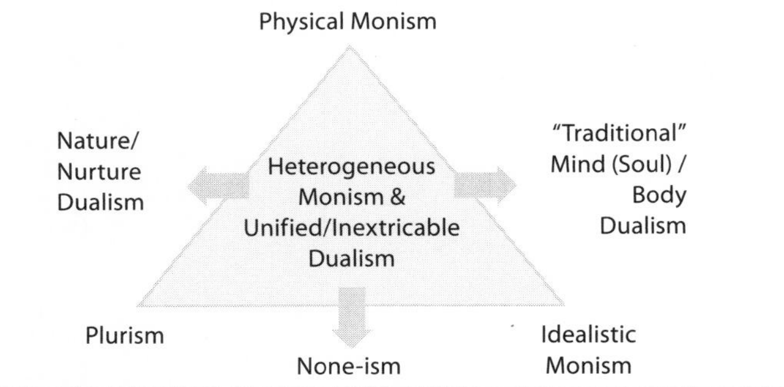

Figure 4.1.

two sides of reality are one individual. Not only do evangelical Christians define themselves as somewhere inside the triangle but the U.S. social contract requires the same and that point of commonality can serve as a basis for bioethical conversation. The individual matters and his or her physical condition matters.

In the midst of crises, day-to-day approaches to morality are tested. At such times, often in response to theodicy problems, people attempt to tinker around the edges or to use theodicies that serve a passing purpose. The tendency is quite strong to resolve—or seemingly resolve—the difficult moral concern without recognizing the far more numerous ethical difficulties thereby created. This is particularly evident in the unfortunate reliance in secular bioethics on theodicies developed to protect autonomy or utility. Sometimes deductive arguments about metaethics are used without considering the problems with the starting assumptions and, more importantly, disregarding the serious problems that would result if the arguments were actually applied in real life.

Sometimes positions are staked out on the basis of one's own emotional need. In order to avoid the existential pain that is generated by an inadequate theodicy, partial information is used to rationalize away anomy and justify immorality. Perhaps an anecdote about an almost unbelievably extreme case, or poor social research about what most people would "want" if they were suffering in a given manner, is used, all the while ignoring the naturalistic fallacy problem and questions of statistical validity in order to avoid thinking about the meaning of suffering.

The West, especially the United States, often avoids the problem of suffering or finesses it by shifting to proclamations about the "person" in order to compel certain moral conclusions. If a person must look like a middle-aged academic teaching at an elite East Coast university, then many will not qualify and their suffering will not count nor need to be explained with a theodicy. Yet, the term *person* actually resolves little unless used in the strict sense of the American social contract. All humans are persons and their suffering counts because they count.

The moral question then becomes not who is a person, but what is the obligation to the human "entity" before us? Under the social contract, some obligation should be extended to any human being living within the borders of the nation or holding U.S. citizenship anyplace in the world. While other moral obligations may exist (specifically for acts of charity) to those elsewhere, this is not necessarily within the shared thin value system of the U.S. social contract. Christians have duties that go beyond the boundaries of the nation-state, but they cannot demand the same of others unless there is consent through legal procedures.

In bioethics, when the question of "personhood" is the subject of a debate one can be almost certain that those who are unquestionably biologically alive, but at the edge—such as following severe injury or illness—are at risk of having care ended or even of facing active termination of their lives. The word *person* is generally used as a synonym for member of the social contract, but is then redefined in some difficult situation in ways that have nothing to do with the biological condition of humanness in order to exclude the most vulnerable rather than acknowledge they are, presumptively, endowed by their Creator with a right to life.

The philosophical and bioethics arguments about personhood are finally political claims for or against a right to continue to exist when experiencing suffering or potential suffering. The language debate matters, not intrinsically but because of the moral implications when individuals are threatened by the power of the state, by insurers all but exclusively interested in cost, by health-care providers who interpret persons with disabilities as professional failures, or by family members who lack necessary models for understanding "difference" yet are confronting a sudden, tragic situation.[15]

---

[15]The apprehension among some in the disability rights community about bioethics as a mechanism for dismissing the rights of individuals while, ironically, tending to include a vehement defense of autonomy, is not misplaced. For an excellent (and, sadly, accurate) portrayal of much of bioethics, see Wesley J. Smith, *Culture of Death: The Assault on Medical Ethics in America* (San Francisco: Encounter Books, 2000). For other perspectives, see Mark G. Kuczewski, "Disability: An Agenda for Bioethics," *The American Journal of Bioethics* 1, no. 3 (summer 2001), and the responses in the same volume.

For that reason, evangelical Christians must politically engage how the personhood of people with disabling conditions (as well as those who are marginal in society for other reasons such as poverty or education) are defined. Regardless of all other components of identification, any biologically living individual is a person and a member of the social contract. Parenthetically, this implies that evangelicals should be willing to form temporary political alliances with those with whom they might disagree on significant, but finally less important, moral issues. For example, even if a group of persons supporting disability rights included a clause in their by-laws that encouraged persons to practice sexual behaviors outside of heterosexual marriage as they choose, evangelicals may legitimately form a temporary political alliance with them, yet while insisting that no one holding such views can serve as a pastor or even hold membership within the Christian community.

Importantly, not all redefining of humans out of existence is crass and vicious. Most often it is to resolve an anxiety-creating theodicy dilemma. Decision makers seek to assuage their consciences as much as resolve philosophical questions by defining a problematically disordered life out of existence. After all, the unconscious (or intentional) reasoning goes, this person's disorder is creating disorder in *our* lives—his or her disease or injury, new or ongoing, is causing dissonance, creating daily problems, pushing us toward anomy, which must be controlled even if that means the elimination of the one who is disordered. The person with a disorder is redefined out of personhood. She or he is a producer of near irresolvable liminality and the disorder must be eliminated even if that means eliminating the disorderer. In terms of secular bioethics, this is no more than curtailing the interference of the sick/injured/suffering individual who is, by virtue of his or her condition, depriving others of their autonomy. The ethical decision precedes the philosophical deduction as a post hoc justification.

In the not so distant past, the sickest and most disabled would be hidden or shunned. Jesus is not responding to an abstract question when asked by those with severe skin and nerve disorders to be healed. His was an era in which those with Hansen's disease were lepers.[16] They were placed in their own

[16]Paul Brand, a leading researcher and physician for persons with Hansen's disease, once said that labeling was sometimes necessary in order to aggressively develop treatments and mechanisms for community reentry of persons who have been categorized by those communities. "They are lepers. One does not understand the position of these people in their communities unless one knows that." (Personal conversation between author and Paul Brand at "Paradoxical Problems: Chronic Pain and the Chronic Absence of Pain," Mississippi Methodist Rehabiliation Center in Jackson, Miss., January 13-14, 1995.)

communities, in part to quarantine for public health reasons, but also because the person so diseased was ritually polluted and culturally degraded. Now, rather than deal with such pollution and degradation, the choice is increasingly to simply kill those whose suffering is too difficult to watch.

Though it may initially seem harsh when considering the family member who feels overwhelmed by tragedy, Christians should interfere within the boundaries of the law to protect the vulnerable. Family members have the legal right to abandon sick and injured relatives, but they do not have the right to kill them. Preferably for the sake of the broader community and the functioning of the nation-state, as well as for the Christian's own character, families facing such suffering will be supported and receive needed economic and social resources in order to respond to the changes that occur.

The state and the health-care professionals who would define the person with a disorder as the disorderer, on the other hand, do not deserve such support. Their power must be met with power. The arguments that de-identify or de-person the individual whose life has become disordered require a political response. The similarity of justifications for the termination of those defined as unworthy of life to terms like *lebenunwertes Leben* and *Dasein ohne Leben* is not accidental, for the similarity with the conclusions of such reasonings reach is evident. Honest declarations by those wanting to solve suffering by eliminating the marginal (e.g., "As they are now, they deserve death") would be intellectually refreshing, though morally repugnant, and not as calming to those who might feel guilty or might be ashamed.

Defining someone as having a disorder defines the person as being disordered. This is not intrinsically problematic language. It becomes such when the society connects certain disordering conditions with the loss of social status—even to the point of losing the status, to use the language of contemporary bioethics, of person and, therefore, of rights holder.

CONCLUSION

Debates about the relationship of the body and the soul or mind influence how a society understands the person. The language of consciousness or rationality or interests is used as a substitute for *soul* and results in either a radical bifurcation of the individual or the denial of his or her existence. The subsequent marginalization of persons with serious diseases, injuries or ongoing disabling conditions should come as no surprise. Under the U.S. social contract, this should be opposed. To be simplistic, life is a sufficient proof of life.

While others do have the right to leave relationships or to ignore the suffering stranger, Christians cannot be content with the minimums of the social contract. Their obligations to those with disorders and those who are disordered by the sickness or injury of others is far more substantial. This is true even for those who have been the proximate or immediate cause of their suffering. Christians must be willing to put on the healing balm, escort those in need to the pool of healing and to help them reorder their lives.

5

Moral Anthropology for Bioethics

HUMANS AS DISTINCTLY HUMAN

Species, role and integral identification are offered as three perspectives on how the indivudal is morally understood in the secular West. The first is in social contract (formal political) discourse about rights, the second for consideration of how one functions in given social settings, and the third is the ongoing identification of the individual through time. Identification is bioethically significant especially given the confusion that arises over rights in the abortion and euthanasia debates and over changes in obligation following a serious, disabling event. The distinction is also pertinent when considering the welfare obligations of humans for nonhuman creation.

> When Jesus came to the region of Caesarea Philippi, he asked his disciples, "Who do people say the Son of Man is?"
>
> They replied, "Some say John the Baptist; others say Elijah; and still others, Jeremiah or one of the prophets."
>
> "But what about you?" he asked. "Who do you say I am?"
>
> Simon Peter answered, "You are the Christ, the Son of the living God."
>
> Jesus replied, "Blessed are you, Simon son of Jonah, for this was not revealed to you by man, but by my Father in heaven. And I tell you that you are Peter, and on this rock I will build my church, and the gates of Hades will not overcome it. I will give you the keys of the kingdom of heaven; whatever you bind on earth will be bound in heaven, and whatever you loose on earth will be loosed in heaven." Then he warned his disciples not to tell anyone that he was the Christ.
>
> From that time on Jesus began to explain to his disciples that he must go to Jerusalem and suffer many things at the hands of the elders, chief priests and teachers of the law, and that he must be killed and on the third day be raised to life. (Mt 16:13-21)

PART ONE: THE TEXT

What is Jesus? The initial question of Christianity is always "Who is Jesus?"—the foundation of the faith is a relationship with a real Being. But to determine what implications may arise from that relationship, one is compelled to ask what Jesus was and is. Was he a human? Was he God? Was Jesus the same person when he was infused into the womb of Mary as he was when he questioned the religious elders as a twelve-year-old, and then later as the charismatic figure who sermonized from a hillside to a crowd of the spiritually thirsty? Was he a carpenter, a child growing in the uterus of the virgin, a devoted son to Mary and Joseph, a wandering preacher, a respected rabbi? If Jesus was those things, was he in those roles the same being who claimed the status of deity? For Christians, certainly the answer must be "he was and is all these things." Indeed, to be the Savior he must have been and continue to be in some sense all these things.

"What is Jesus?" The question arose in the early centuries of the church with the debate fully developed during the fourth and fifth centuries in what is called the christological controversy. Arians asserted that there was a time when Jesus Christ was not. The orthodox believers found this doctrinally intolerable because it denied the full deity of Jesus and therefore made the sacrifice of the cross something less than it might have otherwise been. Jesus is, in Christian tradition, both the perfect priest and the perfect sacrifice; if he was and is not divine, then the sacrifice is blemished.

The Docetists, on the other hand, claimed that Jesus was primarily divine, having taken only the external shape, or appearance *(dokesis),* of a human being. The orthodox found this position also unacceptable because it minimized the degree to which Jesus could recognize the sufferings and temptations of human individuals, especially the level of uncertainty and angst associated with death.

The solution of the church, and one that believers claim is evident in the Text, is that Jesus was and is simultaneously of two types: divine and human. His divinity and humanity together provide those who turn to him access to the fullness of the deity. To the faithful, he is the unchanging I AM WHO I AM, even while also having been a human who walked on earth and lived out many familial and economic roles.

In incarnating, Jesus gave up his "rights" as God for his creation's sake. Jesus was (and is) simultaneously fully of our type and of the divine type, thus crossing the gap between Creator and fallen creature. There are numerous scriptural references for the so-called holy paradox:

> In the beginning was the Word, and the Word was with God, and the Word was God. (Jn 1:1)

> Therefore, since we have a great high priest who has gone through the heavens, Jesus the Son of God, let us hold firmly to the faith we profess. For we do not have a high priest who is unable to sympathize with our weaknesses, but we have one who has been tempted in every way, just as we are—yet was without sin. Let us then approach the throne of grace with confidence, so that we may receive mercy and find grace to help us in our time of need. (Heb 4:14-16)

> Your attitude should be the same as that of Christ Jesus:
> Who, being in very nature God,
> did not consider equality with God something to be grasped,
> but made himself nothing,
> taking the very nature of a servant,
> being made in human likeness.
> And being found in appearance as a man,
> he humbled himself
> and became obedient to death—
> even death on a cross! (Phil 2:5-8)

> He is the image of the invisible God, the firstborn over all creation. . . . For God was pleased to have all his fullness dwell in him, and through him to reconcile to himself all things, whether things on earth or things in heaven, by making peace through his blood, shed on the cross. (Col 1:15, 19-20)

Pertinent for this discussion is the claim that Jesus was and is of our type—a biological human and not vaguely so. He was distinctly human and a distinct human. Such a claim does not mean that respect should not be afforded to those of other types, for instance nonhuman primates. It does mean that humanness is, within the Christian understanding, a special category.

Jesus endorsed the distinction:

> I tell you, my friends, do not be afraid of those who kill the body and after that can do no more. But I will show you whom you should fear: Fear him who, after the killing of the body, has power to throw you into hell. Yes, I tell you, fear him. Are not five sparrows sold for two pennies? Yet not one of them is forgotten by God. Indeed, the very hairs of your head are all numbered. Don't be afraid; you are worth more than many sparrows. (Lk 12:4-7)

It is necessary to Christian understanding that Jesus the Christ was fully immutable in essence, that he experienced life in its particularities as does each of us, and that his life was and is a comprehendible story. Becoming human, he demonstrates the significance of humans and reveals what we may become—the children of God.

PART TWO: CHRISTIAN BIOETHICS

To state the obvious, humans are human. The Christian assertion, one shared by most people groups throughout the earth, is that being human is distinctive, that is distinguishable from other forms of life and from information processing machines. Not only are all human beings defined or identified as members of the species, they are also holders of socially prescripted roles and individuals with narratives. Every person is simultaneously an individual unlike any other, a component of many social systems, and one of a species type.

The identification of Jesus also occurs in these three ways—as human and divine types, as a person living out social roles, and as an individual with an ongoing story. This identification is not merely a doctrinal assertion, it is faith. To genuinely identify Jesus as these things is to enter into a relationship with him.

In a broader sense, the same three forms of identification apply to all humans. An individual is a human (of the species), is a human with particularities, and is a particular human. The identification of any person as of the human species or as a holder of roles or an individual with a narrative necessarily demands the other forms of recognition as well, and subsequent moral responses. Though some aspects of these identifications are socially shaped, the possibilities are limited by natural order. In other words, human functioning requires a moral recognition of self and others that is simultaneously natural, socially shaped (nurtured) and a matter of choice.

For purposes of ethical analysis, a question that always matters is, who counts? For evangelicals anyone who is human counts. Anyone who is distinctly human, therefore, should be entitled to care, concern and protection. The indicator of *human* is biological. The sign by which one recognizes a human is present is the biological function of that being. Yet the humanness is not the biological existence, but the bearing of the image of God, which is primarily defined by being the renderer and object of love. Humans exist biologically because such is the nature of existence in this setting of reality, not because it is the nature of humanness beyond this setting. Still, in this material setting, it is a sufficient indicator.

The assumption that being of the human type warrants due moral consideration implies not only that all humans deserve respect, but also that those creatures that are not human are to be treated differently. Or, more accurately, the difference in types requires consideration of whether or not the different creatures should be treated differently. Evangelicals have distinguished sharply between humans and nonhuman animals, and will continue to do so. The distinction follows both from direct references in the Text and from the theological anthropology the faithful accept. Some secular bioethicists seem to use "personhood" language subsequent to and for justifying a moral decision to kill the vulnerable. Evangelicals generally find this unacceptable. All humans are persons; nonhuman animals are not. This does not mean other creatures are not due welfare concern. It does mean that all who are Homo sapiens are morally distinct in their claims on other humans.

That distinctions can be made between, say, rats and chimpanzees or, more noticeably, between worker ants and higher primates is evident in the creation story and should be recognized by the faithful.

> And God said, "Let the land produce living creatures according to their kinds: livestock, creatures that move along the ground, and wild animals, each according to its kind." And it was so. God made the wild animals according to their kinds, the livestock according to their kinds, and all the creatures that move along the ground according to their kinds. And God saw that it was good. (Gen 1:24-25)

Evangelicals should vigorously support the protection of primates not because they are *persons* or have *rights* but because of the duty of humans to assume welfare obligations for other creatures in accordance with the status of their type. Unfortunately, this kind of caring has not been deemed an important moral concern by most believers, but it should be.

The moral argument for evangelicals is not that nonhuman primates are "close" to being human. Any claims about high percentages of shared genetic coding or commonality are neither statistically convincing nor morally persuasive. Being genetically human requires a threshold to be crossed, not a percentage of nucleic acids to be present. Likewise, the claims about evolutionary closeness remain a matter of disagreement among believers and, more importantly, are not morally compelling to either those who favor theistic evolution or who favor six twenty-four-hour-day creation or any position in between since that threshold exists between humans and nonhuman primates. However, evangelicals can and should recognize that all animals are worthy of genuine concern and sometimes strong protection. Further, the vulnerable ecosystems that provide food, shelter and breeding opportunities for these various species/types should be conserved unless humans would genuinely suffer.[1] This need not and should not result in the diminishing of human rights, but in the elevation of concern for nonhumans. Animals, and all creatures from the kingdoms of life:

1. share with humans "creatureliness" or existence that brings joy to the Creator;
2. can serve as examples by way of analogy;
3. join with the faithful in praising our God.

Each distinct type and the distinct individuals of each type are worthy of type-appropriate welfare concern. The following passages are indicative.

> [It is He] who gives food to every creature.
> *His love endures forever.*
> Give thanks to the God of heaven.
> *His love endures forever.* (Ps 136:25-26)

> But ask the animals, and they will teach you,
> or the birds of the air, and they will tell you;
> or speak to the earth, and it will teach you,
> or let the fish of the sea inform you.
> Which of all these does not know
> that the hand of the LORD has done this?
> In his hand is the life of every creature
> and the breath of all mankind. (Job 12:7-10)

> My mouth will speak in praise of the LORD.
> Let every creature praise his holy name
> for ever and ever. (Ps 145:21)

In actual practice, the distinction of types matters not because of the ontological reality but the ethical significance. Two analytical issues often get conflated inappropriately in discussions about type and personhood—identity and identification. In the final analysis, what matters morally is not what one is at any moment, but how one is defined by those around him or her. Or, to

[1]Though various typologies can be drawn, the current trend in the United States seems to be a model of six kingdoms in three domains: archaea (archaebacteria), bacteria (eubacteria) and eukarya, with the latter including animalia (generally heterotrophs), plantae (generally autotrophs), fungi (generally saprotrophs) and protista (generally single-cell eukaryotes).

draw a fine line, the identity of a person (or a thing, for that matter) is a philosophical question, while identification is a social one. Morality is concerned about the former only to the degree that it informs the latter. This explains why some evangelicals are almost incredulous when arguments for partial birth abortion are asserted on the basis of the individual not being a person. On the face of it, the assertion that a human is not a person is convoluted, constructed to exclude voiceless people and eliminate awkward situations by eliminating awkward humans. It is philosophical juggling at the edges of ethics that ignores the obvious.

Of course, in any given case these are not conceptualizations—the ontological and the ethical—isolated from one another. The real ontological status of a person or thing affects how she, he or it may be treated. Still, one does not need to have certainty about ontological status (identity) to have confidence about social location, cultural significance and moral responsibility (identification). The faithful need to reject ontological claims that lead to positions contrary to the morality of the gospel. Christians should have greater confidence about their actions toward another human, as well as other creatures, than about the philosophical and theological speculations about what makes that human a human definitionally. Christian morality is inducted from the Text as read by the community, both historical and current, not deducted from philosophical premises.

Certainly, philosophers and theologians can argue about the mind/body dualism or lack thereof and about the reality of individual continuity through time. Theologians can debate the significance of interim states and the transformation of the physical body into a spiritual body. For Christians, whatever they may choose to think about what occurs after biological death, it is imperative that they not promote any form of dualism that denies the "human = valued person" equation. Morality that is certainly scriptural takes priority over philosophical speculation that is, well, speculation. Having said that, it is useful to rehearse what the range of positions on identity (rather than identification) may be for the follower of Jesus Christ. While Christians should not waste too much time engaging in esoteric debates about the relation of body, spirit and soul, some understanding of the range of ontological claims that can be made is helpful when entering into conversation with others.

From both Christian and Western cultural perspectives, either a practical heterogonous monism or unified dualism—that is, a nonreductionist acceptance of the physically identifiable living human individual and the recognition that she or he is something more than the sum of the parts—is necessary to protect the rights of individuals before the state, before the various institutions with whom they constantly interact and before other individuals.[2] In other words, any given human being remains the same person through life, though conversion-like events and simple developmental and life processes may alter aspects of identification.

Believers need to assert two morally essential claims. First, the human being continues to exist as his or her own unique self following the cessation of biological function. Second, while on this earth the body, soul and spirit—assuming they are even distinguishable analytically—are a unified whole and so living physical human existence is a sufficient marker for the presence of a person.

According to traditional interpretations of the Text, especially centering on the theological anthropology laid out in the opening of Genesis, there are four core human characteristics:

1. All are made of the dust of the earth into which life has been breathed.
2. All are bearers of the image of God.
3. The individual is always a being in relationship, with God, other people, and the natural world.
4. Each has been sinful, and so stands in need of mercy (grace).

According to evangelicals, to convey these truths as one composite truth about what constitutes a human, the Holy Spirit allowed the writing of the book of Genesis in such a way that the creation of humans is presented from two different perspectives (Gen 1:1—2:3 and Gen 2:4-25). A description of the Fall follows which asserts that no one is good enough to be in the presence of God without first receiving his grace (Gen 3:1-24). Further, these stories in the Text are held together narratively by the interaction of individuals as parts of communities; they have the capacity to love and/or be loved (Gen 2:18-24; 3:8-11). This social component is sometimes defined in terms of covenants.

Christian moral anthropology implies a *telos* or purpose in existing. There is a standard against which one is currently evaluated and toward which one

[2]Steven Post, "A Moral Case for Nonreductive Physicalism," in *Whatever Happened to the Soul? Scientific and Theological Portraits of Human Nature*, ed. Warren S. Brown, Nancey C. Murphy and H. Newton Malony (Minneapolis: Fortress, 1998).

should aim, conducting one's life so as to conform to that standard. Some evangelical traditions emphasize this standard as being innate in Creation, while others emphasize the standard arising in Jesus Christ. Catholics and Calvinists tend to emphasize the former, while sectarian holiness and Anabaptist evangelicals tend to favor the latter. However, this is only a tendency, only a matter of emphasis, as all evangelicals would assert that believers are being what God wants them to be when they more perfectly, by the power of the Spirit, imitate Jesus Christ.

The notion of purpose or *telos* becomes problematic for persons whose primary worldview is the hyperindividualist model provided by late modern Western culture in either subjectivist or utilitarian forms. Those living in ICUs, surviving with certain serious disabilities or, potentially, genetically engineered to be intellectually inferior are easily disregarded as having no purpose. To evangelicals such individuals do have a *telos*. Though sorrow and sadness are associated with loss of capacity or having abilities that are less than those maintained by the majority, the individual human (regardless of how disabled) is not only the holder of an individual purpose and dignity but is part of the communal purpose and dignity of the family, church, broader community and species.

To avoid becoming adherents to just another version of hyperindividualism, evangelicals, especially those in the so-called West, should be careful about using forms of genetic vitalism to argue against abortion and the euthanizing of the disabled. The use of such arguments tends to make biological life the ultimate good, when it is actually a good only because of the ultimate good of an eternal relationship with Jesus Christ. Still, this ultimate goodness has resulted in biological life being a penultimate good, one that should be vehemently protected.

A stronger moral argument than "vitalism," and one more consistent with the evangelical moral anthropology, is to assert that the biological body is not the sum of life but is a conclusive indicator of humanness and that humanness itself is worthy of protection.[3] The language of "humanness" is preferable to that of "person" because it acknowledges the different aspects of being human without assuming a radical mind-body dualism with the word *person* serving as a substitute for *mind*. The moral threat that arises from the use of "person"

[3]The term *vitalism* is used perjoratively against persons who are prolife. See Lawrence Nelson, bioethicist and attorney for May Wendland, "The New Vitalism (Protection or Disrespect? Courts and the Conscious Incompetent Patient)," plenary presentation, American Society for Bioethics and Humanities, Annual Meeting, October 25, 2002.

(or its utilitarian equivalent: *interest*-bearer) language is that those at the margins, too disenfranchised to speak for themselves, will be simply dismissed out of existence because of their supposed diminished personhood. While the same is possible with *human,* it is less likely because being a member of the species is biologically defined nominally, as either-or, by multiple criteria any of which may or may not be present without denying humanness.

The entity in the womb or the unconscious body in the bed is clearly Homo sapien. And, once the possibility of twinning is past, the being is not only distinctly human, but is also uniquely a given human. If the being is of the human type (species identification), then it can and should be assumed that she or he has roles relative to others (role identification) and has begun or continues a story (integral identification). Further, evangelicals must assert that human existence itself is a good, even when it is experienced by the individual or by those observing it as burdensome, difficult, awkward or as "life unworthy of life."[4]

Perhaps the clearest, most indisputable examples of this dismissal of human worth are partial-birth abortion, infanticide, and the extermination of the seriously disabled. The moral repugnance of these activities cannot be hidden behind euphemisms like "a comfortable exit" or "merciful release."[5] To the Christian, these beings have souls or are souls. And, though biological life is not the ultimate end, the final *telos* is to be reached through this existence. For Christians, the near-neonate and the neonate and those with a severe brain injury are not potential persons, but are humans. They do not merely possess minds; they are souls.

When the question of personhood is the subject of a debate in bioethics, one can almost be certain that somebody wants to change or eliminate obligations to somebody else even though that somebody else is unquestionably biologically alive. The somebody else is inevitably at the edge of social value (as defined by lost abilities, high medical costs, etc.). Even though she or he is not dying in the near-term, she or he is defined as "as good as dead." This is possible because, though the boundaries of life are restricted by the biological

[4]*Lebensunwertes leben:* one of the phrases used by Nazi exterminators based at Tiergartenstrasse Vier (T-4) to dismiss the humanness of persons with disabilities.

[5]For more examples see Rita L. Marker and Wesley J. Smith, "Words, Words, Words," International Task Force on Euthanasia and Assisted Suicide <http://internationaltaskforce.org/fctwww.htm#1>. Based on "The Art of Verbal Engineering," *Duquesne Law Review* 35, no. 1 (fall 1996): 81-108. See also Ian Dowbiggin, *A Concise History of Euthanasia: Life, Death, God, and Medicine* (Lanham, Md.: Rowman & Littlefield, 2005) on how the word *euthanasia* was redefined, away from the historical notion of a *telos,* to what is now called mercy killing, as initaited by Samuel D. Williams in the 1870s.

possibilities, the precise cultural line between living and dead is socially constructed according to various organizational and community needs, as is the category "person."

The individual who is deemed different or as having a new identity as "less than a person" is often culturally and socially degraded. When some disability rights advocates declare that they are not dead yet, they are actually demanding that they not be defined as "less," for degradation is not just embarrassing or shaming.[6] It simultaneously deprives individuals of their rights (in this social contract society) and relieves others of their familial and cultural obligations.[7]

Indeed, according to some bioethicists, reidentification of someone as less than a person may not only relieve care obligations but also create new obligations to terminate. Ultimately, the assertion that human identity is lost, that the real person is gone, that the soul has departed the breathing body, will shift the argument from a *right* to die to a *duty* for individuals to cease being. The descriptive becomes prescriptive.

In Christianity, the identification of a human being is first of all the identification of the individual by God. From the beginning of one's existence one is a social creature somehow in relationship with the Creator. Humans are created to be loved by and to love God. In most current forms of Christianity, including most expressions of evangelicalism, this is understood as meaning that humans are free to love God and free to not love him. Second, identification is only proper when the individual recognizes in some sense who she or he is relative to the Eternal One, with *recognition* understood as more than a cognitive event. The individual comes to love God. This recognition is a dramatic change in self-identification. The moral anthropological significance for evangelicals is simply this: identification is simultaneously fluid and stable. Third, identification as loved by God and as his image-bearer (an unchanging status), when yoked with the individual's acceptance of that love (becoming his child, a new status, yet in continuity with who one was before), alters how one identifies others. Put more simply, one is always the object of God's love; one is converted through faith to the knowledge of that love; and, one responds morally with others in a growing self-expression of that love.

The implication for this argument is that all human beings are of value.

---

[6]See "Not Dead Yet" at <www.notdeadyet.org/docs/contact.html>.

[7]See, for example, Ernst Tugendhat, "The Role of Identity in the Constitution of Morality," in *The Moral Self*, ed. Gil G. Noam and Thomas E. Wren, with Gertrud Nunner-Winkler and Wolfgang Edelstein (Cambridge, Mass.: MIT Press, 1993), pp. 4, 9, 13.

Bearing the image of God is indicated by physical existence, even while physical existence is not the sum of the image of God. All are equal before God, even though they may not be equal in all ways relative to each other. All have been tainted by sin and graciousness from God is available to all. This equality of image-bearing and brokenness is evident in one of the oldest passages in the Text:

> If I have denied justice to my menservants and maidservants
> when they had a grievance against me,
> what will I do when God confronts me?
> What will I answer when called to account?
> Did not he who made me in the womb make them?
> Did not the same one form us both within our mothers? (Job 31:13-15)

For Christians this means that those at the boundaries of social value—the unborn, those with mental illnesses and so on—must be loved. The believer is to recognize his or her commonality with those who suffer, especially those who suffer unjustly at the hands of others who would deny the reality of their existence. It also means that while Christians cannot expect that those at the margins also be loved by those of the world, their right to exist and to be treated with dignity must be protected.

Christian love, in this case, manifests itself in three distinct ways. First, Christians must offer special respect to all who are human. Believers must constantly recognize that they have sinned, that they are dust and that those on the margins are bearers of the image of God. If the faithful are going to err morally, they should overemphasize their own sinfulness and earthly fragility and overestimate the extent to which the image of God is borne by the other.

Second, respecting the other while recognizing the social location of the believer can lead to political advocacy. The evangelical, excepting those who are members of strict separatist groups, should be involved in changing laws or encouraging adherence to laws that protect people on the margins. While some evangelicals have made strong arguments for a libertarian approach to civil moral legislation, this cannot mean that the vulnerable have choices made for them that actually define them out of existence. Love properly expressed in civil settings often looks a great deal like justice.

Third, the faithful must offer care as an expression of love. Evangelicals are frequently berated as hypocrites. More often than not, this arises from those who choose to take seriously neither the beliefs of evangelicals nor their own behaviors. Still, the accusation can ring true if evangelicals do not actively and personally participate in care for those on the margins and, almost as importantly, for those who care for those on the margins.

Christians may question the functionality of the imprecise moral reasoning of subjectivism while the highly secularized of the world may be dismissive of the faithful for their moral confidence. In both cases, the attitudes may get expressed in simplistic characterizations. Regardless, it is not the attitudes that finally matter but the moral action—this is particularly true when it comes to how people are defined and the extent of protection rendered by the state. While much day to day moral activity among the faithful, secularized individuals, and persons of other religions takes place without considerable ethical analysis, whenever the state becomes involved (or might become involved) the precision of language about the status as a human person becomes imperative. Entitlement, rights and obligations hinge on precisely defining who counts, how and when—and humans count.

PART THREE: CHRISTIAN BIOETHICS AND THE WORLD

Most Western nations, their artifacts of a regal past or Marxist regimes aside, operate under some form of social contract. Most late modern social contract states are deontological in their reasoning, not virtue teleological. The assumption is that persons are due respect on the basis of intrinsic human dignity. This is not dissimilar from the Kantian claim that all human beings are ends in themselves, not simply a means to the ends of others. In other words, human individuals can have their own *teloi* (or not) as they choose, but the state and the culture will not assume there is one that is preferable to all others —at least not within certain constraints.

What the state does have to assume for the functioning of the social contract is that through time the same individual lives a given life. Various claims about human ontology are possible, but the idea that a given human is many persons through time or none at all would make the social contract nonsensical. A historical transition occurred when natural law thought gave way to natural rights; the former is teleological, the latter is not. Still, natural rights and the social contract rest on the idea that the individual is a contract maker and all contract makers not only gain benefits but have responsibilities that are, of necessity, ongoing.

The moral order of most of these social contract countries is increasingly thin, in that individuals and mediating institutions can have their own values and *teloi* that are not shared by other citizens and residents of the nation.

While it might be argued that culture is always "thick," the operations of the state (at least in United States) are assumed to be "thin."[8] Basically, a minimal super-culture functions in such a way that various cultures in the land and individuals who are part of one or more of those cultures can be held together as a civil society. Admittedly, there are values that allow for the functioning of the structures of such a super-culture, but the tendency is toward a thinner content of values—except those that legitimate the structures themselves. Pluralism and procedures increase, and shared *teloi* and character virtues decrease. This works quite well unless, for instance, the shared culture becomes so thin that conflicts over the definition of human or the nature of the social contract become irresolvable.

Precision in defining who counts matters precisely for the sake of the procedural rules. As an example, persons with serious debilitating birth defects have been and continue to be pushed to the margins of society. However, the Americans with Disabilities Act (ADA) has made a counterargument by defining these human beings into the regular procedures of U.S. law. In social protests against definitions of societal membership that exclude them, persons with serious disabilities have increasingly made their presence known. The ADA was and is an effort to morally and socially normalize persons with disabilities. To a lesser extent, the earlier Social Security Disability Insurance did the same.

If there is any thickness to the culture of the late modern West, it is in the definition of who counts, of what a person is, of where the boundaries of humanness lie, but even that is growing thinner and thinner. The U.S. social contract is *speciesist*, to use a popular (and often pejorative) word in bioethics. Or, to use a term from political philosophy, practical political ethics should be humanist. The formula is

> *Homo sapien* = person = identifiable individual = morally significant as carrier of intrinsic rights

Speciesism, that is the distinct dignity of the human individual, gave rise to powerful abolitionist and feminist arguments in the nineteenth century, and continues to be significant in disability rights campaigns. This equation has in the past sometimes been denied, such as with ethnospecific slavery, ethnic cleansing of indigenous people groups, the modified utilitarianism of social Darwinism and the eugenics movement. Christians and those accepting the

---

[8]Clifford Geertz, "Thick Description: Toward an Interpretive Theory of Culture," *The Interpretation of Cultures: Selected Essays* (New York: Basic Books, 1973).

U.S. Lockean-Jeffersonain contract agree that the human person is irreducible. Yet both understand that human identification is more than the yes/no of humanness.

Philosopher David Heyd is concerned with identity as "gradual process, rather than of a yes-or-no state."[9] His concern is correct. His solution is problematic. Identity—or more properly "identification"—is not a choice between essentialist and mutable models; at least with human identification, both essentialist and mutability claims are valid. As Amélie Rorty noted, philosophers and, long before them, people simply living their day-to-day lives have used multiple definitions of identification.[10]

In daily existence people define others in three general ways: (1) in terms of the roles they fulfill, (2) the history they have and the future they expect, and (3) as humans. At the end of modernity, persons are best understood as being identified from three coincidentally existing perspectives rather than from a dialectic or a trialectic of identification. The humanness is unchanging; the roles come and go; the history is the ongoing narrative of the socially-located individual. If one is present, then all are present, even if not readily observable, for these are perspectives on the single being, not three different beings nor three different definitions of being.

Species identification is the recognition of a biological human as a "person." This is membership in the human race, with the term *membership* being intentionally selected. In the West, and increasingly throughout the world, such membership entitles one to rights. Notoriously, the United States did not always consider all individuals fully human and, therefore, they were not entitled to basic human rights (e.g., the Dred Scot case). Much of the debate about abortion is framed along this line, though the reality of the fight seems to include as much about the role of women in society as the identification of the preborn as a human. Species identification questions tend to be framed using deontological language. One either fits into a category, and therefore has rights and responsibilities, or one does not. Not only do some try to limit this identification so as to not apply it to those with significant disabilities, others try to expand it. Animal rights arguments, as opposed to those using animal welfare language, try to expand the concept of person or of interests beyond the species so that rights are afforded to all in a given order or all in a given

---

[9]David Heyd, *Genethics: Moral Issues in the Creation of People* (Berkeley: University of California Press, 1992), p.162.

[10]Amélie Oksenberg Rorty, *Mind in Action: Essays in the Philosophy of the Mind* (Boston: Beacon Press, 1988).

taxonomic kingdom. Paradoxically, the seriously disabled sometimes have this protection diminished or eliminated (not infrequently justified on the basis of a philosophical argument in which "personhood" substitutes for humanness).

Role identification is based on the multiple identities one assumes or has given on the basis of performance or association with specific tasks and/or transient relationships. One can have roles such as a parent or a spouse that are significantly modified or abandoned or accepted through time. The moral language of role identification tends to be utilitarian in that the role is frequently associated with performance-evaluated tasks or affective because it involves friends and family.

Identification by roles is common in face-to-face interactions. Adults are asked what they "do" with the understanding that their employment somehow defines who they are. College students are identified by their majors and the courses they take. Roles are numerous, often transient, sometimes overlapping or conflicting—parent, employee, sports fan, guy who sits at the end of the counter and drinks coffee each morning, or the patient with pancreatic cancer. Roles are discontinuous and, when the focus of moral identification, allow the initiation and termination of some types of moral obligation. Roles are often, in Western society, understood in a contractual manner.[11]

Both species identification and role identification are valid means of morally identifying individuals, but they are inadequate by themselves or, even, together. It is necessary to link with these two a third form of identifying individuals as those with continuity through time—the narrative or historical

[11]Two seminal works on identification with roles are George Herbert Mead, *Mind, Self, and Society: From the Standpoint of a Social Behaviorist*, ed. posthumously by Charles W. Morris (Chicago: University of Chicago Press, 1934); and Erving Goffman, *Presentation of Self in Everyday Life* (Edinburgh: University of Edinburgh, 1956). Two other important theorists on social construction and roles are Peter Berger and John Shotter. The questions these social theorists raise center on the function of role and the function of dialogue and/or dramatic presentation in how one is identified. At least in the case of Shotter and Mead (and, arguably, in Berger), the dynamic of interaction creates a different reality than that described by the sum of the parts. This ongoing interaction may over time provide a narrative continuity. Various feminist authors have also strongly asserted the need to understand persons as embedded or as part of a narrative. See also the narrative arguments of Christian ethicist Stanley Hauerwas.

Elsewhere, in describing different ways of understanding identity, Amélie Rorty along with David Wong include "social role identity" by virtue of "socially defined institutional roles or being cast to play a certain kind of role in the unfolding of social dramas" (Amélie O. Rorty and David Wong, "Aspects of Identity and Agency," in *Identity, Character, and Morality: Essays in Moral Psychology*, ed. Owen Flanagan and Amélie O. Rorty [Cambridge, Mass.: MIT Press, 1990]). An earlier and somewhat similar argument is Erving Goffman's concept of roles.

understanding of the individual as the "same" being. This *integral identification* is transformable but continuous.[12] A classic example of identification being continuous but transformed was Phineas Gage. Often cited in bioethics and rehabilitation literature, Gage was injured when an iron rod, propelled by an explosion at a railroad work site in 1848, went through his lower cheek into his brain and out the top of his skull. The reportedly congenial Gage recovered from the injury excepting lost sight in one eye and, far more importantly, a noticeably altered personality. Gage was defined as no longer Gage by at least some of his acquaintances. And, yet, he was. In spite of the changes, he was recognized as the same person, but now radically altered.

Integral identification is the narrative of the specific individual, the thread of continuity from the beginning to the end of life. This concept is accepted by virtually all persons even when debating the starting and concluding points of that narrative. Using these three aspects of moral identification simultaneously prevents risks to persons with disabilities that arise from excessive forms of dualism, physicalist or idealist monism, "noneism," or plurism.[13]

This model leads to several moral conclusions. First, the body and soul (or mind) are a single unit. Second, even though vitalism does not sufficiently explain how people should be identified, physical existence does work as a sufficient indicator of the presence of a human. Third, the marginal of society matter even when they cannot fulfill "normal" roles as they continue to exist biologically and warrant identification as humans; they count as holders of the basic right to life and should be protected by the social contract. In sum, any denial of a human "counting" as a human to the extent that would lead to a "slaughter of the innocents" should be rejected out of hand as contrary to the U.S. social contact or Christian core values or both. Even in a "thin" culture, this understanding of human is necessary not only to protect those at the margins but for everyone's well-being. Any might, under some circumstances, be moved to the edge of society—if not for reasons of physical disability, then for reasons of ethnicity, religion or age. Each and every person's worth is the assumed base of the social contract and the very reason for the existence of the state.

If moral identification is only made on the basis of political personhood

---

[12]Integral identification might correspond to recognition of the "soul" for Christians, but I would prefer to keep the three concepts of species, role and integral identification together as the means of identification on the horizontal, or earthly moral level, and let debates about the vertical concept of identity take place outside of ethics.

[13]See chapter five.

(species identification), then strict defining by a solitary cognitive characteristic could readily allow some individuals to be defined out of the human race and deprived of rights. While less common with adults having acquired disabilities, such is certainly not infrequent with newborns that have disabilities. Defining neonates and postneonates as not "persons" because someone

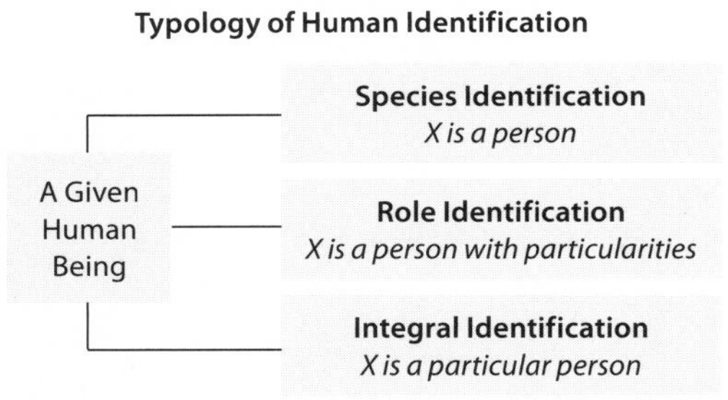

Typology of Human Identification

A Given Human Being	
	Species Identification *X is a person*
	Role Identification *X is a person with particularities*
	Integral Identification *X is a particular person*

Figure 5.1.

decides their intellect is insufficient can be used to rationalize killing and thus assuage the guilt and mitigate the shame of family members and health-care practitioners. Though less likely, the reality of the risk for older children and adults of being so identified as nonhuman is significant enough that some disability rights advocates vociferously claim that they will not accept being treated as nonhumans.

If moral identification is only made on the basis of roles, then as roles are suddenly lost or severely altered, the relationships can be discontinued. If role identification dominates notions of species identification, then the diminished or lost functional capacity for a given role or roles may result in the person being defined out of the human race.

If moral identification is made only on the basis of integral identification, then the opposite risk tends to arise: that persons who are biologically dead will remain on "life-support" machinery for no reason. Similarly, persons who have experienced major disabling events may not receive proper care, because the losses in some capacities are denied.

All three of these approaches to moral identification should function "trialectically." In the 1960s Joseph Fletcher composed a list of criteria for personhood that reflects an extraordinary bias against those with disabilities. Versions of his arguments remain popular in some academic circles and are used to eliminate tragic circumstances by eliminating obligation. For instance, a severe spinal cord injury may lead to a spouse, say the wife, to say that her husband is no longer the man she married. He cannot perform sexually, he cannot respond in the typical manner of a father with young children, he cannot return to the same kind of employment, his presence will radically alter the functioning of the house. All of these may be true. Still, these do not make him not the man she married. Should she decide that she is going to end the relationship, she still needs to obtain a divorce in that the state "believes" he is the same man.[14] Certainly from a Christian perspective, she remains obligated as a spouse regardless of the severe role transformation. Spouses through divorce and, though less likely, parents and children through simply ignoring the relative have the right to deny their moral responsibility for a severely disabled person on the basis that she or he is not the same human due to role failure. They are wrong in doing so. Even so, this is not as immediately threatening to the individual as being defined as nonhuman or nonperson, even though it readily leads to social isolation and marginalization. If role identification dominates notions of species identification, then the diminished or lost capacity to function in a given role or roles may result in the person being defined out of the human race. If the loss of role capacity results in the loss of advocates, then it is easy for others to define the injury or illness survivor as a nonhuman.

To expand this application, when a child is not yet out of the mother's womb, but is clearly viable, the vast majority of people in the United States recognize that a human being is being killed in abortion. When a child with a serious but treatable disability is denied the opportunity to receive a medical procedure that is standard for "normal" babies, it is apparent that a human is being passively euthanized. Such deaths, whether by commission or omission, present a significant problem for a social contract society. After all, the only thing that matters fundamentally in the United States is humanness. It is being human that precedes the social contract itself and serves as its foundation. The thinnest claim for humanness always calls forth from the state the provision of some degree of protection, unless the civil notion of human is not

[14]It is not uncommon to hear a spouse say of a traumatic brain injury survivor or spinal cord injury survivor, "he is not the man I married." For more on traumatic brain injury see James R. Thobaben, "The Social and Moral Identity of Traumatic Brain Injury Survivors" (Ph.D. diss., Emory University, 1994). The dissertation and an earlier presentation on "Traumatic Brain Injury as Conversion" at the Society for Scientific Study of Religion in 1987 serve as the basis for this chapter. See also William J. Winslade, *Confronting Traumatic Brain Injury: Devastation, Hope and Healing* (New Haven, Conn.: Yale University Press, 1998).

centered on biological humanness as the indicator and some other criterion is arbitrarily applied by the powerful.

The state, certainly the United States and probably all other social contract defined civil governments, are claiming that

- humanness is an intrinsically valuable condition;
- in some sense all persons join the contract without rational consideration;
- there may be more than one level of membership, but the minimal level includes a right to life;
- location within the physical boundaries of the state creates a contractual obligation for the state to protect.

In terms of specific issues, it is incoherent for a social contract state, operating with the cultural claim that humans matter, to not actively oppose attacks on the lives of members. Without the protection of individual persons, the grounds for the contract cease to exist, the powerful are in control, the reality is war of all against all. By all practical evaluations, people with serious disabilities are still recognized as *people* with disabilities and the child who is viable in the womb is certainly dependent on his or her mother, but is still a *child* with such dependence.[15] At minimum, the state should oppose

- partial birth abortion, or the abortion of any child who is viable given the state of current technologies or who, unimpeded and unassisted except by normal natural developmental processes, would mature into an autonomous individual;
- euthanizing disabled persons with any level of function;
- "rights" for nonhuman animals, though the state should mandate welfare based on the obligations of the humans and not on the nature of the nonhuman animals since to do otherwise would threaten the operating assumptions (intrinsic value to the human) upon which the social contract state is based.

[15]Importantly, though the notion of rational autonomy remains an important concept for social contract theory, and comes into play in U.S. bioethics such as with advance directives and the right to chose providers, this autonomy operates at political and legal levels, not at the pragmatic level of care delivery. Newborns do not rationally decide to enter the social contract. Dying people may choose to exit, though not without implications for everyone around them and for other vulnerable persons in the society. No doubt, many who enter the United States as immigrants (legal or illegal), and many born in the United States do not understand that they have become part of a contract that protects their lives, but they have.

At the end of modernity, the use of coincidentally existing species, role and integral identifications can assist in protecting the rights of humans. The humanness is unchanging; the roles come and go; the history is the ongoing narrative of the socially-located individual. If one is present, then all are present. Many common moral dilemmas in health care arise by erroneously assuming that because a person is incapable of fulfilling different roles, the individual has ceased to be the same person or to be human altogether.

CONCLUSION

Ontological questions are important, but need not and cannot finally be resolved in a pluralistic society. Rather, the real question for morality is not what is the identity of the individual, but how will the individual be identified? Logical deductions about the body/soul in Christianity or the body/mind in Enlightenment-based thought are important, but they do not provide practical moral guidance. Likewise, empirical findings, including those drawn from neurological studies, cannot finally resolve what constitutes a person nor whether or not she or he will have her or his rights or be treated respectfully.

Theological and philosophical speculation that does not take into account the moral implications of the arguments is irresponsible and should be rejected out of hand. This does not mean that all reasoning should be prejudged by a desired outcome. It does mean that the moral consequences of philosophies and theologies are powerful indicators of the legitimacy of the reasoning. The resulting moral conclusions may not demonstrate the correctness of an argument, but they can prove when the argument is completely contrary to the foundational moral claims of the social contract state or to the faith and therefore must be intrinsically flawed.

A better starting point is consideration of how people actually do identify one another morally. To use an analogy, the measuring machine for bioethics should be normed to the reality of human experience and the foundational values of the culture. This does not mean that theology, philosophy, or neurosciences should be disregarded, but that the moral identification of the human cannot be reduced to a philosophical deduction, a biblical prooftext or the most recent finding published in *Science* or *Nature*. It is, instead, necessary to recognize the moral identification of human beings on the margins of society as being human, particular humans, and humans with particularities.[16]

---

[16]Amélie Rorty suggests at least four meanings of identity are operating when the question of who one is is asked. Using somewhat simplified language, these are: What constitutes hu-

For all with social power, and for Christians especially, to engage in discussions about what defines the real individual human without considering the possible negative consequences on real people in hospitals, nursing facilities or in homes is irresponsible. Furthermore, to do so reveals an epistemological error. There is no good reason for a Christian community or individual to base his or her moral claims on extensive deductions about the nature of persons when the Scripture itself speaks more directly to the moral matter. In the case of persons surviving traumatic injuries or illnesses who are altered in personality, the starting point should be the moral assertion. Christians know that humans with severe personality altering injuries or illnesses deserve care and respect, so what is asserted about person or, more properly, moral identification must be compatible with this ethical position.

The model as presented above allows that (1) humans exist in time, (2) human identification is mutable, and (3) change is neither the same as cessation nor the same as constancy, but something that is both. This model morally assumes that (1) the marginal of society (be it economic, political, mental, or physical) matter to the extent that they count, (2) such people should "count" and (3) moral reasoning that demonstrably leads to the "slaughter of the innocents" is contrary to either the U.S. social contact or Christian core values or both.

---

manness? What distinguishes humans? What keeps a person the same person through time? What cluster of characteristics constitute the essential self? (Amélie Rorty, "Introduction," in *The Identities of Persons*, ed. Amélie Rorty [Berkeley: University of California Press, 1976], pp. 1-2). Her analysis is outstanding, but these do not represent the most important political question (the life and death question): who owes what to whom? As outrageous as this may sound to people weaned on autonomy and emotivism, the obligation of persons to those with disabilities and those with disabilities to the society is binding, for it is tied to the core operating assumption of the American social contract: humans matter.

6

Moral Identification and Disability

HUMANS AS UNIQUE HUMANS

The distinctness of humans lies in their being created in the image of God. The uniqueness of each human lies in their identification before God and others. Identification can be converted. The individual simultaneously remains the same person while becoming something new. The religious imagery can be used in bioethics to gain a better cultural, sociological and psychological understanding of persons who go through significant disabling events. In doing so, the unique individual can be recognized as changed even while some former relational obligations remain intact.

> They went across the lake to the region of the Gerasenes. When Jesus got out of the boat, a man with an evil spirit came from the tombs to meet him. This man lived in the tombs, and no one could bind him any more, not even with a chain. For he had often been chained hand and foot, but he tore the chains apart and broke the irons on his feet. No one was strong enough to subdue him. Night and day among the tombs and in the hills he would cry out and cut himself with stones.
>
> When he saw Jesus from a distance, he ran and fell on his knees in front of him. He shouted at the top of his voice, "What do you want with me, Jesus, Son of the Most High God? Swear to God that you won't torture me!" For Jesus had said to him, "Come out of this man, you evil spirit!"
>
> Then Jesus asked him, "What is your name?"
>
> "My name is Legion," he replied, "for we are many." And he begged Jesus again and again not to send them out of the area.
>
> A large herd of pigs was feeding on the nearby hillside. The demons begged Jesus, "Send us among the pigs; allow us to go into them." He gave them permission, and the evil spirits came out and went into the pigs. The herd, about two thousand in number, rushed down the steep bank into the lake and were drowned.
>
> Those tending the pigs ran off and reported this in the town and countryside, and the people went out to see what had happened. When they came to

> Jesus, they saw the man who had been possessed by the legion of demons, sitting there, dressed and in his right mind; and they were afraid. Those who had seen it told the people what had happened to the demon-possessed man—and told about the pigs as well. Then the people began to plead with Jesus to leave their region.
>
> As Jesus was getting into the boat, the man who had been demon-possessed begged to go with him. Jesus did not let him, but said, "Go home to your family and tell them how much the Lord has done for you, and how he has had mercy on you." So the man went away and began to tell in the Decapolis how much Jesus had done for him. And all the people were amazed. (Mk 5:1-20)

PART ONE: THE TEXT

"We are Legion." With this the man declared himself to be his disease. He described himself as his disorder. He conceived of himself as illness. Jesus asks—not directing his question to "normality" but to that which had mastery over the normal—"What is you name?" Regardless of the interpretation at the end of modernity, it is quite clear that 2000 years ago Jesus and the man himself understood his condition to have taken control over who he was. The man was possessed.

It is likely, given the description, that the man's behaviors made it extremely difficult for him to function in the community. But it is also likely that his community's response exacerbated the man's condition. They had tried to chain him, either out of fear of what he would do to the innocent, concern over what he would do to himself or out of superstitious terror about the infectiousness transmission of the demonic. If the first and last were not legitimate concerns, certainly self-injury was; the man either by recklessness or with masochistic intention injured himself over and over again. The demon-possessed man was not only disheveled and naked, but covered with scabs and open wounds. In ancient Israel, he was as ritually (and perhaps physically) unclean as one could be.

Identifying himself as the disordering spirits, he accepted a place at the margin of society—until Jesus came. The Christ recognized that the roles the man fulfilled—both as object of disdain and pity to the villagers and as site of inhabitation for the evil disease—were not the only roles he could hold in the social order. Jesus' healing simultaneously restored him to his previous life and made him new.

To give the man normalcy required the challenging of that which had become the norm for the community. Marginalization, after all, defines margins; it sets the edges of the community, his being at the margin helped define the standards of the community. He, being the possessed, helped establish for the village the boundary of the good and the right and the pure—or, at least, the pure enough. Some kind of social boundaries are necessary and, in fairness, the villagers did not kill the man, recognizing at least to some extent that he was not to blame—or not completely to blame—for his disorder. Still, Jesus found the social construct unacceptable. The marginalization of the demon-possessed man legitimated the social order and if that order had to be challenged to provide a reasonable life for the man, then Jesus was prepared to do so.

The people of the village recognized this. Jesus threatened their community's values when he sent the demonic powers into swine. The village, probably dominated by Gentiles given the rearing of hogs and designation as part of the Decapolis, found their safety away from threatening Jewish authorities.[1] Jesus, though not having formal political or religious authority, had destroyed their animals and so it may have appeared to them that Jesus represented the broader society's status quo. Ironically, they were marginal themselves. They—both the beasts and the people —were ritually unclean to Jews and insignificant to the Romans and could find safety by being left alone. Jesus did not leave them alone. He did not send the demons into one or two but into two thousand of their animals. This effectively destroyed the economic base for a portion of that village for that year if not for years to come.

Any restoration of persons to the divinely intended norm of being valued as image-bearers will threaten a social order that promotes marginalization of the vulnerable. Healing is always destructive in some way. To declare that persons with disabilities are part of the divine moral norm (that they "count") or to claim that the unborn deserve a right to life even though such does indeed impede the free choice of the mother is to challenge a social order that discounts the validity of humans. Such discounting of individuals usually occurs in order to maintain or to establish power and control by taking advantage of the socially weakest.

A moral response to such necessarily requires the reidentification of the marginalized, perhaps through his or her own new self-understanding, but always with others seeing their moral responsibilities as changed because they

[1]The community was one of those called the Decapolis, cities settled by warriors of Alexander. They were both non-Jewish and apparently resentful of the Romans. Some commentators believe the city was actually Gergesa not Gerasa, as the former is close to the sea and the latter a distance of over a day by foot.

reidentify the individual. The Scripture is replete with stories of the reidentification of individual humans. Indeed, Christianity hinges on the idea that in accordance with their own proper appropriation of God's love and acceptance, any and all can be reoriented, transformed. Such a transformation, then, calls for others to view the individual in a different, if not entirely new, way. These are conversion stories, manifesting a simultaneously fluid and stable identification. The three most important records of transformation in the Scripture are the story of Abraham, the story of the Exodus, and the story of Paul of Tarsus. These were people who were changed as surely as the man from whom the legion of demons was cast.

Yahweh spoke to Abram, telling him to leave his country, leave behind his relations, and leave the gods his father and mother had worshipped. And God made a promise. Abram was to be great on the condition that he made this transition or, more accurately, transformation. Abram was asked, in other words, to leave behind his former self-identification; that is, he was asked to repent not only of sins but to reject that which was past. This was the initiation of conversion.

God demanded that Abram fully accept the responsibilities of the covenant, including the bearing of the physical mark of covenant—circumcision. Abram had reidentified himself in accordance with his reidentification by Yahweh, literally taking the new name of Abraham. As significantly, the writer of the Text reidentified him as well, even while telling the story as a continuing narrative.

Importantly, this change does not affect only Abram. When his name is changed, he is told by the Lord that the name of his wife is to change also and that she will be blessed in accordance with this transformation. This is true of all radical reidentifications. Some obligations and relationships remain unchanged, some are ended, and some are altered. In this case, the couple remained married, but they began to share in a new self-understanding. Specifically, they saw themselves under Yahweh, which generated new understandings of each other and themselves.

The question arises when examining the conversion of Abraham and Sarah, were they the same persons after their transformation as they were before? Certainly, they reidentified themselves. They understood each other differently, including having different obligations to each other. Their social setting was radically changed and, if they had gone back to Haran, it is unlikely they would have been readily accepted by the family they had left behind. Still, there was a continuity that can be, and is, narratively traced in the Text—and presumably it was by them.

In the exodus, a people that had a history traceable back to Abraham had been redefined by oppressors. They were a displaced people, enslaved by powers beyond their control. Moses came and revealed that the God of their father Abraham wanted to reclaim his people after four hundred years. The assigned social identification as an oppressed people was intentionally rejected. The miraculous was sought.

Some have argued that this was the first time that these various tribes assumed a common, albeit loose, self-identification. While that may be open to debate, what is true is that this is the first time the name I AM WHO I AM is revealed. Clearly the people are identifying themselves, as are others who see them, as the people of Yahweh.

The early Christians adopted this image of reidentification when they claimed that their own individual transformations were part of a broader conversion into a new people.

> But you are a chosen people, a royal priesthood, a holy nation, a people belonging to God, that you may declare the praises of him who called you out of darkness into his wonderful light. Once you were not a people, but now you are the people of God (1 Pet 2:9-10).

When Saul of Tarsus first started to seek out those of the Way—those who had had their own identification altered by becoming followers of Jesus the Nazarene and, therefore, were perceived as a threat to Judaism—his purpose was to destroy them. Indeed, Saul was responsible (or, at least complicit) in the killing of the first Christian martyr, Stephen. Seeking out more Christians for the sake of persecution, Saul began a journey to Damascus to attack the rapidly growing sect in one of its new centers. While traveling, Saul had a vision of Jesus. This was not a vision of a generalized "Christ-Spirit," but of Jesus of Nazareth. The change of identification was so dramatic that, like Abram and Sarai, Saul apparently took a new name—Paul—and asked that others now see him a differently identified individual. Not surprisingly, the acceptance of the reidentification of Saul/Paul by the early church came hesitatingly. To do so meant he would have to be treated differently, that their moral responsibilities would change. In fact, it took a divine intervention to hasten the acceptance of Paul's ethical reidentification (Acts 9). For Paul and for the early church, this experience could not be understood in abstract philosophical terms, but only as an event within the broader story of the Messiah coming to earth, which demanded that persons be understood (identified) in new ways.

Abraham's and Sarah's journey, the Exodus, and the Damascus Road transformation all resulted in new identifications. Evangelical Christians and their predecessors assert that such new identifications have salvific significance. The ontological status of the person (and, in the case of Israel and the church, the community) is radically changed even while remaining continuously connected with that person or community of the past. Christians assert that conversion makes one a "new person" while, at the same time, ask that the changed human be recognized as the "same person." For this reason, Paul speaks of himself as "a new man," while referring nonetheless to his pre-Christian past with the first person pronoun.[2]

In Saul's, Abram's, and Sarai's cases this reidentification involved the adoption of new names. In the other, the case of the Hebrew people, a new name was revealed, that of Yahweh. In each case there was a reconsideration of all social relationships and a new perspective from which to judge the course of the future. Transforming events are central in the Christian narrative and central to evangelical self-understanding. Obviously, then, the concept of conversion or transformation is central in evangelical ethics.

Christian conversion, with its assertion that somehow one can be identified as something totally new and yet somehow the same, implies a specific moral anthropology. A person continues to be the same person in the sense of having a continuous narrative, though through many changes in roles and relationships. Christians go further and claim that this continuity exists because God identifies the person as a specific person or as "having" or "being" a soul. Identification as human, as a human with particularities, and as a particular human allows both constancy and change.

PART TWO: CHRISTIAN BIOETHICS

The demon-possessed man spoke of himself as being the demons. Was he right? Is there a true self of each individual? Can an individual person recognize his or her self, or are humans inevitably self-deceived? Is the I that I perceive internally the same as the me that others see?[3] Does it matter how

---

[2]See 2 Corinthians 5:17; Galatians 6:15; Ephesians 4:24; Colossians 3:10 on new person. See Galatians 1, Philippians 3:4-7; 1 Timothy 1:12-16 on Paul's continuity with his past as Saul of Tarsus.

[3]This is the standard epistemological question of social interactionism. The classic work in that school is George Herbert Mead, *Mind, Self and Society: From the Standpoint of a Social Behavior-*

other people see the me, or can each person declare his or her identity and compel others to accept it as such? In more contemporary language, was the man called Legion an invalid, a cripple, a person with disability, mentally ill, eccentric, simply different, or should he be identified in some other way? Was he all of these and a man possessed by demonic forces as well?

From a moral perspective, how people act certainly depends on how they understand their own identity. Yet, for bioethics, most difficult moral questions actually hinge on how others identify who or what one is. In the case of an ongoing disabling condition, Christians should see a person as one who is simultaneously not his or her health condition and one who has the condition as part of who she or he is.[4] To pretend there is not an impairment is denial. To define another only in terms of that impairment is to deprive the individual of the respect she or he warrants as an image-bearer. How this balance is maintained goes a long way in determining how one is treated.

Given how this society, and indeed almost all societies throughout history, view persons with disabling conditions, recognizing such an individual's worthiness may require a reconsideration of how that person is morally identified. As elsewhere noted, there is a great deal of inconsistency in the interpretation of the individual at the end of modernity. The most popular arguments for continuity in identification come from the state with the social contract, from the religious with their understanding of the soul and from persons favoring developmental theories of the person. The conceptual problem for ethics is how continuity is maintained through radical change and how change is described when life is viewed as a continuous process. This is nowhere more difficult than in considering the apparent discontinuity of traumatic disabling injury and the dissimilarity from "normal"—as the population norm—of persons who have severe genetic or congenital disabilities.

Most major changes in humans are developmental. Individuals mature anatomically and physiologically, and to do so is normal and desirable. People also develop psycho-socially—though the degree to which this is determined by genetics, environment, unpredictable circumstances and choices is open to

---

ist, ed. and with an introduction by Charles W. Morris (Chicago: University of Chicago Press, 1962).

[4]When responding to a question about eternal life a close friend, who happened to have quadriplegia, said that he really did not know how to think of himself in heaven—whether he would or would not be in a wheelchair—but he was confident it would make no difference. He said he did not really know how to think of himself as an adult without picturing the chair, as that was all he had ever known. As the conversation continued, another question asked was, How will we recognize Christ? One answer given was, By his majesty and by his wounds.

debate. Some have asserted that how one understands personal purpose and meaning changes in a developmental manner. *Development* is a useful structural concept; it is reasonable to generally claim that physical and emotional maturity, at their proper stages, are relatively preferable to immaturity.

Development is not the only way that people change. People can be transformed through dramatic, radical—as down to the root—conversions. Both development and conversion are normal aspects of human life as an ongoing process. Both can move toward or away from what is healthy, broadly defined, for the individual and for the community. Arguably development can be negative, if the deterioration of the body with aging and the apoptosis of cells are taken into account, though generally the concept development implies a positive direction. Conversion can be either positive or negative.

Evangelicals, needless to say, assert that conversion to Jesus Christ is the one truly positive, unadulterated conversion. They might also assert that conversion out of, say, a street gang into a nonviolent life or from being a greedy white-collar criminal to a kindly school teacher with conventional employment might be relative goods, regardless of the religion of the individual. Other changes besides the religious can be understood as conversions. One is "converted" whenever there is a sudden alteration in how reality is interpreted or in how one fits into reality.

Consequently, the best language to explain a disabling change may be that of *transformation* or *conversion*. In the case of serious disease or sudden disability, the conversion is usually seen—at least initially—in negative terms. The transition, as with all dramatic conversions, must be followed by a period of support and entry into a new community of concern (or the conversion of the injured person's community so that it receives the individual who is disabled). The early transition period is the time when the individual is most vulnerable to falling into anomic despair. Yet, at least in some cases, it can also be the beginning of a positive, new time of life.

While adjustment and acceptance are spiritually desirable ends that the now disabled person should seek, the change goes beyond an internal attitude shift. Who the person is in the eyes of others changes as well. The Christian who faces a major illness or disabling condition should expect those changes and make sure the attitude shift is toward greater reliance on God. This does not mean that all things—including terrible injuries or illnesses—are good, but that all things can be used for good (Rom 8). The attitude results from genuine belief in the power of God to be victorious regardless of the evil one brings upon oneself, that others cause or that random circumstances generate. While Christians cannot demand those of the world to recognize the sameness and the change in a transformed person to the same degree, they can expect some recognition that the individual is due civility. The faithful are expected to respond to a higher degree in both respect and the recognition of dignity, even with a radical transformation in life, and even if the physical and cognitive changes appear to be quite negative.

The Christian viewpoint is that suffering, though not an intrinsic good, is an opportunity for spiritual growth. The status of disabled is not therefore elevated anymore than the status of poor ought to be. Further, when poverty or physical disability can be alleviated, the faithful believer is obligated to assist as appropriate in making such possible. Still, when the believer is tested by anything, including physical or mental disability and concomitant social degradation, she or he can be transformed for the better. From an evangelical perspective, the redemption of suffering is a foreshadowing of the final redemption of the soul that God offers to all. Earthly suffering is relativized by the hope that eternal suffering has been alleviated for the one who accepts God's grace through Jesus Christ.

> Therefore, since we have been justified through faith, we have peace with God through our Lord Jesus Christ, through whom we have gained access by faith into this grace in which we now stand. And we rejoice in the hope of the glory of God. Not only so, but we also rejoice in our sufferings, because we know that suffering produces perseverance; perseverance, character; and character, hope. And hope does not disappoint us, because God has poured out his love into our hearts by the Holy Spirit, whom he has given us. You see, at just the right time, when we were still powerless, Christ died for the ungodly. (Rom 5:1-6)

The positive response to a disabling event is not limited to the person who has suffered from a disease or debilitating injury. Those around that person should also recognize the conversion and, if need be, convert themselves to properly respond with support and respect. The books of 1 and 2 Samuel describe the friendship of David and Jonathan. When Jonathan died in battle, David felt a strong obligation to care for the son of Jonathan.

> Jonathan son of Saul had a son who was lame in both feet. He was five years old when the news about Saul and Jonathan came from Jezreel. His nurse picked him up and fled, but as she hurried to leave, he fell and became crippled. His name was Mephibosheth. (2 Sam 4:4)

> When Mephibosheth son of Jonathan, the son of Saul, came to David, he bowed down to pay him honor. David said, "Mephibosheth!" "Your servant," he replied. "Don't be afraid," David said to him, "for I will surely show you kindness for the sake of your father Jonathan. I will restore to you all the land that belonged to your grandfather Saul, and you will always eat at my table." Mephibosheth bowed down and said, "What is your servant, that you should notice a dead dog like me?" So Mephibosheth ate at David's table like one of the king's sons. (2 Sam 9:6-8, 11)

Mephibosheth had a severe acquired disability. He was, as a consequence of this disability, unable to serve in the military and, in spite of the death of his father, not permitted to serve as a royal leader. Though it cannot be said with certainty, the disability might have limited Mephiboseth's possibilities to become king even if his father had survived and Saul's dynastic line been established. The priesthood was closed to those who were not considered whole, and it can be safely assumed that the people would have viewed Mephiboseth's physical "incompleteness" as a sign of inadequate leadership skills or even of spiritual incompleteness. Perhaps this was what Mephiboseth himself meant by referring to himself as "a dead dog"—though it is equally possible that he was verbalizing his recognition that David was king and his claims to special royal privilege had come to an end, unless David restored them. Generally in the Scripture, persons with disabling conditions are persons of worth, though limits in function are recognized; sometimes in the Old Testament social status is lesser. Questions of such persons as being nonhuman generally did not arise, though the matter of lower social location did, until Jesus changed that cultural order.

Scripture clearly asserts six things about persons with disabilities, especially as one moves from priestly qualifications in the Pentateuch through the familial-like obligation of David (1000 B.C.) to the declarations Jesus made about persons with disabilities and healings (ca. A.D. 30):

1. They are persons of worth.
2. They are unique individuals, not simply members of a category *disabled* or *crippled*.
3. They have characteristics that limit in one or more specific areas, given the "normal" range of activities for a person of a given age and social location.
4. Physical and spiritual suffering are evils that can be transformed into opportunities for the manifestation of divine goodness, even while some of the consequences of those expressions of evil may remain.

5. Obligations to cure or care for those who have disabilities cannot be avoided.
6. Obligations for persons with disabling conditions to provide concern and service to others remain, though specifics may change, regardless of limits on certain abilities or capacities.

A shift occurs with the teachings and miracles of Jesus. In the Pentateuch it appears that the inability to meet priestly qualifications has less to do with functional inabilities than with the perceived "incompleteness" or "unholiness" of the individual. He (always a *he* in the case of the priesthood) was morally identified as inadequate, as a person of lower status, a lower level of social membership. Though respected as humans, it is clear that unless an exception was made as with Mephiboseth, the social status was lower. Persons born with disabilities were deemed sinners or the product of particular sinfulness or simply not worthy of full social consideration (Jn 9). Persons with acquired disabilities were culturally degraded and their own particularly grievous sinfulness was assumed to be the cause of their condition. This was true even though the book of Job (one of the earliest books written in the Text) made clear such assumptions could not and should not be made—the author of Job asserts this while noting that such degradation, even by one's friends, is common. Jesus rejects that "common" response.

Evangelicals must defend the "right" of a human to exist, regardless of the physical or mental condition of such a person, and regardless of the kinds of changes that individuals go through following disabling events. To use the language introduced above, the individual's species identification warrants such as she or he is an Image-bearer, *imago Dei.* Christians are morally required to protect, care for and respect the vulnerable. The faithful should always recognize that they were orphans until God adopted them; that they were lost until Christ put them on the Way; that they remain always in need of protection from those who hate, abuse or casually disregard. The central argument for caring for any in need is drawn from the Old Testament and then amplified by the elevation of mercy, justice and humility to the cosmic level through the offering of Jesus Christ.

Because God has helped the believer by exercising justice, mercy and humility toward him or her, so the believer is obligated to help others. As the Scripture constantly notes, certain people are more vulnerable than others, primarily because they are either physically at a boundary of life or culturally at the edge of the society or both. These people are frequently mistreated because they are defined out of existence or out of social significance—often the two are indistinguishable. They are identified as having lower cultural status or not having morally significant status at all. Sometimes this occurs at the onset of life, sometimes as one physically deteriorates and sometimes following a sudden change. Regardless, the obligations of protection and respect remain. This caring for those who have been converted by a physical disorder should be based on a mixture of social virtues: justice, mercy and humility. Some key prophetic passages can serve as examples: Isaiah 1:15-20; Jeremiah 9:23-24; Ezekiel 22:23-31; 34:15-16; Micah 6:6-8.

It has been asserted that there should be, based on Scripture, a deference toward those with disabilities in the same way that liberation theologians have argued that there is a divine bias toward the poor.[5] While the specific liberationist arguments may not find great acceptance among evangelicals, especially the implying of a greater divine love for the poor or disabled than for others, the basic moral assertion does—or should. The believer should have an awakened sense of obligation, powerful obligation, to render concern and care to those in need of the community of faith as an expression of brotherly love and to those outside as an example of Samaritan-like neighborly love. The believer's spiritual conversion should help him or her recognize the significance of the cultural conversion and its commonly negative implications for the person with a significant disability.

However, liberationist arguments per se tend to use analytical models that finally do not serve believers well, either those with or without significant disabilities. First, liberationist thought is always rooted irrevocably in the specific community. Indeed, there are communities of persons with disabilities, but there are few. In other words, if liberationist thought is to be honestly appropriated to any degree it must been done so for specific communities, like "the blind" or "the deaf."[6] While done to empower, this is not ultimately ac-

---

[5]Paulo Freire, *Pedagogy of the Oppressed*, trans. Myra Bergman Ramos (New York: Seabury Press, 1968); Leonardo Boff, *Church: Charism and Power: Liberation Theology and the Institutional Church*, trans. John W. Diercksmeier (New York: Crossroad, 1985). A preferable understanding of liberationist thought is found in the work of Gustavo Gutiérrez, *A Theology of Liberation: History, Politics and Salvation*, trans. and ed. Sister Caridad Inda and John Eagleson (Maryknoll, N.Y.: Orbis, 1973), especially in the revised introduction. Still, liberationist thought does not prioritize the moral good in the same way as evangelicals; even in with the nineteenth century social activist evangelicals, the first concern always remained conversion to Christ. For a liberationist argument applied to disability, see Nancy Eisland, *The Disabled God: Toward a Liberation Theology of Disability* (Nashville: Abingdon, 1994).

[6]Of all the groups centered around disability issues, those with severe hearing impairments have come the closest to actually living in a liberationist mode. It seems that this has, indeed, occurred because there is a distinct language that allows community stories to be told in ways

ceptable in evangelical moral reasoning because persons of all levels and types of abilities are supposed to be part of one community under Christ—effectively a new "ethnic" group to which persons with or without significant disabilities who accept Jesus Christ as Lord belong. Other important differences, of course, remain, but they do not function as the primary characteristic of social identity.

Second, and following on the first point, liberationist arguments and praxis are not first of all about the obtaining of individual rights or rendering personal care. Liberationist thought is about the fulfillment of the cultural community of the marginalized. Evangelicals should be concerned about the inclusion of the marginalized in the faith community and the protection of their rights in civil society. The ADA has been correctly termed one of the most sweeping pieces of civil rights legislation in history. It is an assertion that persons with disabilities have the right to function as individuals in American society. After all, the legislation is called The *Americans* with Disabilities Act specifically because the basic group identification is with being American, not being disabled. Christians can and should support individual political rights and, it will be argued below, rights to basic health care and daily living support. However, this is not the same as assigning people into pseudo-ethnic groups according to disability. Indeed, Christians must reject such, even while encouraging support groups and advocacy for rights.

> As you come to him, the living Stone—rejected by men but chosen by God and precious to him—you also, like living stones, are being built into a spiritual house to be a holy priesthood, offering spiritual sacrifices acceptable to God through Jesus Christ. . . .
>
> But you are a chosen people, a royal priesthood, a holy nation, a people belonging to God, that you may declare the praises of him who called you out of darkness into his wonderful light. Once you were not a people, but now you are the people of God; once you had not received mercy, but now you have received mercy.
>
> Dear friends, I urge you, as aliens and strangers in the world, to abstain from sinful desires, which war against your soul. Live such good lives among the pagans that, though they accuse you of doing wrong, they may see your good deeds and glorify God on the day he visits us. . . .
>
> For it is God's will that by doing good you should silence the ignorant talk of foolish men. Live as free men, but do not use your freedom as a cover-up for

---

that those without the impairment *and* the ability to sign cannot comprehend. For more on the limit that language places upon community formation, see George A. Lindbeck, *The Nature of Doctrine: Religion and Theology in a Postliberabl Age* (Philadelphia: Westminster Press, 1984).

> evil; live as servants of God. Show proper respect to everyone. (1 Peter 2:4-5, 9-12, 15-17)

Faithful Christians see an indication of how the believing community should respond to Christians who have been converted by injury or illness in the story of David and Mephibosheth. This is primarily a story not about David's obligation to Mephibosheth but about his obligation to Jonathan's family member. The son of his deceased friend is to be treated as family, regardless of the disability. Similarly, the believer is to treat those who have entered his or her spiritual family (that is, have become brothers or sisters in Christ) in a like manner. This comes as an expression of familial love.

Believers are also to treat others with respect and care in light of their particular needs and in full recognition of the particular abilities those others bring. These obligations of justice, love and humility are first toward other believers, yet care and respect should be extended beyond to all persons, especially those in need. This is one of the implications of all humans being bearers of the *imago Dei*. They are not only human beings entitled to rights, they are individuals in relationships who may not have a civil right to be loved, but are due love from believers.

PART THREE: CHRISTIAN BIOETHICS AND THE WORLD

The United States since its formal founding has never been and never will be a Christian society. Having said that, it has been culturally, socially and politically shaped by the Christian faith. This religious influence has led to a sociopolitical understanding of individuals that has resulted in humans being valued as humans. When this understanding has actually been applied in political action, it has led to the protection of human rights as "endowed" by the Creator, "unalienable" and "self-evident."

The American notion of civil society is based in part on assumptions about original sin and conversion that seem principally derived from revivalist-evangelical theology. This is not to deny the substantial influence of the Enlightenment thought nor Native American models of governmental discourse and wilderness pragmatism nor British common law nor market individualism. Still, the influence of evangelical doctrine and behavior is noteworthy; after all, the United States and evangelicals began at the same time and have "grown up" together. The secularism of America was not originally nonreligious, but multireligious national disestablishment. In the early years of the Republic, the multiple religions were really multiple denominational forms of

Protestantism and the Protestant understandings of original sin and conversion have had a profound impact on the culture that remain evident today.[7]

Americans, following (to at least some significant degree) on these two doctrines—original sin and the reality of conversion—tend to (1) be suspicious of too much power being held by one individual because all humans have their failings, and (2) believe that individuals can make radical changes. These are yoked to the Enlightenment social contract idea of human rights. It is the second doctrine, conversion, that is most pertinent when considering the transformation that occurs following a postchildhood disabling traumatic injury or illness. Such injuries are culturally more similar to evangelical religious conversion than to any of the other analogues with which they are usually compared.

Evangelicals, because of the importance of life transformation in evangelical spirituality, readily understand that somehow the converted person is both a new and the former person. Because of U.S. history—the role of deistic humanism, revivalism, Calvinism, and market utilitarianism in the founding of the nation-state—progress and transition are simply assumed. Individuals can solve problems with inventions and that includes reinventing themselves—by moving to a new region, or taking a new job, by starting over.

There is for both evangelicalism and for the United States an identification dialectic—actually a three-way dialectic, or trialectic—that must be maintained without resolution into any unity except that unity of a specific real human being: the individual is human, is a particular human, and is a human with particularities. Such a claim about human nature is not often formally expressed, but does pragmatically operate nonetheless. The trialectic of species, integral and role identification allows for transitions after which someone is new and the same simultaneously.

As discussed above, the first question of identification in a social contract society is species identification. This is a general category applied to individuals: is one individually human or not, and what does that imply for the obliga-

[7]Catholicism was also very influential, but in highly limited areas of the early United States (e.g., Maryland). Also, Catholicism and Russian Orthodoxy were influential in areas that would be later annexed, though not until the mid-nineteenth century. Judaism and Anabaptist forms of Protestantism had relatively little impact beyond local communities. Quakers were influential, but at the time were also very Protestant and evangelistic, unlike most forms of the Society of Friends today. Native American religions may have been influential in some areas, but seem to have had little effect on the European American culture. Though later the multireligious nature of the United States would include Catholicism and Judaism as strong presences in the "public square" (and, eventually, traditional and modified forms of Eastern religions, Islam and Eastern Orthodoxy), initially Protestantism was most culturally influential.

tions of the state? The other aspects of identification are more particular. How are roles tied to identification? How is one the same person from birth until death, or (more accurately from an evangelical perspective) from the initiation of an individual human life in the womb until the end of eternity? The way people treat others depends on this threefold identification.

Humans can be identified as having species, role and integral identification. Humanness, or species identification, remains constant. Roles come and go. The integral identification is a narrative that flexes and turns, but is nonetheless continuous. Sometimes, when the roles come to an end, the integral identification, while continuing, is radically reconsidered. A person can change so much—even while remaining the same human being—that she or he has a transformation of identification. The person is converted.

An American can readily claim, "I am who I am, though I am not the same person in the same way year to year, day to day, even moment to moment." When transformation of the individual occurs as an expression of physical, cognitive or emotional development, it is readily accepted and often applauded. Though seemingly less true than in the past, even those changes associated with age-typical physiological, anatomical and mental decline are accepted as simply a part of the reality of the individual and the community in which she or he lives. When a traumatic injury or illness occurs that radically transforms the individual and severely impacts his or her immediate community, this ready acceptance is lacking, which makes sense. Such injuries and illnesses are often tragic, in that potential is lost and expectations are drastically altered. The same is often also thought to be true at the birth of those with genetic and congenital disorders. The question is how to recognize the reality of some degree of tragedy while not seeing the individual as tragic.

The trialectic of sameness and change is the practical reality most persons experience at a day-to-day level. Others will usually identify a human individual as being the same person in spite of some significant changes. For instance, generally Widow Smith, at seventy years of age, is considered, in some defining way, the same person as Baby Smith was sixty-nine-and-a-half years earlier. At the same time, she is not the same person since her gross physiological and anatomical characteristics may bear greater superficial similarity to seventy-two-year-old Ms. Jones than to the baby who lived seven decades earlier. Nonetheless, both biologically and socially there is a continuity that encapsulates all the changes.

Yet when a tragic event occurs such as a serious injury or illness, in the

West at the end of modernity, the altered or out-of-norm individual may be interpreted by health-care professionals, the state and family out of existence. They try to decide whether the individual is a person and, therefore, a member of the contract warranting protection and care. Sometimes they may also insert some discussion of utility. The family members, on the other hand, may refer to roles and stories. The discussion tends to center around the idea of who the posttrauma, transformed individual is, or what the person is. The family may ask, Is he the same person? The practitioners and state ask, Is he a human being at all?

The history or narrative of a person binds his or her life into a unity, even with distinct moments marking transitions from being identified as a person of one sort to a person of another. This is the same person, even while a different sort of person. The communities to which one belongs may or may not accept the conversion. If they do, they must adjust as the individual adjusts. The only other option is extreme marginalization.

The practical concern with identification is not ontological, nor epistemological, but relational or moral—how persons understand their obligations and relationships. For serious disabling conditions (for instance like traumatic brain injury), this means how the now altered individual is interpreted by others who have previously had obligations to that person. The question here is not how the survivor responds, but instead how the others view their own obligations to the converted. The greatest threat to the individual is the claim that the person ceases to be following a disabling event.

The society as a whole is quite conflicted over how to understand those who are born with disabilities and even more so with those who suddenly acquire them. Having a sizeable population of persons with significant disabling conditions is relatively new and that, in part, explains why the language of serious health-related reidentification is so awkward. In the past, for instance after the American Civil War, there were large numbers of amputees and for most of the nineteenth and early twentieth centuries, there were many who were disabled by various diseases, especially leading to blindness and deafness. Still, having a noticeable segment of the population with significant disabilities is fairly recent. The growth in the proportion to the broader population is associated with the presence of dangerous equipment, the significantly increased efficiency of emergency medical technicians and emergency room personnel, the development of rehabilitation and the availability of antibiotics. The visibility of such persons has also increased, in part because of the patients' rights movements. Because the presence of persons with significant disabilities is new for many in the society, the cultural tools needed to interpret and respond to such persons are often inadequate.

In addition, disability is not one thing. In the United States, because of the tendency to define people with dichotomous categories, like Republican/ Democrat, it is easy to do the same with disability. This tendency is exacerbated by people who tend to define *disabled* by the presence or absence of a parking permit. Persons may be categorically lumped together, but there are significant variations between visual, mobility and affective functional limits, and even more within each of those categories. Like immigrants, it is sometimes convenient for institutional reasons to recognize the commonality of marginalization due to a physical impairment. Forms will sometimes have categories like Asian or Pacific Islander, but it is important to understand that Koreans, Japanese and Thais are different culturally and have further distinctions within those subcategories. So with disability there are many differences between categories and within categories for any given individual. Individuals are particular people, though categories are useful when considering needs and the distribution of social resources.

Rather than develop new models or look for traditional models that might be more useful, those confronted with suddenly disabled family members and those in the broader society have tended to fall back on interpretive schemes that only increase the marginalization of persons who are already pushed to the periphery by physiological and anatomical limitations and the physical and social structures of a society not fully equipped to include them. The dominant and inadequate models are denial, death, regression and degradation. To these, conversion as an interpretive model should be added; it is generally less demeaning and less threatening, but acknowledges significant transformation.

Persons with serious acquired or newly recognized disabilities often are interpreted differently by different persons, leading to different moral consequences. If the significance of the change is denied, then the person will be expected to achieve impossible standards or may be shielded from accomplishing in new arenas of life. Family members may argue that one should keep a positive attitude or may choose to ignore scientific facts about the survivor's condition. Initially, this may support the hope that is so important to motivation in rehabilitation or to adjustment. The difficulty is not that persons hope for a better physical outcome. Rather, when denial prevents a transformation in moral identification that accounts for changed roles and allows new perspectives on the future, rehabilitation and reintegration into society may be inhibited.

Paternalism/maternalism is similar to denial in wanting to buffer the individual from the consequences of disability, and accepting the seriousness of the condition but not recognizing potential. The newly disabled individual is protected, perhaps excessively, on the grounds that she or he has *regressed* or is now stunted. Parents who have an offspring with an acquired significant disability not uncommonly see that child, even if an adult child, as a preadolescent. The parents may revert to behaviors that were useful when the son or daughter was last so dependent, rather than in an age appropriate manner that also takes into account the disabling condition. This identification can lead to overprotection that actually curtails activities that would promote the growth and development of the individual.

If the seriousness of the disabling condition is considered irreversible and significant then the survivor may be defined as a nonsurvivor, as good as dead. Family members, friends and health-care professionals may abandon the "living corpse," declaring that the previous person has ceased to exist. "John the swimmer is gone"; "we are not in a hospital, but a funeral home"; "I'd rather be dead than like that" are frequently expressed in conversations of persons in rehabilitation center lobbies. Claiming disability is the same as death releases family members, friends, practitioners and the state from obligations to the survivor. After all, the reasoning might go, why spend effort and funds on the dead or the as-good-as-dead? This is extremely problematic under the U.S. social contract. No individual is functionally dead who is yet alive, and no living person should be deprived of fundamental rights unless that person has threatened the contract (such as an imprisoned murderer). A person with a serious disability does threaten a community like a family or group of friends to the extent that broad reexamination of relationships and obligations will be required but does not threaten the social contract. Importantly, even if the individual is considered effectively dead by the family, while morally reprehensible from a Christian perspective, it is not the same as the state depriving one of contract-protected rights.

The person with the acquired disability may be identified as living, but less than human or at least less than a person. The individual may be defined, somewhat paradoxically, as imprisoned in a broken body. Or, the disabled individual may be defined as a malingerer. Either way, she or he is culturally degraded. Strict dualists who emphasize the exclusive significance of memory, interests and willful control over daily activities in defining personhood may offer to free the imprisoned person through euthanasia or, at best, insist on institutionalization in prisonlike environments. Those who are noneists or plurists will simply deny the reality of the individual's existence as a valued individual. Each of these responses to moral identification has, obviously, moral implications.

Persons with acquired disabilities and those born with disabling conditions almost without exception begin the transformation of identification within a medical context. They are defined as patients and the disability as sickness. As such, they are excused from responsibilities, and those around them will assist with daily living tasks even if inconvenienced. However, as the disability is progressively understood as permanent, the survivor may well be increasingly perceived as a malingerer or as a prisoner. She or he is seen as not trying hard enough or needing liberation. Heroic pictures of persons who have gone on to accomplish extraordinary feats are offered not as encouragement, but as an expectation. Escape or be condemned for not doing so. Not inevitably, but often, this leads to discouragement for the survivor and disgust on the part of others. The sense of disgust can be exacerbated by the presence of atypical (not for the injured, but for the not-yet-disabled public) behaviors and characteristics (e.g., drooling) that may elicit a pollution avoidance response. Survivors may even be seen as disease vectors (the sick as carriers) or vectors of the truth of human fragility, reminding others of their own physical vulnerability. Or, they may be defined as imprisoned in their malfunctioning bodies. Should the disability be a result of a poor decision, the survivor may be deemed as justly deserving his or her imprisonment. Depending on the availability of appropriate housing and the attitude of the surrounding community, persons may actually be placed in institutions that are not entirely unlike prisons.[8] The "convict" or "disease carrier" may be seen as being a bad influence, a cause of sadness or disgust on the part of the observer, or simply ignored as culturally invisible. Less likely, though more threatening, some might desire to "free" the person from the prison of the body or eliminate the disease vector through active euthanasia. The person with the disability is defined as polluted—literally with disease or psycho-socially—and the response to the person will be pollution avoidance. The now culturally degraded individual will be avoided, shunned, quarantined or, in the most extreme cases, exterminated.

[8]The literature on "total institutions," based on Goffman is helpful, even though sometimes exaggerated. Erving Goffman, *Asylums: Essays on the Condition of the Social Situation of Mental Patients and Other Inmates* (New York: Doubleday, 1961).

A better understanding of severe disabling injury or illness is to interpret it as a conversion event—a moment of both change and consistency. As noted above, the concept of conversion remains common in American culture (even if the language is less familiar than in the past). In the United States, the structural similarity of serious acquired disability and evangelical conversion provides a basis for understanding humans with disabilities following traumatic injury or illness as persons still warranting full moral consideration and concern. This does not mean that it is necessary by Christian morality or the American social contract that the individual bearing the image of God have life extended by any and every means. Still, a model of conversion can prevent the devaluation of those with nonterminal disabilities who too readily are defined as being essentially dead or so diminished as to be unworthy of existence by those with power over their lives.

In table 6.1, the tripartite moral identification is on the vertical axis with the dominant interpretative analogues for disability on the horizontal. The cells in the bottom row describe likely responses when one particular aspect of moral identification is emphasized using a particular analog.

Table 6.1. Moral Identification and Interpretation of Severe Disability

	Denial	*Death*	*Regression*	*Degradation*	*Conversion*
Species	Same	Same/Lost	Same (though could diminish)	Demoted	Same
Integral	Same	Lost	Stunted/ Stagnant	Transformed	Transformed
Role	Same	Lost (gain as living corpse)	Lost (gain as child)	Lost (roles only at social periphery)	Lost and Gained
Response to Others	Deny/ Avoid	Grieve/ Abandon	Treat as Child/ Act as Parent	Treat as Prisoner/ Pollution Avoidance	Accept or Reject as Sectarian Convert

With most conversions, as with most acquired disabilities, the crisis event occurs suddenly, even if the circumstances leading to it actually were cumulative. Often religious conversions appear to occur out of the blue, so to speak. Similarly, traumatic brain injuries, spinal cord injuries and some severe disabling illnesses occur rapidly, usually without significant physiological or anatomical precursors. As with religious conversion, the person with a serious acquired disability tends to lose friends and has to redefine relationships within the family. As with religious conversion, the person may be rejected, especially as she or he redefines life purposes. If the person is not rejected, then usually the family itself is converted to some degree or becomes tolerant of the new subculture in which the survivor wholly or partially participates.

This is not an argument against mainstreaming, but a recognition that for both treatment and social justice reasons it may be necessary to participate in specialized communities with others who understand the particulars of medical, daily living and cultural needs. First, she or he spends time in rehabilitation. Special language is used. Special clothing sometimes is worn. Special behaviors are demanded. Even special attitudes are now expected. Second, and more importantly, if she or he becomes involved with advocacy organizations, she or he will be participating in a sectlike community. The group reinforces values that distinguish it from the outside world which tends to either ignore or have an antagonistic attitude toward those with disabilities.

While not denying the spiritual validity of religious groups with high clerical authority or the therapeutic value of clear rules and patterns for some, control over persons with disabilities should be at the least restrictive level. As with religious conversions, the new convert may be subject to inappropriate control by leaders in one or more of the new communities entered. Supervision over the supervisors is an appropriate task of the state or a state surrogate. To extend the metaphor, as with religious liberty, the newly disabled person should be free to associate with whom she or he chooses. Yet, as with religious converts, it may well be that the survivor will prefer the company of those who better understand his or her circumstances.

Assuming the person with the disability maintains the ability to function in the world, she or he often modifies her or his understanding of what constitutes human interaction. Thus, sometimes the transformation is more than metaphorically a religious conversion; it can be a genuine change in worldview. An existential reexamination is forced on the survivor and on the family members of that survivor. This compels a re-identification of the person with the acquired (or newly recognized) disability.

If a conversion model is adopted, then the person with the acquired disability will be generally interpreted as the same and as new. Further, if the person is identified as converted, then obligations to the individual remain at some level. For instance, rather than walking away from a marriage since the survivor is not the person once married, the spouse should recognize that she or he is divorcing or remaining married to the same person—though the same person now radically changed.

In a society in which liberty is one of the primary values, the right to be impolite or even nondestructively immoral—while not ensconced in the Constitution—is nonetheless one that should be protected. What is not a right is to become so callous as to not treat someone as a fellow member of the contract. This means that each individual must be treated as an individual and as a particular—a unique, ongoing—individual. Each individual is a person with a name and a history, with obligations and obligations due.

Not only should family and friendship obligations be recognized, so should those of the state. Christians can legitimately work toward legislative protection and provision for persons who have been converted by a major illness or trauma. The now-disabled person, or for that matter the one who is genetically or congenitally disabled, remains a holder of rights and is entitled to reasonable protection from those who would deprive him or her of life, liberty and/or property. One specific example of this would be provision of least restrictive housing when housing is required by law.

Still, the state should not be used to end immoral but not immediately destructive choices or those decisions that might have a high probability of being so. In other words, Christians have to tolerate and should expect the use of incorrect interpretive analogs. Still, Christians should do all they can to support families so at least such poor choices are not encouraged. Further, Christians can work with the state to facilitate the opportunity and provision of resources for decisions that will provide positive long-term opportunities for the individual who is disabled and for his or her family.

The vast majority of persons who have to adjust their daily living due to a disabling condition do not have such significant cognitive or affective disorders that they are in any way impeded from functioning in society. To the contrary, without devaluation by society and with reasonable accommodations, most are fully capable of engaging others and being full members of society. The changes they have experienced or differences from "normal" should be recognized without denying the continuity of individual life.

CONCLUSION

In a social contract society all persons matter as distinctly human. Ideally, each should also matter as one who is a unique individual. Some in American society prefer to deny either the distinctly human rights that each is owed or disregard the unique worth of each on the basis of some disabling condition. This must be actively opposed. Even the most disabled are social beings and their interaction, as minimal or different as it may be, is important for a social contract society.

While it would be wonderful to declare that reasonable care and respect of persons with serious disabilities shows what strong, gracious community exists among all Americans, that is not the case and need not be. If someone wants to be impolite or disregarding to another, disability or not, that person should have the right to do so. People may disregard the distinctive individuality of anyone they choose. They may not deny, though, the reality of humanness in a person with a serious disabling condition. For a social contract society to draw a line that intentionally includes even the most severely disabled is extraordinarily beneficial for those at the boundary who get included and for everyone else. It says, regardless of the cultured elite, the political powerholders and the masters of the marketplace, that individuals count. They can be disregarded, ignored as anonymous sufferers, even mocked by those with poor taste or little sense, but they cannot be defined out of existence.

Human individuals are distinctly human, they are morally identifiable as a member of the species, and that, under the U.S. social contract, means that certain rights (including the right to life) should be protected by the state. Individuals are not only distinctly human, they are unique humans. They live through various discontinuous roles as they live out a continuous narrative. The casting out of the demon in the healing story was unquestionably a conversion event. As such, it changed the individual and the communities of which he was a part. Jesus named the demonic and, in so doing, initiated the proper reidentification of the exorcised man. With that reidentifcaiton came the recognition of some ongoing and some new obligations to the man as well as some ongoing and some new obligations on his part.

Identification can matter a great deal. For instance, if someone is identified as no longer a person but a corpse, then the moral response will be quite different than if she or he is seen as a living being. Putting this process in the framework of moral identification, the injury or illness survivor does remain a human being. The person maintains species identification. Many, perhaps most, roles in which the individual had participated are lost or severely altered. This is true for all persons throughout their lives, though the suddenness of the change following traumatic injury or illness is different from most transformations. Certainly one could disagree whether this is the same person in some metaphorical sense, and even what obligations remain given the significant alterations in role capacities. But with the continuity of integral identification, those changes in moral obligations would need to be justified with due consideration of the same person, though radically transformed, being the object of those obligations. The narrative of the individual is continued, though with a sudden and harsh or even tragic change in the storyline. For believers this narrative should always include being loved by those who follow Christ.

7

Sickness and Being Sick

HUMANS AS VULNERABLE

Illness is simultaneously a physiological/anatomical experience and a cultural categorization with typical responses (the sick role). It is perfectly legitimate for believers to seek healing of physical problems, yet Christians should redefine the sick role in accordance with the faith they hold and the virtuosity they are called to live.

> Some time later, Jesus went up to Jerusalem for a feast of the Jews. Now there is in Jerusalem near the Sheep Gate a pool, which in Aramaic is called Bethesda and which is surrounded by five covered colonnades. Here a great number of disabled people used to lie—the blind, the lame, the paralyzed. One who was there had been an invalid for thirty-eight years. When Jesus saw him lying there and learned that he had been in this condition for a long time, he asked him, "Do you want to get well?"
>
> "Sir," the invalid replied, "I have no one to help me into the pool when the water is stirred. While I am trying to get in, someone else goes down ahead of me."
>
> Then Jesus said to him, "Get up! Pick up your mat and walk." At once the man was cured; he picked up his mat and walked.
>
> The day on which this took place was a Sabbath, and so the Jews said to the man who had been healed, "It is the Sabbath; the law forbids you to carry your mat."
>
> But he replied, "The man who made me well said to me, `Pick up your mat and walk.'"
>
> So they asked him, "Who is this fellow who told you to pick it up and walk?"
>
> The man who was healed had no idea who it was, for Jesus had slipped away into the crowd that was there.
>
> Later Jesus found him at the temple and said to him, "See, you are well again. Stop sinning or something worse may happen to you." The man went

away and told the Jews that it was Jesus who had made him well.

So, because Jesus was doing these things on the Sabbath, the Jews persecuted him. Jesus said to them, "My Father is always at his work to this very day, and I, too, am working." For this reason the Jews tried all the harder to kill him; not only was he breaking the Sabbath, but he was even calling God his own Father, making himself equal with God. (Jn 5:1-18)

PART ONE: THE TEXT

Prior to healing the man at the pool of Bethesda, Jesus asks him if he wants to get well. What a peculiar thing to say. Is Jesus claiming that the man might not wish to have health? Or is he noting the inadequacy of the accepted instrument of healing, the supposedly miraculous pool? Or is he mocking the culturally accepted means, the physicians, who had proved so ineffective that the man had made his way to these waters? Or is he providing the man with a possibility for health that goes beyond the disorder by which he and his community have defined the man's existence? Is Jesus offering health and healing that include, but are not limited to, the damaged physical body? Is he redefining the concept? It would not be unreasonable to suggest that Jesus meant all these.

The pool of Bethesda was east of the center city with small buildings and pavilions built nearby. The name means "house (or place) of mercy" or, perhaps, "house of grace." It was known primarily for its reported healing capacities, though built to supplement the water supply within the city, apparently by Herod the Great. While thought by some critics to have been nothing more than an image created by John to convey some spiritual truth, the site has been discovered, including the five porticos—one on each side and one in the middle separating two sections of the pool. It is approximately 350 feet long, 200 feet wide and 25 feet deep. Needless to say, the man had come to the pool with some hope of cure, but for reasons only partially revealed in the story, had not been able or had not chosen to avail himself of the "technology" of the day.

This passage about the paralytic immediately precedes the Scripture of the healing of a royal official's son. The man at the pool's edge does not have that kind of family. Possibly there is no one left as they are all dead, or perhaps they live at a great distance. Perhaps they simply are poor and cannot afford the time necessary to wait with the man for the propitious moment. Or maybe they simply do not want to, out of self-centeredness. The possibility also should not be rejected out of hand that the man at the pool has alienated his family—with some believing he is a malingerer and others, while accepting the physical reality of the disorder, having grown weary of the man's weariness.

In the period of the New Testament writing, a serious health disorder defined the individual culturally and socially. Disease was something the person had and the disease had the person—as a form of possession. The man at the Bethesda pool was apparently socially disconnected, likely due to his disorder, and had come to define himself as others did by that disorder. Regardless, Christ's response to the man after the healing is a recognition of responsibility: "Behold, you have become well; do not sin anymore, so that nothing worse happens to you" (Jn 5:14 NASB). This was a matter of theodicy not only in the sense of explaining the cause of suffering but also in the sense of how one responds to suffering. Jesus seems to be telling the man, "You are healed. Well and good, but understand that you must respond to this healing. And understand that you should have responded to the illness differently, as well. Still, you are healed. Now change."

Before the healing at Bethesda and that of the royal official's child is a passage recording Jesus' declaration that his food—that which he offers to those who believe—is something greater than earthly food. In the same sense, John means for the reader of the Bethesda miracle story to understand that the health of which Jesus speaks is more than having a normal anatomy and physiology, that is, one functioning in a manner typical of one's sex and age.

The two healing stories are followed by Jesus' statement about his authority and, by extension, his status. Religious leaders sought to kill him because, as the Gospel writer puts it, he "made himself equal to God" (Jn 5:18). Certainly Christians have understood this confluence of healing miracles and self-declaration as evidence of the divinity of Christ. But for bioethics, it begs another question. Jesus the deity on earth is asking the man at the Bethesda pool to approach illness and treatment in a new way. Health is more than physical well-being, but it is usually that as well. Still, if being sick involves more than physiological and anatomical problems, then should not the response of the believer to such illness go beyond passive acceptance of medicines? In other words, what does it mean to be sick, to assume the sick role?[1]

---

[1]Talcott Parsons made the term *sick role* popular. See Talcott Parsons, *The Social System* (New York: Free Press, 1951), esp. chap. 10, "Social Structure and Dynamic Process: The Case of Modern Medical Practice."

PART TWO: CHRISTIAN BIOETHICS

The man Jesus served at the pool of Bethesda did not yet believe in him. Indeed, the man's experience of physical and cultural suffering apparently initiates a relationship with Christ. After he is healed he is told not only to enjoy his new physical health but to be prepared to suffer differently when physical and other kinds of difficulties arise in the future. Those who are in relationship with Christ are to suffer illness and injury differently than those who are not. The Gospel calls for an attitude unlike that suggested by many of those of the world.

Paul provides instruction in consideration of his own response to suffering:

> To keep me from becoming conceited because of these surpassingly great revelations, there was given me a thorn in my flesh, a messenger of Satan, to torment me. Three times I pleaded with the Lord to take it away from me. But he said to me, "My grace is sufficient for you, for my power is made perfect in weakness." Therefore I will boast all the more gladly about my weaknesses, so that Christ's power may rest on me. That is why, for Christ's sake, I delight in weaknesses, in insults, in hardships, in persecutions, in difficulties. For when I am weak, then I am strong. (2 Cor 12:7-10)

St. John Chrysostom, an ancient figure in Christianity, in his homilies on the Bible, states about this passage and Paul's thorn:

> There are some then who have said that he means a kind of pain in the head which was inflicted of the devil; but God forbid! For the body of Paul never could have been given over to the hands of the devil, seeing that the devil himself submitted to the same Paul at his mere bidding; and he set him laws and bounds, when he delivered over the fornicator for the destruction of the flesh, and he dared not to transgress them. What then is the meaning of what is said? [It was an] adversary.[2]

Yet, some early voices asserted Paul's thorn was, in all probability, a physical malady and that Paul's words indicate the necessity of using even physical suffering as an opportunity to live out the Christian life. As an example, Tertullian notes that elation "was being restrained in the apostle [Paul] by 'buffets,' if you will, by means (as they say) of pain in the ear or head."[3] And

---

[2]St. John Chrysostom "Homilies On Second Corinthians, 20-30," trans. the Rev. Hubert Kestell Cornish and the Rev. John Medley, rev. the Rev. Talbot W. Chambers <www.ewtn.com/library/PATRISTC/PNI12-8.TXT.>

[3]Tertullian "Of St. Paul, and the Person Whom He Urges the Corinthians to Forgive," chap. 13, trans. S. Thelwall, in the Ante-Nicene Fathers translations of *The Writings of the Fathers*

according to Ireneaus it was physical suffering serving as a means to teach the immortality of God by the mortality of human flesh.[4] Reading the "thorn" as a physical problem is accepted as possible, if not probable, in most evangelical circles, with the possible exception of some strict Pentecostal groups.[5]

Using Paul as an example of the Christian pattern for responding to one's own illness, the believer's behavior should be marked by at least two characteristics: perseverance and proper prioritization. These can be understood as the two sides of Paul's declaration that "to live is Christ, and to die is gain" (Phil 1:21 KJV). Continued earthly living in the midst of suffering does require perseverance when such joy is ahead in heaven. Still, it is not only possible, but desirable, because when properly prioritized earthly living itself is recognized as a joy—albeit a lesser one.

Perseverance is hope enacted or active patience. The Christian should never confuse acceptance of physical frailty and finitude with fatalism. Resignation is not a Christian virtue. An honest understanding of one's health condition should never leave the sick Christian relishing in a supposedly spiritual way that is actually masochistic. Being *dis-eased* is not an intrinsic good. Rather, biological life is a good, and Christians should act as if it is. This includes living through suffering and maintaining biological life with the use of reasonable health care. Because the ultimate good is an eternal relationship with God, this life gains its penultimate value.

One of the great mistakes in contemporary bioethics is to accept the false dichotomy that biological life is to be valued above all or it is to be valued as nothing as soon as it is significantly damaged. For believers, human life is extraordinarily valuable—to rightly value life, even one's own, is virtuous—but to love this existence disproportionately or, likewise, to hate it even though it was given by God makes one "vicious" (in the sense of being *vice-ful*). Jesus tells believers to hate their life relative to their love for him, not to despise the gift of life that has been given (Mt 16). Earthly existence is always an almost, but not most, significant good. Such an evaluation of priorities elicits perseverance, but conditioned by the ultimate goal or good that is sought. This

---

down to A.D. 325, ed. Alexander Roberts and James Donaldson, rev. A. Cleveland Coxe (1873; reprint, Grand Rapids: Eerdmans, 1978), vol. 4, p. 87.

[4]Ireneaus *Adversus Haereses* 5.3, New Advent Website (Catholic Encyclopedia), <http://www.newadvent.org/fathers/0103503.htm>.

[5]Ronald Russell, "Redemptive Suffering and Paul's Thorn in the Flesh," *Journal of the Evangelical Theological Society* 39 (December 1996): 559–70.

means seeking all reasonable means to work cures and to address disabling injuries and illnesses.

As for medical therapies—be they medicines, surgeries, physical therapy or any demonstrably effective technique—the Christian patient need not try everything, but there is a need to try what is reasonable. Medical "futility" for the Christian can only be defined by the lack of therapeutic reasonableness for further treatments and that should be a consistent evaluation for other persons in similar conditions. Age, disability status, ethnicity, or moral culpability for one's sickness or injury should not come into play when deciding how hard the believer should try to get better. This does not mean that an evaluation may not include consideration of likely outcomes. More succinctly, treatments may be futile, but people never are futile.

Yet, it is not just taking medicines or seeking appropriate treatments that constitute the proper way for a Christian to be sick or injured. As perseverance is hope enacted or active patience, the believer is called to enact that hope by the way she or he lives with illness. Patience is, indeed, a virtue and believers should develop this virtue by the grace of God, regardless of circumstances. The Christian patient should make every effort to recognize that many of the burdens inflicted upon him or her in the midst of receiving treatment are not actually directed at him or her personally. Rather, they are generalized wrongs and the Christian should learn to bear wrongs.[6]

The bearing of wrongs is most needed when practitioners and others begin to treat the sick or injured believer as if the latter merely fulfills the role of sickness-bearer—as the disease carrier in a certain room or the old woman who should be in a nursing home or the baby wasting resources others might use.[7] The wrong that must be carried is not the biological sickness, but rather the bearing of being identified only as the carrier of the sickness, or only as the one who is a problem or a burden.

Such categorizations reflect conflicts within health care and, indeed, the society at large. And precisely because they do represent cultural struggles, the Christian patient may sometimes need to take a stand and make demands but must not do so selfishly. Often one is treated wrongly when she or he is viewed as simply another unit in a utilitarian calculus—an interchangeable part in a health-care delivery machine. Christians may respond to such trivi-

---

[6]Sidney Callahan, "To Bear Wrongs Patiently," in *With All Our Heart and Mind: The Spiritual Works of Mercy in a Psychological Age* (New York: Crossroad, 1988).

[7]The classic discussion of this is in Paul Ramsey, *The Patient as Person: Explorations in Medical Ethics* (New Haven, Conn.: Yale University Press, 1970).

alization of human suffering. The Christian patient can assert his or her rights, but only when it is for the moral good and will serve others. In other words, the believer should assert his or her rights primarily when denying those rights will spiritually hurt the one acting irresponsibly or when a pattern of injustice would be established or reinforced. At all times, it is a call to the Christian patient to be more than civil and polite, but actually defiantly gentle in the face of wrongs.

Patience is further required in that some suffering is not a matter of general wrongs or even individual harshness or error, but simply the progress of the disease and injury. In a fallen world, the Christian should exemplify how to suffer, seeking to imitate Christ, with graciousness and kindness and respect. Pain and even the immanence of death are not excuses for acting harshly or becoming bitter. Patience is a virtue to be learned and, though not to be sought, suffering when it comes can be used toward the end of personal training in that virtue. This does not make the suffering good, but allows the suffering that is bad to be used for a good end.

Patients, minimally, must be willing to take the physician's advice or to seek services elsewhere. Christian patients must go further, treating practitioners as persons worthy of respect who need to see the gospel lived in that patient's life. This does not mean that believers must accept intentional or even accidental abuse. The Christian may request, with an appropriate tone, his or her rights as a member of the social contract. Yet certainly the faithful should not become irritated or angry over what might be considered inadequate hotel amenities during a hospitalization, or even by the bad manners of practitioners, as that would indicate wrong prioritizing within one's life. Christian patients should be persevering as believers called to a peculiar vocation in a particular moment.

It is not only one's own spiritual well-being that is served by perseverance; such behavior is evangelistic. The first apologetic is always the life of the believer. Perseverance is a powerful witness to the spiritually defeated and exhausted and patience is an encouragement to those who are trivialized and ignored by others. The evangelistic task is not to be relinquished even while facing sickness, injury and death. The standard has been set for evangelicals since early in the revivalist movement, for instance, by believers like William Turner. Turner, a man now virtually unknown and little recognized even in his own day, undoubtedly influenced generations by changing the lives of at least some in the hospital on the night he died. John Wesley reported about the events in 1748:

> I buried the body of William Turner; who, towards the close of a long illness, had been removed into Guy's Hospital, though with small hope of recovery. The night before his death he was delirious, and talked loud and incoherently, which occasioned many in the ward to gather round his bed, in order to divert themselves. But in that hour it pleased God to restore him at once to the full use of his understanding; and he began praising God and exhorting them to repent, so as to pierce many to the heart. He remained for some time in this last labour of love, and then gave up his soul to God.[8]

For all human beings, the initial question when confronting illness or injury tends to be "why?" For the Christian, this must always be immediately succeeded with the question "how?" How should the believer suffer, how should the Christian be a patient? To put it another way, being physically sick is a religious vocation for the believer. It might not and should not be relished. The sickness itself can be resisted. But the religious role as a sick person is not to be repudiated. Contrary to the denial counseled by the so-called name it, claim it healers or by heterodox groups like Christian Science, or the fatalism of those with reductionist philosophies, or those advocating a hyperautonomy that decries any limit on what is their life anyway, believers are to accept and serve at all times and in all circumstances. As Paul describes in 2 Corinthians 12, a position of weakness need not render the believer spiritually impotent. The demand is that Christian living—even in illness and with injury—is supposed to be for his purpose. It is not an expectation Christians should have of those of the world. A religious vocation can and should not be imposed on those who are not on the Way.

PART THREE: CHRISTIAN BIOETHICS AND THE WORLD

In being sick and in receiving health care, the expectation for the believers is different from what should be expected of the world. While the believer is to be virtuous in fulfilling the temporary vocation of sickness, those of the world need only meet the deontological expectations of rights and duties arising out of or verified by the social contract. It has been claimed that those of the world should be virtuous in the midst of their suffering.

> But who would qualify as a "virtuous patient"? On first reflection, a virtuous patient might be conceived of as someone who is passive and compliant—manifesting stoical qualities which are at odds with the emerging emphasis on the

---

[8]John Wesley, *Journal*, December 24, 1748.

> "expert patient". The expert patient is proactive, assertive, informed, and not afraid to challenge medical authority. However, these two conceptualisations of patient character are not necessarily entirely at odds. Virtue is a much richer concept than modern usage of the word implies. It encompasses many qualities of character and intellect, and virtue in action is a subtle concept.[9]

While virtue, perhaps, might be preferable, it cannot and should not be expected under the American social contract. Nobility is not necessary to be a good citizen, but only clear adherence to the procedures and standards of the contract. The pursuit of happiness is no more nor less than the pursuit of each individual's self-selected *telos* (or, more likely, *teloi* as persons tend to vary within as well as between themselves).[10]

Certainly there are some evangelicals who bemoan the loss of moral consensus. It has been correctly noted that "[w]hen the Enlightenment's confidence in a rational unity is broken by the fragmentation of postmodernity, a polytheism of moral vision is reborn."[11] Yet it is important that the recent past is not romanticized. As has been frequently noted, the "good ol' days" were not good for those suffering under ethno-specific slavery or ethnic cleansing. Nor were they particularly good for those with serious illnesses or disabilities. The most basic social problem with moral polytheism in health care today is not that there is a lack of agreement on certain moral matters, but that (1) such disagreement is itself deemed preferable, (2) that those values necessary for the social contract are relativized (specifically the valuing of individual human life) in the name of that preference, and (3) important values that may not be intrinsic to the social contract, but are nonetheless highly functional, are disregarded. Each of these social moral problems gets played out in responses to sickness.

Increasingly those of U.S. society, using deontological reasoning, have generally agreed that patients do not need to accept treatments. It is a matter of liberty or, to use the language so popular in bioethics, of autonomy. In

---

[9]Alastair V. Campbell and Teresa Swift, "What Does It Mean to Be a Virtuous Patient? Virtue from the Patient's Perspective," *Scottish Journal of Healthcare Chaplaincy* 5, no. 1 (2002): 29 <http://www.bioethics.it/pdf/pu_5/virtue_ethics.pdf>.

[10]A critique of late modernity or postmodernity (depending on how one draws the lines between eras) was anticipated in the writings of Kierkegaard, especially *Purity of Heart Is to Will One Thing: Spiritual Preparation for the Office of Confession*, trans. Douglas V. Steere (New York: Harper & Row, 1948). He warned against multiple *teloi* as generating anomie.

[11]H. Tristram Engelhardt Jr., *The Foundations of Christian Bioethics* (Lisse, Netherlands: Swets and Zeitlinger, 2000), p.xvii. See also his earlier work, *The Foundations of Bioethics* (New York: Oxford University Press, 1986), p. xvi. I am sympathetic with both works and believe that, even with the significant reference to postbiblical tradition, they are quite useful for evangelicals.

fact, under most circumstances, to render a medical therapy against the expressed will of a competent individual is battery. Refusals of treatment should be tolerated, even when immoral, because the freedom of the citizenry under the social contract must be protected. Such should be tolerated even when the vast majority of persons, including Christians, deem the action grossly erroneous. And so, the refusal of a blood-transfusion by a Jehovah's Witness or of antivenom treatment by a snake-handling Pentecostal-Holiness Protestant should be respected. There are exceptions—most notably when the individual patient is not competent by mental limit or age or is being coerced. But, in such a case, the state is protecting the life of the nonautonomous member of the contract, rather than preventing the autonomous contract-maker from making a decision.

Unfortunately, not only is tolerating expected, but affirming another's decision—immoral or not—is increasingly deemed a cultural requirement in health care. In fact, such acceptance is as close as some in secular settings get to declaring a particular behavior virtuous. This should be opposed for Christian and U.S. social contract reasons. The practitioner should be able to disagree with a patient's morality, even while acknowledging the permissibility of the patient to seek other professional services. This is the other side of the patient's liberty. Admittedly, the practitioner is in a relationship with the patient that tends to be imbalanced in power, but that does not mean the patient is powerless nor that she or he is free to act in any manner or make any demand on another person. The patient too must recognize that the nature of an institution may require that the best way to honor his or her freedom is by discharge, as conceding to the patient's wishes would fundamentally violate the character of the institution or practitioner. While premorbid behaviors that contribute to the patient's condition should not be a reason for discharge, present behaviors can be. An AMA (against medical advice) discharge is sometimes the most moral choice for a practitioner to make and for a patient to accept.

Patients are entitled to the service guaranteed by whatever service contract they have, including certain expectations about the behavior of professional providers. More importantly, they are entitled to the rights that are protected under the U.S. social contract. Patients can and should make demands to reasonably protect their life, liberty and property. This includes receiving generally available treatments for disorders without which the patient would die or be severely sickened or disabled.

Normally, persons can only demand of another that she or he simply do no harm, but in the case of special contracts, parties have specific duties—such as those generated by organizational location or professional role. The question of health care as a right is addressed below; but, with or without a formal right, once in the health-care system, the individual who is vulnerable to the knowledge-based power and even physical power of the providing organization and professionals is entitled to protection from abuse and neglect. The patient is entitled to standard care from the provider and the providing organization, and the individual patient or his or her advocate can demand such care. While politely asking tends to be more efficient, an underlying willingness to use coercion is implied in all contracts.

Relationally, the patient is not entitled to anything more than civility. Civility includes mutual respect and basic politeness. The patient who lacks humor and kindness—or more generally, civility—need not be affirmed, and if genuinely and continuously harsh need not be tolerated. Such lashing out may be understandable, but it is not excusable. Still, evangelicals should fully support the right of a patient to act in a manner contrary to his or her well-being.

There are five clear moral imperatives for the patient-provider asymmetric contractual relationship in the U.S. health-care system. From the patient's perspective these are:

1. The patient may defend his or her own liberty (and thereby that of other patients) under the social contract; this includes, but is not necessarily limited to, specific practices and procedures outlined in most professional society ethics codes:
   - to receive information and copies/summaries of charts
   - to accept/refuse care
   - to confidentiality (assuming legal competence), except by law or welfare of another individual or public interest
   - to continuity of care between and among providers and institutions
   - to available care, dependent on and limited by the distributive choices of society[12]
2. The patient must accept the freedom of providers:
   - by not asking for illegal treatments or actions

[12]These are modified from the "Fundamental Elements of the Patient-Physician Relationship," *Code of Medical Ethics* (Washington, D.C.: American Medical Association, 1992).

- by respecting the right of the provider to not turn tolerance of the patient's behaviors or beliefs into affirmation

3. The patient may expect reasonable service, including professional competence; again, this is not only for one's own sake, but for the maintenance of justice under the broader social contract.
4. The patient must recognize boundaries and expectations of service contracts.
5. The patient and provider must maintain civility, including during disagreements and moments of confusion.

None of this would need to be outlined were it not for the fact that the patient is simultaneously vulnerable and a moral agent, using and purchasing professional services and products. To understand how this imbalance can be negotiated, thus protecting the liberty of both the patient and the provider, as well as tending to improve the health outcome, one is well served by understanding the sick role. The sick role helps define both the patient and the provider's response to him or her.

Talcott Parsons, in the early 1950s, described the behavior of sick persons and the behavior of others toward the sick person as "the sick role," a generally acceptable form of deviant behavior. Parsons was a structural-functionalist; that is, he thought society exhibited relational and organizational patterns (structures) that allowed social functioning. Most pertinently, all individuals tend, so Parsons argued, to exhibit social patterns through living out limited sets of options or roles. Occasionally, individuals deviate from standard roles and these must be controlled. The social management occurs in the development of deviance roles that help set social boundaries and help normal people in coping with abnormal situations—in this particular case, sickness or injury.

> [I]llness is a state of disturbance in the "normal" functioning of the total human individual, including both the state of the organism as a biological system and of his personal and social adjustments. It is thus partly biologically and partly socially defined. Participation in the social system is always potentially relevant to the state of illness, to its etiology and to the conditions of successful therapy, as well as to other things.[13]

[13]Talcott Parsons, "Social Structure and Dynamic Process: The Case of Modern Medicine," *The Social System* (New York: Routledge, 1991), p. 290.

The sick role has four basic aspects:

1. The sick person is exempted from normal social role responsibilities.
2. The sick person requires care as she or he cannot immediately or without the help of another address the deviant condition.
3. Being sick must be undesirable for the patient and his or her family and friends.
4. Technically competent help must be sought.

The exemption from normal tasks is temporary but real. The patient is allowed to temporarily deviate from the normal by dressing in clothing that indicates his or her condition, by skipping work, etc. There is generally no penalty for being sick as it is considered beyond the control of the sick person and, therefore, not a matter of moral culpability. The one clear moral obligation is seeking treatment, be that through professionals at pharmacies dispensing over-the-counter drugs or high-technology treatments in tertiary-level university hospitals, or something in between.

Numerous theorists have built upon Parsons' work. Criticisms have been raised, but the model is still useful. A Parsonian influence can be found across medicine, from therapists helping with daily living skills to social workers working in hospitals to the World Health Organization. How someone is sick depends in part on the capacity of the individual socially, psychologically and spiritually to cope with illness and injury. For that reason, scales of illness and incapacity sometimes include consideration of psycho-social measurements. For instance, the International Classification of Functioning, Disability and Health (ICF) takes into account the social location of individuals and attempts to measure the psychological needs and strengths of persons who have disabilities.[14]

Negatively, the Parsons' model tends to explain the doctor-patient interaction in terms that are similar to parent-child. In part, this was because he wrote prior to the rise of patient's rights in the 1960s, a time when physicians often were paternal and nurses maternal and such was actually encouraged. In part, he uses this language because he was influenced, though to a limited extent, by Freudian psychoanalysis. Also, Parsons was influenced by the soci-

[14]The ICF was derived from the ICIDH-2, named after the first version, the International Classification of Impairment, Disability and Handicap. The name change reflects a desire to alter the cultural interpretation of disability. Of course, as the classification is used for pooled numbers of people, it will also be used for classifying individuals.

ologist Max Weber; Parsons' description of the "power" of the practitioner to heal is similar to the charismatic power of a religious priestly authority in Weberian sociology.

Another problem with early versions of the theory is that it is too narrow; in reality, patients act out the role in different (sometimes very different) ways. In part this is due to the modeling of sickness they appropriated, but also because they may have different goals in receiving care. Also, the role itself can be abusive. Ideally, health care for a given individual should not be a contest between the individual, the broader society, the state, the family caregiver(s), the practitioners of different stripes or those with vested interest. Sometimes an emphasis on the role of being sick is used to trump the various concerns, a way of avoiding negotiation of freedoms and responsibilities.

Another negative about the application of the sick role is that too often it is assumed to be a nominal level categorization, that is, either-or—either healthy or sick. Parsons did not assert this, but the common use seems to do so. The magnitude of sickness or severity matters, as anyone can attest who has seen how handicapped stickers get used by those who claim to be so severely sick they cannot walk an additional ten feet in a parking lot yet can shop for hours. Indeed, the magnitude differences and categorical distinctions of sickness can be seen clearly in how the term is or is not applied to persons with disabilities. Some have special contractual relationships with practitioners, but may not have a current infection or injury that needs ongoing treatment. When such persons are deemed sick as compared to healthy but disabled people, they may well be further marginalized.

Positively, the sick-role theory allows an understanding of illness that goes beyond anatomical mechanical failure, microbial invasion or physiological malfunction. There is a recognition that not allowing the person who is deviant because of sickness to be cared for will require that she or he is defined as deviant for other reasons—reasons that will lead to inappropriate condemnation. The label of malingerer when falsely applied is a form of blaming the victim. It is appropriately assigned when the patient or the providers gain secondary benefits from the illness or injury that outweigh the embarrassment and inconvenience of the label.

Though the Parsonian model could be applied to other cultures, a careful reading of Parsons' argument reveals underlying Western social contract assumptions. The patient has rights associated with the approved deviance—specifically that she or he will be relieved of some responsibilities and treated with kindness and care. She or he has these rights because of a vulnerability of sickness. That vulnerability comes in the form of weakness associated with the physical condition and relative to the power of practitioners. In this, one hears echoes of Adam Smith's argument about human sympathy.

The patient has duties accompanying these rights—to treat the condition as undesirable by not malingering and seeking competent help. And she or he must submit to physical inspection in order to verify that such is the case. The practitioner, then, is not only a paternal/maternal figure but also a social gatekeeper. Again, as Adam Smith argued, if it is believed that the concern and care generated by sympathy are being abused, then the patient's benign deviance is redefined as malicious deviance and is condemned.[15]

Arguments still rage about the use of sickness categories as a means of controlling persons (intentionally or not). In the nineteenth century, for instance, sickness designations were used by women and against women to maintain certain components of the status quo. Some claim that this was an effort by powerful classes to control the weak (the "alienated"). Perhaps. But if it was, the endeavor was far less conscious than sometimes implied. The control seems to have been primarily an expression of the broader social control of women *and* the general lack of medical knowledge that led to a deference to cultural prejudice about health.

Poor urban women were subjected to truly abominable public health hazards, through sweatshop employment, atrocious sanitation and poor nutrition. The lack of diagnosis and appropriate treatment was used to keep these workers in production and prevent claims against owners. A wealthy urban woman, on the other hand, might have a "sickness" that endorsed her position as the cultural balance to her husband and, thereby, cemented the social location of both. Female adults were diagnosed with hysteria, a "disease" that was supposedly scientifically verified by Sigmund Freud at the turn of that century, and with melancholic-related female invalidism, believed to be sometimes caused by the cumulative effect of familial traumas. Even the very real disease of tuberculosis became a legitimation of the cultural definition of the refined woman as frail. Consider, for instance, the poetically masterful, but spiritually depressing works of Edgar Allen Poe[16] who seems to define the ideal woman as all but a living corpse.[17] It should be noted that this use of the defining of

[15]Adam Smith, *The Theory of Moral Sentiments* (Indianapolis: Liberty Fund, 1982).

[16]The classic Poe references can be found in "Annabel Lee."

[17]See the informative but biased Barbara Ehrenreich and Deidre English *Complaints and Disorders* (New York: Feminist Press at the City University of New York, 1973). The work provides

women as sick or not sick appears to have been far less prevalent within rural communities.

Having agreed with those who assert that the understanding of disease is socially constructed, it is essential to acknowledge that this does not make it any less real. Both the social constructs and the initial biological disorder are realities. To suggest that an infection with hepatitis A is not a real experience is not only philosophical hubris, it is immoral in that it may deny, through social constraint, access to treatment. The best understanding of disease, from the evangelical perspective and under the U.S. social contract, is that it is both/and—both a physical reality and a socially constructed category of experience. Further, from the evangelical perspective it is both a temporal experience and an eternal event, affecting the whole human.[18]

To continue using the example of women's health, breast cancer is a disease that brings with it large cultural components. This is exacerbated at the beginning of the age of genetics. With a genetic diagnosis, some women are choosing to have prophylactic mastectomies.[19] Is this based on the statistically reasonable fear of the disease and subsequent death or is it tied to cultural understandings of the disease and body image or both? Does a genetic risk factor, even a high one, constitute a disease state? Is a person sick or diseased when a gene is present but the disorder is not otherwise manifest? What percentage of risk warrants such a designation—a 25 percent risk for the disorder?

---

a fine overview of the skewed orientation of American health care in the nineteenth century. Also, it has a good bibliography for initial study of the subject. Unfortunately, the authors were not rigorous in providing references to cited works nor in offering alternative explanations to those they favor. Still, for the reader who can step back from the flaws, the work is useful.

[18]Jennifer Fosket, "Problematizing Biomedicine," in *Ideologies of Breast Cancer: Feminist Perspectives*, ed. Laura K. Potts (New York: St. Martin's Press, 2000), emphasizes the social construction of the categories of disease. She makes the useful argument that women with breast cancer may have a "bifurcated consciousness" (a concept not unrelated to the Marxist notion of the "false consciousness") in using both the biomedical constructs of the disease of breast cancer and those arising from women with the experience of breast cancer. She also relies on secondary analyses of Foucault's argument about the "clinical gaze" in *The Birth of the Clinic: An Archaelology of Medical Perception,* trans. Alan Sheridan (New York: Vintage Books, 1973). In doing so, she correctly asserts that power is necessary for the authority to define disease and, reciprocally, assist in the maintenance of that power. Still, there is not a sufficient consideration of the other component of reality, the cells that are growing without restraint. The women may be bifurcated not out of confusion but because both components of reality are correct and must be held in tension.

[19]In other words, the gene for a given disorder (the genotype) is present but not expressed—yet (the phenotypic expression of the disorder has not occurred, but the probability is high enough and consequences grave enough, that some choose to have a preventative operation, even taking into account the risk of the procedure).

50 percent? 99.9 percent? Is there an advantage in knowing? Sometimes there is, because it can lead to effective treatment, but the label can also marginalize the person in the family, at work and through the society.

A lot of money is associated with designation (e.g., research), as well as the alteration of social status. To see the impact of defining one as sick or a condition as sickness, the following list should be considered. All of the following are described as disease somewhere in the medical literature, popular health articles or advertisements for treatments of the past century:

- Alcohol abuse/alcoholism
- Slightly below average intelligence
- Retardation
- Obesity
- Baldness
- A big nose
- Poverty
- Masturbation
- Old age
- Chronic but not life-threatening disability
- Spouse abuse
- Nazi holocaust
- Opposing the Soviet state
- Irrationality
- Disagreement with practice of homosexuality
- Homosexuality [20]

The language of disease, injury, sickness and illness remains quite inconsistent in the medical and bioethics literature. Sometimes these words are viewed as near synonyms; at other times they are radically distinguished. What is important is to recognize that sickness is both a biological and a sociocultural experience. And, arguably, the two can exist distinctly from one another in a given person's life.[21] Certainly, some socially assigned illnesses

[20]Portions of this list are drawn from H. Tristram Engelhardt, "The Social Meaning of Illness," *Second Opinion*, no. 1 (1986): 26-39.
[21]Ibid.

are not physiologically or anatomically based and, likewise, the body may be disordered relative to a biological norm and yet not considered "diseased."

As an example of how the language of illness can be transformed for the purpose of obtaining power, one can look at the cultural debate about homosexuality and AIDS in the 1980s. Homosexual practice has been considered at various times an immoral choice, a legitimate self-expression, a psychological disorder due to parental failure and a genetic tendency. At times the sickness designation led to imprisonment or even murder. Now in the United States some argue that a biological causal factor validates the behavior while in the past it was a reason to see the practice as a manifestation of an illness. From a Christian viewpoint, both are incorrect. The first is the so-called naturalistic fallacy in that it claims that what is, ought to be.[22] The latter allows a prejudice against a biological aspect of the person over which she or he has no control. The Christian claim is that biology is not destiny; there is always a component of choice in behavior—the moral issue is actions of word and deed, not orientation. Interestingly, the reverse of earlier discrimination now occurs, as those who consider homosexual behavior immoral are dismissed as "homophobic." As consequence of their being "sick," they can be disregarded or, in extreme cases, considered polluted and, therefore, socially excluded.

From the 1980s on, AIDS was culturally defined not so much as a sexually transmitted disease (STD) far more likely to impact the sexually promiscuous but as a mysterious epidemic like the plague in the Middle Ages. This was, in part, the use of sickness language in a broader effort to socially legitimate homosexual behavior. Similar efforts to use diseases as a means of changing cultural values have been made previously, but none with the same apparent success in social transformation. HIV/AIDS was deemed an indiscriminate disease, which is not true etiologically as it is strongly associated with certain behaviors (such as sexual promiscuity or casual intravenous drug use). Though not curable with public health techniques, treating the disease as virtually unavoidable did not help limit the spread in the earlier days of the epidemic.

Regardless of how the disease may have been used politically, the implications of HIV/AIDS now go far beyond Western debates about the morality of homosexuality. Huge populations suffer from what is a pandemic. The health-care systems in many nations have been found inadequate and incompetent (the blood donation process in the People's Republic of China and the denial

[22]G. E. Moore, *Principia Ethica* (London: Cambridge University Press, 1922).

of the HIV/AIDS relationship by some in South Africa in the 1990s serve as examples). Those who are infected and subsequently redefined as vectors to be avoided need the care of believers and anyone willing to recognize the extraordinary impact on the social order and economics of developing nations. In other words, the sick role must be redefined, the cultural experience of the disease reordered, so that proper public health preventions can be used and drugs can be made available for those who are already infected.

The sick role is frequently applied imperfectly. As noted, the malingerer willfully abuses it. Also, it can be partially appropriate, such as with alcohol abuse in which there may be poor decisions, genetic factors and physiological degeneration, such that the initial willful abuse of alcohol should be morally condemned while the later should be medically treated. A greater problem arises when someone is marginalized by virtue of being defined as sick. They might be quarantined as vectors or dismissed as malingerers or even killed as the disease itself. The Nazis used the sick role against persons they considered deviant for other reasons—those who had disabilities, and then Jews and Roma (gypsies). In a less dramatic, but nonetheless perverse, way persons who disagree on moral positions are sometimes defined as sick—as homosexuals were in the past and as those who disagree with homosexuality are now homophobic—and pushed to the cultural margins. Arguably, those who are mislabeled as sick or who are infected with a disease but have additional, unrelated characteristics assigned to them because of it have a moral duty to reject the social designation.

CONCLUSION

The patient-physician relationship once was primarily covenantal, but now it is essentially a contract—albeit one requiring extraordinary trust given the lack of knowledge and vulnerability of one of the parties. These weaknesses, as well as the physical illness itself, require obligations on the part of providers, but do not eliminate social duties for patients. The proper recognition of the sick role allows the person of the world and the evangelical believer to assert, in the United States, that patients

- may defend their own liberty, and others may defend their liberty and the liberty of everyone to make decisions when competent;
- must accept that freedom extends to providers, though it is limited by their professional status and obligations;

- may expect reasonable service, including professional competence, as the most significant of those professional duties;
- must agree to reasonable participation (e.g., in the form of compliance) in the service contract;
- must maintain mutual civility, for the sick role does not take one out of all societal obligations, nor does professional take priority over social membership.

The society may expect and must facilitate these. On the other hand, the society cannot demand that all persons go beyond civility in bearing wrongs. It is not up to Christians, beyond their own example and in gentle conversation, to demand that those who want to complain about being sick or want to relish being defined as sick (assuming the society is not bearing an extraordinary cost for such) should change. Jesus recognized the secondary benefits of being sick when he asked the man at the pool of Bethesda if he wanted to be well. Jesus offered healing. He did not demand the arrest of the man for malingering.

The faithful should become advocates for the just treatment of patients, even while being willing themselves to patiently and with perseverance bear wrongs when they are patients and face physical suffering. For better or worse, evangelicals will sometimes view with disdain the behavior of those of the world who relish their sickness or barely maintain civility while they are sick or who use sickness for political purposes. Hopefully, this is not an expression of spiritual arrogance, but of sadness over the sin because of what it does to the sinner. Evangelicals, though, should not tolerate the mislabeling or abuse of the sickness designation as a means of social control.

8

Family and Congregational Caring

HUMANS AS FAMILIAL

The first layer of health care is familial. While the family can be the source of extraordinary physical and emotional pain, generally it is a reproductive and productive unit that protects, educates and provides basic health care to its members. Christians consider the family a natural institution, that is, part of the created order, and a relative good. Further, Christians believe that this institution can express redemptive love and, therefore, they should go beyond the mere normal expectations of Western culture in providing care to their family members. They should not expect the same sense of obligation among those of the world, even though the family in that setting as well is generally one of the most efficient sites for health care.

> It was just before the Passover Feast. Jesus knew that the time had come for him to leave this world and go to the Father. Having loved his own who were in the world, he now showed them the full extent of his love.
>
> The evening meal was being served, and the devil had already prompted Judas Iscariot, son of Simon, to betray Jesus. Jesus knew that the Father had put all things under his power, and that he had come from God and was returning to God; so he got up from the meal, took off his outer clothing, and wrapped a towel around his waist. After that, he poured water into a basin and began to wash his disciples' feet, drying them with the towel that was wrapped around him.
>
> He came to Simon Peter, who said to him, "Lord, are you going to wash my feet?"
>
> Jesus replied, "You do not realize now what I am doing, but later you will understand."
>
> "No," said Peter, "you shall never wash my feet."
>
> Jesus answered, "Unless I wash you, you have no part with me."
>
> "Then, Lord," Simon Peter replied, "not just my feet but my hands and my head as well!"
>
> Jesus answered, "A person who has had a bath needs only to wash his feet;

his whole body is clean. And you are clean, though not every one of you." For he knew who was going to betray him, and that was why he said not every one was clean.

When he had finished washing their feet, he put on his clothes and returned to his place. "Do you understand what I have done for you?" he asked them. "You call me 'Teacher' and 'Lord,' and rightly so, for that is what I am. Now that I, your Lord and Teacher, have washed your feet, you also should wash one another's feet. I have set you an example that you should do as I have done for you. I tell you the truth, no servant is greater than his master, nor is a messenger greater than the one who sent him. Now that you know these things, you will be blessed if you do them. (Jn 13:1-17)

PART ONE: BIBLICAL ANALOGUE

If unfamiliar with the practice, the first moment is one of awkwardness and insecurity.[1] Questions about being ticklish or having a strong foot odor or perhaps unsightly toenails run through one's mind. The first feelings and thoughts when one's feet are washed are those of embarrassing intimacy. Caregiving must be intimate, often embarrassingly intimate in the late modern West with its persistent emphasis on individualism, youthfulness and physical health. It can be difficult in any society when caregiving requires the crossing of commonly accepted cultural boundaries.

Jesus told Peter on the night he was betrayed that he would wash the feet of his followers.[2] When Peter objected, Jesus said that Peter, if he persisted, would no longer be part of him and his ongoing story of salvation. If the disciple would not allow care to be rendered, then he was not a follower. Jesus went on, indicating that if any of the disciples would not be a giver of care in the manner of Jesus, then that so-called disciple was not a true follower either. A willingness to give and receive care is part of what it means to accept a proper place within the story.

There has been speculation through the centuries as to what was Christ's intention in the exchange between Peter and himself. Especially confusing is the fact that when Peter concedes that Jesus should wash his

[1]For a discussion of the analogical significance of foot washing, as well as other teachings of Christ, see William C. Spohn, *Go and Do Likewise: Jesus and Ethics* (New York: Continuum Publishing, 2000), pp. 50-71.

[2]The phrase "on the night in which he was betrayed" is purposely used since that is the language of the Eucharistic ritual. Some traditions understand the washing of feet as a sacrament (for instance, most Anabaptists) or as a significant act for the leadership (the annual papal washing in the Roman Catholic Church).

feet, but asks that all the rest of him be washed too (for he is entirely unclean), Jesus says that only the part needing genuine, significant care will be administered such.

Perhaps the cleansing reference is solely a sacramental clarification. Perhaps Jesus was denying a whole washing of Peter because baptism does not need to be conducted over and over. Perhaps the intent of requiring some cleansing was to convey a truth about their spiritual disciplines, telling the believers that in this world they are bound to get spiritually dirty and should continually return for cleansing.[3] Maybe the whole incident is about the spiritual cleanness of the church, not the purity of any given individual. Perhaps this was an expression of the servanthood of Jesus and about a duty to participate in a specific ritual. Or, perhaps this had nothing to do with theological assertions about baptism or keeping clean from the sins of the world; it was just an event of that night.

The passage above begins with the statement that Jesus will demonstrate his love. Not only will he die for the body as a sacrifice, but also he will serve his bride in an atypical way, given the traditions and cultural patterns of that day. He will serve by doing that which indicates low status and which crosses boundaries established for ritual pollution avoidance.

For Christians, serving is not merely a right action; it is character expressed in practices. One of those practices is caregiving for the sick and the injured. Evangelicals believe they are called not only to a priesthood of all believers but also to the continual expression of holiness. Holiness means "purity that sets apart" and the evangelical expectation for such is essentially an appropriation of not only the Reformation notion of the priesthood of all believers but also the monasticizing of all believers in the appropriation of the counsels of perfection. This commitment to Christian living in daily life appeared in proto-Protestants such as Brethren of the Common Life (from which emerged *The Imitation of Christ*) and following the Reformation by Anabaptists and Pietists before the rise of revivalism/evangelicalism, and then the Wesleyan revivals and especially the Wilderness revivals (i.e., the Second Great Awakening). In other words, all believers are called to the vocation of living as Christian servants. This includes an obligation to care for the sick and injured.

[3]This is often called the problem of dirty hands. Christians can get their hands dirty in pragmatic compromise as long as they are not morally stained in the process.

PART TWO: CHRISTIAN BIOETHICS

Like footwashing, caregiving often involves full engagement of the senses, the affections and the will in a manner that precludes reduction of the practice to rational philosophy. Dirty feet smell, as do gangrenous wounds and the bed sheets of the incontinent. Healers, those of lesser social status and immediate family members have traditionally touched such unclean (culturally polluting) objects. Not always, but often, the very act of such physical contact transforms the caregiver, allowing him or her to recognize that which some might see as a carrier of filth is actually a bearer of the image of God.

Christians are obligated to love all persons as bearers of that image. Each individual is deserving of respectful care. Yet, the relational nature of caregiving means that it cannot be rendered to all, by all, equally. Caregiving should be love practically applied. It is limited to those in need. It is limited by the capacity (resources, skills, etc.) and proximity of the caregiver, and it is limited by a differential in duty according to family relationship and friendship. Limits are necessary if care is to be efficacious for anyone.

In practice, the evaluation of the call to care occurs more often as a response to a gut feeling or sense of sympathy or emotion of concern than it does rational analysis of social and physical location, of condition and capacity. But only relying on feelings can create moral problems. First, it is too easy to disregard one's feeling of sympathy because of competing interests until the heart is hardened. Second, one can respond too easily, without due consideration of limits, creating what might be called *codependency*. Third, relying only on feelings can cause one to focus almost exclusively on the one who is most attractive or most similar to the potential caregiver. As has been noted often, whitetail fawns (which are not endangered in the least as a species) readily elicit more sympathy than some endangered species of frogs or increasingly absent pollinating bees. Likewise, other humans that look more like oneself (some sociobiologists argue this is for genetic reasons) are more likely to generate sympathetic feelings. Believers are to go beyond such feeling limitations—or perhaps they are to expand their feelings of genuine concern.

To determine the appropriateness of any given expression of Christian caring, the boundaries or limits that cannot or should not be passed must be discerned. Arguably, this is not as much a cognitive event as a matter of holy habits developed through time. In other words, in actual practice the loving believer does not stop minute by minute, asking what level of care a given person may deserve, but rather acts in accordance with the moral practices she or he has developed in the community of faith. Nonetheless, there are occasions when such conscious analysis is required and it is based on what can be described as limiting factors. In particular, how one cares is altered at least by (1) geographical proximity, (2) relational proximity, (3) condition of the sick or injured person(s) and (4) capacity of the caregiver. The limits of care establish the call to duty, which differs for the believer and those of the world.

First, how does the Christian know the limit to neighborliness—that is, duty based on geographic proximity? It may be best to begin with the opposite. If one always diverts one's eyes, or if one is consistently willing to "step over" the suffering ones who are near, then clearly the morality is weak, as perhaps is the faith. *Caritas/agape*, which for ethical discourse should be understood to include enacted compassion, includes first the obligation to not avoid and then the obligation to render care. Though extraordinarily unlikely, living in a community in which there are no apparent sufferers (i.e., visible on the by-ways) is (1) self-deceptive, because they are there even though hidden, and (2) indicative of enough wealth that the range of proximity can and should be expanded.

The parable of the Good Samaritan is an example of geographic proximity eliciting response. (Chapter nine explores this parable further from the perspective of the professional.) It seems to suggest that the neighborliness of the Samaritan was contingent upon seeing the need. For the believer, seeing the need is a responsibility. One is morally compelled to look, or at least morally compelled to not not look (to use the double negative intentionally).[4] While some have argued that everyone is our neighbor, the implication of Jesus' words seems to be that everyone is potentially a neighbor, but geographic proximity calls forth action in a peculiar and particular way. Neighborliness in the Christian sense might be defined as proximity calling forth hospitality.

Second, there is no denying that the duty to care within a given range of geographic proximity varies significantly on the basis of the prior relationship. If a child is sick or injured halfway around the world, many parents with the means will travel to be with that child and render care. On the other hand, if a child one does not know is dying of disease on the other side of a large city,

[4]See Michel Foucault, *The Birth of the Clinic: An Archeology of Medical Perception*, trans. A.M. Sheridan Smith (New York: Vintage Books, 1973) on the concept of the "clinical gaze." While evangelical scholars are generally, and appropriately, suspicious of the penetration of certain philosophical approaches into the community of faith, this material is analytically useful. The Samaritan gazes, but not as a clinician; rather, as a neighbor with true sympathy (a sense of suffering, but not one that disables, but that leads to response).

there is a lesser degree of obligation. Arguably, one might provide care by facilitating the direct caregiving of others with monetary support and/or endorsing specific legislative or diplomatic activities, but abdicating on other tasks to render direct care is not required and might be wrong on the basis of the cost of lost opportunity to perform other moral responsibilities. As the intensity of the relationship lessens, the sense of an obligation to care also lessens, though immediate geographic proximity would continue to create some degree of obligation for the believer.

To use language that is somewhat problematic but may be heuristically useful, the Christian obligations arising out of the "covenant" with all Creation are not the same as those arising from specific or special covenants. Consequently, the duty to those in relational proximity may take precedence over those in geographic proximity. Relational proximity is the degree of familiarity coupled with shared values. Often, intense feelings of shared values is called *familial*—shaped by what is expected or desired for biological relatives. Familial language is transferred analogically to other relationships. So, in the particular case of Christians, another believer should be understood as brother or sister. This does not necessitate common possessions of goods, but it does create a higher level of obligation than those of the world might generally extend to a friend.

When the believer determines that the person is within the relational range of obligation, she or he must extend care, even if problematic, assuming the other limits to caregiving are not exceeded. This proximity can be understood using a parallel moral concept, that of subsidiarity. Whenever possible, the lowest level of social organization should be the site of caregiving. Thus, for the infant with a cold, the parents should provide care, with other family members participating within the limits of their abilities. Similarly, older adults who need care should be provided that care within their homes or the homes of their near-relatives for as long as possible. Then, if care cannot be properly given, other resources and services should be sought. If, for example, a move to a skilled nursing facilities is appropriate, this must be with the understanding that obligations of care do not cease as the larger, more complex organization assumes some responsibility.

For Christians, the understanding of the obligations inside the family should be covenantal, not contractual. A covenant goes beyond the obligations of a mere contract so that a spouse remains bound to husband/wife even if the latter becomes sick or seriously injured and cannot perform various familial tasks. Likewise, the parents remain obligated to the children (even if they are born disabled) and the children to the parents (even though they become invalids by the standards of the society).[5] Even the superficial reversal of the child/parent relationship should become an opportunity to offer respect for the older generation and an acknowledgment of the worthiness of even the most "decrepit" to receive care from the faithful. The American emphasis on autonomy and notions of privacy have now ironically led to some wanting anonymous caregivers rather than their own relatives; Christians should do all they can in their own families to reverse this trend. The biological family relationship is so important that Paul speaks of a so-called Christian who ignores the physical needs of his or her family as "worse than an unbeliever" (1 Tim 5:8). The biological family does not take precedence over the values of the redeemed, but it is the site of the highest duties of the created order.

Though somewhat simplistic, models of family in the West can be differentiated using a cross-tabulation of the valuing of the individual and cohesion of the family unit. The Christian family should both value the family and the individual members as individuals. Models of the world in the West tend to endorse individuality at the expense of family cohesion. Most American families are segmented. Relations are maintained on the basis of service provided in the market sense, not in the sense of Christian servanthood. While it is true that families are economic units and that individuals do have rights that are not lost by virtue of being part of a family (e.g., freedom from physical

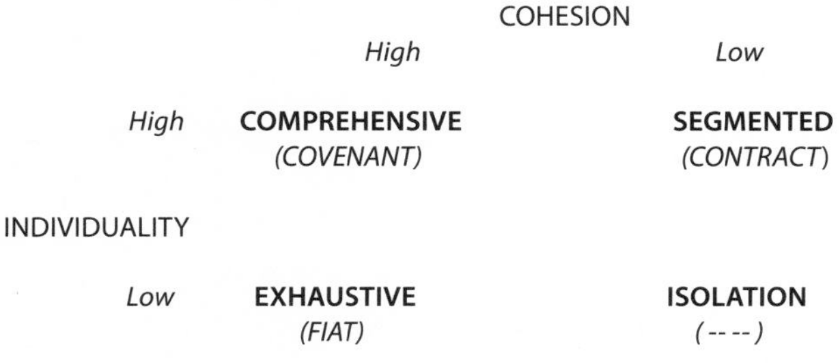

Figure 8.1. Family structure in the West

[5]The faithful should counter the social devaluing of persons who are seriously ill or disabled. In the world there is an "intimate connection between illness and indignity . . . invalid. To be an invalid, then, is to be an invalidated person . . . not valid." Thomas Szasz, *The Theology of Medicine: The Political-Philosophical Foundations of Medical Ethics* (Syracuse, N.Y.: Syracuse University Press, 1988), p. 19. Note, though, that Szasz goes further to argue against much in the standard practice of psychiatry and for suicide as a basic right, essentially on libertarian grounds.

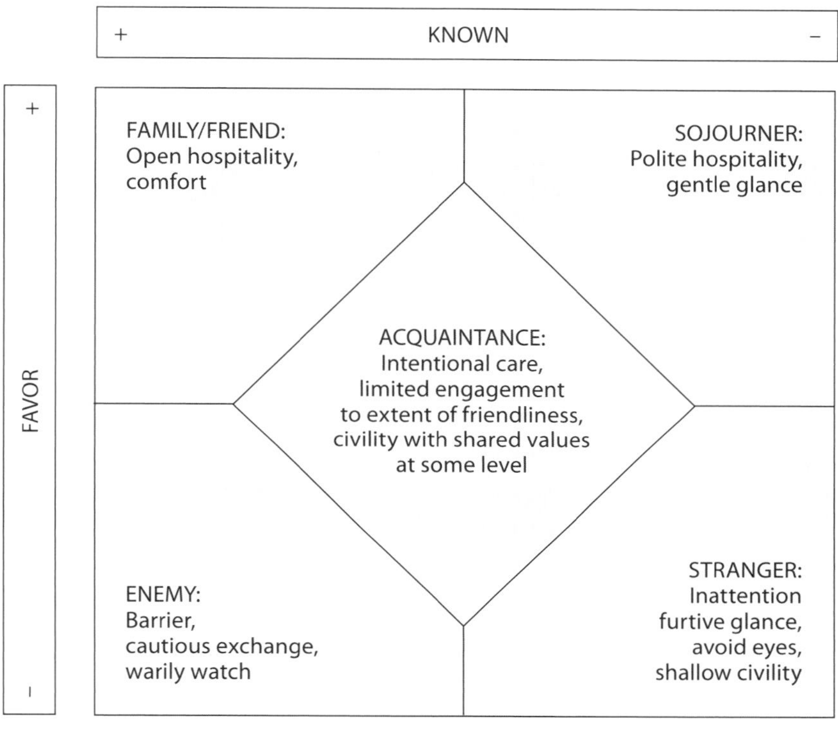

Figure 8.2. Relational proximity generated by familiarity and trusting favor

abuse), they are not to be understood primarily as contractual.

A covenant validates both the well-being of the individual and the well-being of the family as a community. Admittedly, what should be covenantal can become oppressive with the family ruled by the fiat of one parent or the other. Some evangelical families with strongly legalistic interpretations of Scripture may tend toward this exhaustive orientation, but contrary to media portrayals, this seems extraordinarily rare.

At the other extreme, sadly, are those persons who have no family cohesion or no family at all and little strength of individuality. These are the lonely, the abandoned and, in the extreme, the homeless (not necessarily the shelterless, but homeless).[6] These are people who require special care by the faithful and the provision of the concern of the church as a surro-

[6]This image is borrowed from Keith Wasserman, director of Good Works, a ministry to the rural homeless in Athens, Ohio.

gate family. They live isolated lives, with no effective authority, accountability or support.

Besides the biological family and the church fellowship, an obligation exists for those who are friends and even acquaintances, though the degree of relationship will alter the degree of assistance. Christians may, and should as appropriate, reach out to provide direct care to those who are known as friends and acquaintances, even if not of the faithful. Besides being an obligation for one seeking to conform to the image of Christ, it is a powerful witness. Relational proximity and geographic proximity come together in the case of friends and (usually) even more intensely with family. Again, Christian responsibility never completely dissipates even for the stranger, or sojourner in geographic proximity.

Thus there seem to be five basic categories of relationship obligations for caregiving that believers should recognize in spite of the values of the world and the cultural trends in health care (see fig. 8.2). The believer should take seriously his or her obligation to his or her own biological family. There should be more intentional care within the church. In both of these cases, some significant shared values and geographic or relational proximity define friend. The believer may have acquaintances that are outside of the church, outside of extensive shared history or blood that would create relationship, or geographic proximity. The individual believer and the community of faith must reach out to nonbelieving sojourners who are within the range of their care, a range that should be far broader than that of the worldly. Concern for the stranger who is out of immediate organizational and geographical proximity remains a general concern, though it will not necessarily manifest itself as specific care given to a specific person. Christians should always seek to minimize "strangeness" and accept sojourners or acquaintances. Finally, the enemy who stands in need and geographic proximity also requires a response—though with greater caution. The first of these, and perhaps acquaintance to a lesser extent, can be properly called affectional caregiving.

The third major limit on caregiving after geographic and relational proximity is the condition of the sick or injured individual. The level of illness/disability becomes a limit when requirements for technology or expertise exceed that possible within the home. Eventually the condition of the person may exceed the care possibilities of professionals, as well. Truly futile procedures—that is, treatment that will not be effectual because of the recipient's condition—are never required. The Christian, however, remains obligated to give compassionate, supportive care even when medical treatments are no longer effective.

It is important for believers to not confuse medical condition with moral condition. There should not be a distinction as to whether the sick person deserves his or her illness or not. For some of the world, deservingness (to coin a term) by the sufferer might be a limiting factor in care; it should not be for the Christian. While past behavior can be considered as an indicator of how resources will be used, it cannot in and of itself determine caring duties. Persons with self-inflicted wounds or alcohol-related injuries, for example, are not excluded from the Christian care obligation. Believers should also be aware that some in need may be other caregivers. When sickness and injury occur the impact is social. For instance, the parent of a child with severe leukemia may actually hurt more emotionally or even spiritually than the child, who suffers more physically, but these are differences that do not diminish the significance of the suffering for anyone involved.

The fourth and final major limit on caregiving is the capacity of the caregiver. Sometimes care should not be given, at least not by a particular person. One is not obligated to render care when such is simply beyond the capacity of the giver to give, or when it is finally self-destructive. This does not mean costly, for all caregiving is costly, but actually destructive to the potential caregiver. This should not become an excuse for the believer. For instance, it is true that family members sometimes know more about the day-to-day caregiving needs of a person with a specific disorder than do most professionals and, in such a case, the family member should not defer to the supposed expert simply as a way to avoid responsibility. For most persons the moral risk is not rendering self-destructive or futile care, but too little care. The believer should err toward caring service with this *prima facie* standard overruled only for a clearly understood limit of capacity.

Even considering the limits of geographic proximity, relational proximity, the needs of the patient and the capacity of the caregiver, Christians still generally have deeper obligations than those of the world. Though open to debate, the apocalyptic passage in Matthew 25 seems to indicate that. Notable about this passage is that those who do the good, as well as those who fail, are not aware that in doing so they are serving the Christ.

> "When the Son of Man comes in his glory, and all the angels with him, he will sit on his throne in heavenly glory. All the nations will be gathered before him, and he will separate the people one from another as a shepherd separates

> the sheep from the goats. He will put the sheep on his right and the goats on his left.
>
> "Then the King will say to those on his right, 'Come, you who are blessed by my Father; take your inheritance, the kingdom prepared for you since the creation of the world. For I was hungry and you gave me something to eat, I was thirsty and you gave me something to drink, I was a stranger and you invited me in, I needed clothes and you clothed me, I was sick and you looked after me, I was in prison and you came to visit me.'
>
> "Then the righteous will answer him, 'Lord, when did we see you hungry and feed you, or thirsty and give you something to drink? When did we see you a stranger and invite you in, or needing clothes and clothe you? When did we see you sick or in prison and go to visit you?'
>
> "The King will reply, 'I tell you the truth, whatever you did for one of the least of these brothers of mine, you did for me.'
>
> "Then he will say to those on his left, 'Depart from me, you who are cursed, into the eternal fire prepared for the devil and his angels. For I was hungry and you gave me nothing to eat, I was thirsty and you gave me nothing to drink, I was a stranger and you did not invite me in, I needed clothes and you did not clothe me, I was sick and in prison and you did not look after me.'
>
> "They also will answer, 'Lord, when did we see you hungry or thirsty or a stranger or needing clothes or sick or in prison, and did not help you?'
>
> "He will reply, 'I tell you the truth, whatever you did not do for one of the least of these, you did not do for me.'
>
> "Then they will go away to eternal punishment, but the righteous to eternal life." (Mt 25:31-46)

Actual practices should be spawned by these obligations. For example:

- The church should assist families in providing care through informal or organized respite programs. Each person caring for someone with severe disability or serious illness should be offered a "sabbath" from care when the family caregiver can go to the store, or the library, or participate in some ministry of his or her own.[7]
- If a person has the space in his or her house, the church should support the member of the congregation who takes someone sick or seriously disabled into his or her own home. While more common with infants, there is no reason that persons of other ages might not be similarly served. This could

[7]James Thobaben, "Long-Term Care," in *Dignity and Dying: A Christian Appraisal*, ed. John Frederick Kilner, Arlene B. Miller and Edmund D. Pellegrino (Grand Rapids: Eerdmans, 1996), pp. 191-207.

be the health-care equivalent of Habitat for Humanity or hospice for the not-dying, with one family assuming the primary burden, but with significant support from the fellowship.

- Congregational financial and volunteer support of existing Hospice organizations is an appropriate expression of caregiving for the dying.[8]
- A parish nurse program is another model of service. Again, this requires financial support by the church, but more importantly, the development of a network of care to support the nurse who is hired or who volunteers.
- Prior to serious illness or disability, the church can serve with some form of accountability and care along the lines of the Stephen Ministry that reaches out to individuals to make sure their needs are not ignored.
- Christian churches should also do what they can to provide space to family and disease/disability-specific support groups. Such groups will not always be made up of believers. Sometimes they may deal with topics that are not congruent with the moral positions of the church (e.g., sexual behavior out of marriage). The church should set standards for the use of its facilities that prevent immoral behaviors on the grounds, yet the church is well-served by supporting organizations that overall act in a manner that is in agreement with the Christian value of person regardless of illness or disability.
- It is also important that Christians not only agree to serve, but actually serve. For instance, believers should be aware that most caregiving is provided by females, but this should not be interpreted as a "natural" or "spiritual" requirement. Males and females should accept caregiving tasks. This does not mean there should be no "division of labor" for efficiency. It does mean that Jesus did not only die in a heroic manner; he acted like a servant bathing the feet of those in need.

The experience of divine love and capacity for serving as a conduit for that love means the faithful should be held to a higher standard than those of the world, at least by themselves. And, though it is often a bitter pill to swallow, believers must accept the mockery of the world when they hypocritically do

[8]Generally speaking (though not always) Christians should feel comfortable participating in the Hospice movement. It was founded as a Christian movement and even when the organization is not specifically Christian, there is almost always service provided for Christians, though in some areas of the country some questions of value compatibility might be appropriately raised.

not excel. Jesus demanded exceptional practices arising from love.

> You are the salt of the earth. But if the salt loses its saltiness, how can it be made salty again? It is no longer good for anything, except to be thrown out and trampled by men.
>
> You are the light of the world. A city on a hill cannot be hidden. Neither do people light a lamp and put it under a bowl. Instead they put it on its stand, and it gives light to everyone in the house. In the same way, let your light shine before men, that they may see your good deeds and praise your Father in heaven. . . .
>
> I tell you that unless your righteousness surpasses that of the Pharisees and the teachers of the law, you will certainly not enter the kingdom of heaven. (Mt 5:13-16, 20)

The ethical obligations for Christians extend to all, but do not extend to all in the same manner or to the same degree. First, they must caregive in the family and, closely following, within the immediate church community. The acquaintance, sojourner, stranger or even enemy who is presented by the closeness of physical location follows, though the long-term obligation may differ, especially if there are others who should assume the task. As the type of suffering and the level of expertise increase, so does the believer's duty. While there are limits, believers must look different than the world as they, by the Spirit, imitate the holiness of Christ. Perhaps the night before the crucifixion was when geographic proximity and relational proximity combined with the moment of the apostles' greatest actual need and the infinite capacity of Christ to serve yielding the example of Jesus washing the feet. Believers are required to follow.

PART THREE: CHRISTIAN BIOETHICS AND THE WORLD

A family is a group of genetically related persons, or persons who act as if they are genetically related. As such, a family normally functions as a reproducing and producing unit. In other words, the family is the common site for the appearance of a new generation and an economic unit in which individuals usually pool income and divide labor. As a unit of production and reproduction with members having various functions, the family is a political institution with members having varying degrees of power within different arenas of production and reproduction. In different societies, families assume different forms as these reproductive and productive ends are served. Almost without exception the family provides basic health care. This task seems to be part of the natural order.

Even from a late modern perspective, this makes sense. Whenever care is rendered the patient becomes vulnerable, if not already. His or her social boundaries, and sometimes physical boundaries, are relaxed or removed entirely. She or he may be afraid, embarrassed or ashamed. The feelings may be manifest in excessive passivity, extreme anxiousness and even anger. To the extent possible, the sick or injured should be cared for by those with whom she or he is in a preexisting relationship, especially one in which vulnerability is already recognized and accepted. Care, if technically adequate, will be generally superior. For this reason, if no other, the principle of subsidiarity for health-care provision makes sense. In addition, subsidiarity should be valued in secular society in that it provides a mechanism for protecting freedom.

Yet there are, as noted above, limits to family care. There are circumstances in which one should enter or have a family member enter the care of others and, when necessary, the care of the state (for more on the state and the financing of health care, see chapter 11). The state serves as the last resort for the protection of social contract makers, that is, citizens. In such care the individual should expect less freedom, as there are competing claims on the resources of government. As an example, state support for attendants is certainly compatible with notions of subsidiarity, as long as it is understood that choices for those services may be more limited than if paid out-of-pocket.

Of course, it is quite possible that the suffering of another will elicit feelings of guilt or repugnance (a sense that the sick or injured person is unclean or polluting) that will push one out of the range of proximity. Nonetheless, it cannot be denied that those who walk with Christ must be willing to render care, even to the stranger who is nearby. Nor can it be denied that, even if to a lesser degree, so should those of the world.

Subsidiarity, though traditionally a Christian moral argument, does have parallels in secular social theory. It seems, after all, that humans have the capacity to sympathize with others, even those to whom they have no direct relationship, and that that sympathy grows or diminishes in relation to geographic and relational proximity. Adam Smith made a classic presentation of proximity eliciting concern in *The Theory of Moral Sentiments*. Asserting that sympathy is among the most fundamental naturally occurring moral sentiments, he claims that the family is the most natural object of concern.[9] The response to this feeling or sense of sympathy is then shaped, ideally, by virtues of prudence (or what an evangelical Christian might call wisdom), which combine a reasonable evaluation of the circumstances with self-command of

---

[9]Adam Smith, *The Theory of Moral Sentiments* (Indianapolis: Liberty Fund, 1982), p. 219.

one's own abilities and desires.[10]

> And, Nature, indeed, seems to have so happily adjusted our sentiments of approbation and disapprobation, to the conveniency both of the individual and of the society, that after the strictest examination it will be found, I believe, that this is universally the case. . . . These sentiments are no doubt enhanced and enlivened by the perception of the beauty and deformity which results from this utility or hurtfulness. But still, I say, they are originally and essentially different from this perception.[11]

In essence, relational proximity creates a series of concentric circles of sympathy or concern. The closer a caregiver is relationally (assuming geographic proximity remains constant), the higher the moral obligations to care (see figure 8.3). The intensity of obligation increases as one moves closer into the circles of concern.[12] The closer to the middle of the dia-

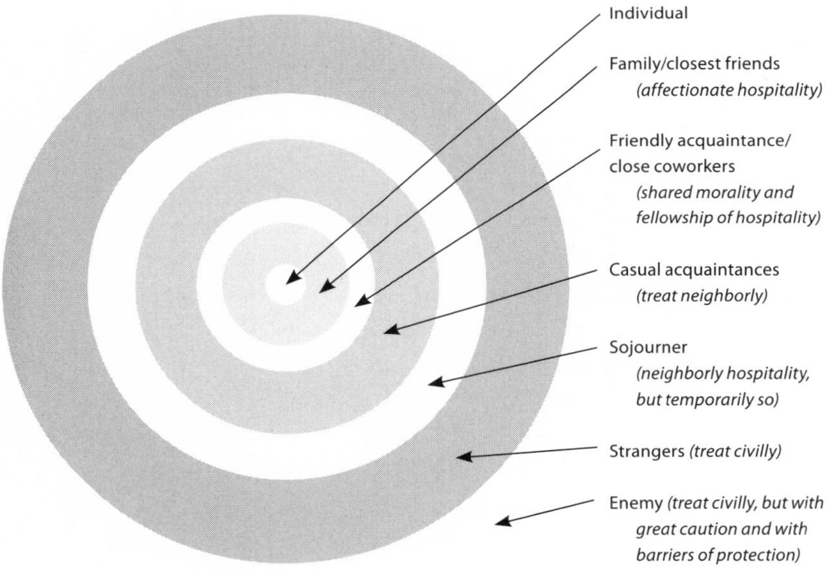

Figure 8.3.

[10]Ibid., p. 189.
[11]Ibid., p. 188.
[12]This model is based on Smith, *Theory of Moral Sentiments,* with additional language from Kevin Wildes, *Moral Acquaintances* (Notre Dame, Ind.: University of Notre Dame Press, 2000).

gram, the more the relationship should be defined by covenant; the further out, the more by contract. In the case of families, immediate family can be assumed to have a higher duty, with parents of children and adult children of elders having higher responsibilities due to the lesser capacities of the ones receiving care. Of course, even if natural and even if the society's "default," familial care cannot and should not nessarily be compelled in a social-contract state.

Moral priority for caregiving in one's family is not accepted in all secular philosophical schools. For instance, some utilitarians assert that the utility calculus requires that all persons be valued equally by each person. Consequently, one's caring for family may be defined by geographic proximity or role obligations, but family members ought not to warrant a sense of higher duty than any other hurting individual.

Yet, even if one could be genuinely impartial in action, it would not be desirable. The only way to be impartial in a world of sorrows is to treat all poorly. One's resources simply cannot meet the needs of more than a few. Further, serving only those one meets will be skewed (e.g., ethnicity, class). Paradoxically, the claim of impartiality as the highest value is, itself, partiality toward a moral approach that disfavors some (e.g., humans with certain disabilities).

Having made this claim, it is important to clearly state that partiality can be inappropriately excessive as surely as impartiality can be deficient. Indeed, in the so-called real world the problems of partiality can be just as horrendous as those of supposed impartiality. The latter can lead to grievous injustices against those with disabilities (as implied by some in the radical animal rights movement), while the former can result in bigotry and, even, genocide. Christians and many others in society can agree that concern must extend beyond the family, and that nuclear families, extended families, tribes and even nationalities cannot become the exclusive objects of concern. Still, most persons would find the assertion that concern and caregiving ought not to be selective as an impractical denial of natural sympathies—in the past, now and for the foreseeable future.

A secular argument for the care of family clearly arises from any reasonable reading of evolutionary theory, though the sociobiological arguments make the case the clearest. The sympathy one has for a family member tends to maximize the survival of the genetic material, which is, phenotypically, the same thing as the survival of the kinship group. In other words, people tend to take care of their own. Christians would agree, though arguing this sympathetic obligation is part of the natural moral law, general revelation or the prevenient grace God provides to all.

Some of the world may claim that, regardless of natural sympathies for family members and those in geographic proximity, there should not be a legal obligation to care. They make the political assertion that all are individuals and obligated primarily to their own self-expression and fulfillment. In practice, the denial of familial obligation tends to mean that needy parents or other family members are disregarded out of selfishness. This disregard is sometimes masked by demands that others provide the care—because those who should cannot or are unwilling.

As problematic morally as abandonment may be, the state can and should be procedurally disinterested, and render the services determined to be appropriate by the society and its agents. That can never replace the needed partiality of affection and the form of care that only those with affection can render, but it does offer some protection for the needy individual. This means that Christians may have to tolerate such familial "dumping" behavior by others as their legal right to be immoral. However, believers do not need to endorse the behavior as good or right, even for unbelievers.

While there are unquestionably cases where affectional level care is not possible or must be reduced in favor of more intense specialized medical care, the obligations of affectional care are never diminished to the point of nonexistence. Christians should be driven by values that extend beyond personal rights and, while possibly endorsing a right to health care, should not be deceived into justifying such as an effort to avoid familial responsibility. Those of the world, on the other hand, may argue that families should not be obligated to care for their own members and the faithful will have to tolerate even while discouraging such in a pluralistic society. Believers cannot compel others to wash feet.

CONCLUSION

Some evangelicals believe that Christians should interact within the political world in an effort to provide a moral influence. Others claim that Christians are a totally distinct community and should have no expectations of those of the world. Regardless, Christians should agree that there is an obligation to the suffering the state cannot meet, and that such suffering often occurs in such a manner that family members or others close to the sufferer can provide care.

Christian caregiving arises within the confluence of need, skills, proximity and particular obligations to render care. While those of the world also sense the need to care for family and the nearby needy, the expectations among those who are Christians should be significantly higher and should include a familial-like, or affectional, care obligation to those of the household of faith. In addition to expansion of affectional obligations, Christians are supposed to also have love for sojourners, strangers and even for their enemies. This means that the highly restrictive limits to care that are operative in the world are unacceptable standards for the follower of Jesus. This does not mean, though, that occasions may not arise when Christians may choose to act through others. Yet even this does not mean that affectional care responsibilities ever end, only that they are modified.

Caregiving is often inconvenient and sometimes costly. It is always degrading relative to the status standards of the world, but has been unquestionably modeled by the footwashing of the Master. It is a requirement generated by the caregiver's prior receiving of care from the Christ. It is a task, however, that has limits. Jesus limited his foot-washing. It was limited to a group within certain proximity and within a certain relationship. Further, it was limited by the needs of the recipient (not all the body, only the feet). Indeed, his offering of care seems to be a model of a necessary spiritual discipline that not only renders assistance to the served, but is a means of grace into the life of the one who serves. If a believer has never directly assisted the sick, suffering or dying, then it is perhaps unlikely that she or he is mature in the faith.

9

Professionals and Truthfulness

HUMANS AS PROFESSING

The Christian "professional" is professing in two different ways—to a standard of practice and to the body of believers. The Christian professional is first a Christian, then a professional, though that should make him or her a better physician, nurse and so forth. Christian professionals may well appear all the more distinct as the traditional notion of covenantal care yields to contractual models.

> On one occasion an expert in the law stood up to test Jesus. "Teacher," he asked, "what must I do to inherit eternal life?"
>
> "What is written in the Law?" he replied. "How do you read it?"
>
> He answered: "'Love the Lord your God with all your heart and with all your soul and with all your strength and with all your mind'; and, 'Love your neighbor as yourself.'"
>
> "You have answered correctly," Jesus replied. "Do this and you will live."
>
> But he wanted to justify himself, so he asked Jesus, "And who is my neighbor?"
>
> In reply Jesus said: "A man was going down from Jerusalem to Jericho, when he fell into the hands of robbers. They stripped him of his clothes, beat him and went away, leaving him half dead. A priest happened to be going down the same road, and when he saw the man, he passed by on the other side. So too, a Levite, when he came to the place and saw him, passed by on the other side. But a Samaritan, as he traveled, came where the man was; and when he saw him, he took pity on him. He went to him and bandaged his wounds, pouring on oil and wine. Then he put the man on his own donkey, took him to an inn and took care of him. The next day he took out two silver coins and gave them to the innkeeper. 'Look after him,' he said, 'and when I return, I will reimburse you for any extra expense you may have.' Which of these three do you think was a neighbor to the man who fell into the hands of robbers?"
>
> The expert in the law replied, "The one who had mercy on him."
>
> Jesus told him, "Go and do likewise." (Lk 10:25-37)

PART ONE: THE TEXT

The Samaritans were closely related to the Jewish people from whom Jesus came, yet there was significant animosity between the groups. As Jewish tradition had it, the Samaritans had betrayed their Hebrew heritage during and following the Babylonian captivity. The Samaritans lived in the northern portions of what was ancient Israel. They had intermarried with other peoples who had been "ethnically cleansed" from their own regions during Assyrian control. On the return of the enslaved Jews from Babylon, the Samaritans refused to repent and seek purification as Ezra, Nehemiah and others demanded. Also, the Samaritans worshiped Yahweh at Mt. Gerizim, reportedly the ancient Bethel site in the north, instead of at the Temple in Jerusalem. Both of the major religious parties of Jesus' day, the Pharisees and Sadducees, asserted that central religious rites had to be held at the Temple. Further, the Samaritans used only the first five books of the Bible (Pentateuch) as the holy Scriptures. While the Sadducees, the priestly party, also relied only on the Pentateuch, the Pharisees considered this practice to be part of the wider Samaritan betrayal, given that many of the prophetic books were written at the time of exile. The Jewish people generally had great contempt for the Samaritans and the Samaritans responded accordingly. The best way for readers of the parable to understand the relations would be using contemporary examples such as the multigenerational animosity of neighboring people groups of the Balkan region.

Jesus recognized the distinctions and elsewhere even accepts them when he comments that the Samaritans worship what they do not really know (Jn 4:22). Still, the differences of ethnicity and religion were less significant in the telling of the parable than are the commonalities between the Samaritan, the Levite and the priest. For all three, there was a religiously-generated moral duty to serve the strickened individual. They all saw the injured party, and all had resources to render assistance.

As discussed in chapter eight, four variables that change the way in which one responds as a believer to the suffering of others are geographical proximity, relational proximity, the condition of the sick or injured person(s) and the capacity of the caregiver. In this case, Christ is telling the teacher of the law that geography as well as relation define the neighbor and that he must expand his understanding of relational proximity.

The scribe to whom Jesus is speaking was trying to justify himself with his exegetical prowess and the precision of his ethical analysis, but the Christ wants him to understand that it is actual moral expression that matters. Jesus initially tells him that he has answered correctly and that since he knows what to do, he should behave in that way.

Testing the edge of moral expectation, as if to discover when the eyes can allowably look away from suffering, the scribe asks for specifics. Jesus responds this time by simply commanding the man to go and do it, go and live the life of servanthood. The vast majority of human moral activity does not arise as difficult cases requiring the drawing of meticulous ethical boundaries. To Jesus, the situation is simple. The sufferer who is near is by definition a neighbor in need, or correspondingly in the parable, the Samaritan is a neighbor to the sufferer—for being a neighbor entails both benefits and obligations.

First, the Samaritan, priest and Levite could hardly have been in closer geographical proximity to the suffering man. The road may have been 15 feet to 30 feet wide. A rough equivalent might be seeing an automobile accident on a two lane gravel country road but choosing to remain in one's own car, insulated by plastic, metal and glass from the reality of suffering. Passing by on the other side and not seeing the sufferer required an averting of the eyes.[1] Human vision does not become as readily accustomed to unpleasantness as does our sense of smell or touch. One may acclimate to certain noxious sensations, but in order to not see suffering one must turn away or define the sufferer as not worthy of consideration.

It may be that this desensitization to the suffering of those who are geographically close is necessary when the suffering is so great as to be otherwise overwhelming. In the case of the parable the suffering may simply be an unpleasantness the priest and Levite wished to avoid. Perhaps they were afraid of stopping or perhaps they did not want the ritual pollution. Regardless, they averted their eyes. There is a vast moral difference between living in a slum, daily walking past beggars with only a nod and a smile, and hiding in a gated community to avoid the conscious recognition that would require a response. The priest and the Levite build the equivalent of an emotional gated community. The sufferer is not part of that community and so can be ignored and his suffering dismissed.

Second, the duty of care depends on relational proximity. This aspect of Jesus' parable might be missed by a late modern reader of the Text. Appar-

---

[1]Using the phrase in a different but related way, see Leon R. Kass, "Averting One's Eyes, or Facing the Music?—On Dignity in Death: A Commentary on Paul Ramsey," The Hastings Center Studies 2 (May 1974): 67-80.

ently, the priest and the Levite are related—of unmixed blood, to use the image that was prevalent at the time—to the sufferer. They are, albeit distantly, all Jews, or at least this is implied. Since they are not "mixed," they should, if anything, have a greater relational duty than did the Samaritan. Further, they are in a position of authority over and, theoretically, formally responsible for the suffering man because of their positions.

Third, the condition of the man is such that he cannot take care of himself. Further, his condition is acute. Without immediate care, he might die. Also significant is the fact that with care he will live. This is not a futile case. The Samaritan provides the initial care and then refers the patient to another practitioner. He assumes ongoing financial responsibility for the injured man's well-being, but another with better skills and supplies is to render the actual treatment.

This leads to the fourth criterion. The good Samaritan is good, not because he provides all the services to the man now defined as his neighbor, but because he assures such care is given by someone with the capacity of providing the care. This capacity includes physical resources, time resources and skills.

Jesus used his story to juxtapose the capacity of the priest, Levite and Samaritan with that of the questioner. The questioner is "an expert in the law," presumably a scribe. He may have also been a so-called lesser Levite and so might have identified with one of the characters in the parable. Levites as a group managed the tasks of the temple. A specific clan of Levites, the descendents of Aaron, fulfilled the higher priestly functions, but they were not usually designated with the term Levite and this man is likely not one of them. This did not mean that the scribe was of a significantly lower social status. To the contrary, a master of the law—especially at that point in Jewish history with the rise of the synagogue—was likely to be quite well respected, and certainly that is what Jesus wants to convey. The scribe was not only a teacher but also was empowered with functioning in what would now be called legal tasks (contracts, wills, etc.).[2] He was probably a Pharisee, the group that shared with Jesus a belief in resurrection and the epistemological legitimacy of all the law and prophets. The scribe would have been expected to recognize that the unwillingness of the priest and Levite in the parable, men who supposedly served God in every moment of their lives, was hypocrisy. And, Jesus wanted the questioner to ask himself if he too was a hypocritical expert. It is clear that Jesus wanted the hearers to recognize that the priest and the Levite—and by extension the question-

[2]Joseph Dongell, Ph.D., Asbury Theological Seminary, private conversation, July 10, 2007.

ing scribe—all had the resources to serve a beaten and robbed man. Therefore, Jesus declared, the scribe was obligated to "go and do likewise."

The leaders who questioned Jesus were not only religious leaders, they were the social elite and that, as much as their religious position, confers them status. Yet, it is not just class and ethnic distinctions Jesus wants to illustrate with his parable. Religious leaders and all with resources and skill should have basic knowledge of moral obligations and, therefore, are doubly responsible when they consciously choose to disregard those requirements. Those who knew better (or should have) had disregarded the real meaning of Mosaic instructions on caring for sojourners and the weak. Invalid arguments based on the lack of sufficient relational proximity had allowed people in close geographical proximity to disregard others in need. Jesus seems to change the notion of neighbor from one based on geography with some degree of prior relationship to one that asserts that geography creates relationship, at least when that neighbor is facing a critical need. This does not alter the responsibility of family to provide help to family, but it does mean that when family is unavailable the "good" follower of Jesus will respond with neighborly love and actual service—assuming she or he is competent to do so.

The unnamed, but good, Samaritan is cited as the model for all faithful followers of the Christ. His response is traditionally and correctly called *right* (a behavioral standard or moral duty), and his character is deemed *good* (the activity of care arises from his moral virtuosity). Still, he also was in a particular place, had particular skills and had sufficient resources. As the virtuoso plays with excellence particular music on a particular instrument for the particular acoustics of a particular hall, so the virtuous moral agent acts in an appropriate manner for distinct circumstances, given his or her abilities, capacities and resources. Even while recognizing the fundamental pattern represented in the parable of the Good Samaritan, it would be inaccurate to assert that the response to the suffering man on the dangerous Jerusalem-to-Jericho road was not both conditioned and distinct.

All the faithful should be good as the Samaritan on the road to Jericho was, but the rightness is additionally shaped by the needs and abilities of those involved. In other words, the believers are always and without exception obligated, though how that obligation is satisfied can vary significantly based on particular circumstances and one's abilities. The short tale establishes a pattern for moral behavior, not only because Jesus taught it but also because it is exemplified in reality by Jesus' life.

PART TWO: CHRISTIAN BIOETHICS

The faithful should take far more seriously their obligations to biological family members than most do in America today. Their actions should also benefit their suffering neighbors in unexpectedly (by the world's standards) gracious ways. The needy stranger and the enemy too should be surprisingly served. In other words, believers have higher obligations to the suffering than do those of the world. Those of the world should be caught off guard by the disarming goodness of believers. If this was not one of the points of the Good Samaritan parable when Jesus told it, it surely would be one of the consequences if Christians lived it.

For all people giving care there must be limits, but Jesus wants believers to extend their concern and their actual care to a place beyond what the world expects. The difference for the Christian—whether family provider or professional provider—is that the boundaries extend more broadly. More people are encompassed in the circles of concern. All caregiving, whether the restricted assistance expected by our natural location or the broader care demanded in the gospel, are delimited by geographic proximity, relational proximity, condition of the needy and the capacity of the potential provider.

Believers, then, must extend their outreach of care beyond limits usually assumed for those categories. If caregiving ever was an exclusively familial activity, by Jesus' command and example, it is not so any longer. If professional caregivers were ever supposed to limit their services to that which would benefit them financially and offer them convenience and comfort, they are not to do so any longer—at least not if they are believers.

Christian health-care providers should see themselves as skilled good Samaritans. This is not the way the world would define the professional class, but believers must understand their professions as vocations, as callings. For Christians, the secular obligations of a professional relationship and practitioner skills are raised to an even greater degree. The Christian professional provider is professing in two ways, both as a member of a guild of the skillful and as a follower of the Crucified. The interactive combination of these professions raises the moral expectations for the Christian professional provider.

Christian practitioners should have a sense of vocation that is simultaneously defined by the faithful community and by the professional guild, which combined create obligations beyond those of worldly practitioners. Evangelicals strongly endorse the idea that their clergy should be responding to divine intention in their employment. So should any professional givers of care who are of the faith. These caregivers should have the same purposeful approach to their work as clergy. To live out the calling is to progressively assume, by discipline, habit and the power of the Holy Spirit, the character of Christ in one's vocation, as if Christ himself lived out his life in such service. The standard should be: if Jesus had been a provider—a physician, dentist, nurse, therapist—he would have been this kind of provider and, therefore, so should the believer who serves in that given profession.

The assertion that all vocations in the economic sense should be vocations in the spiritual sense goes back at least to the Reformation. Luther declared the priesthood of all believers (following on the proto-Protestants such as the Brethren of the Common Life, Wycliffe and Hus who had formed lay brotherhoods and/or begun translating the Text into the common vernacular). This meant that even seemingly secular work could be a special call of God for an individual. In fact, it meant nothing was ever purely secular. The Anabaptists have always understood that vocation is tied to one's commitment to the gospel. Calvin argued that all employment should be for God's glory and that some nonchurch vocations were as special to God as the clergy, specifically the civil magistrate who governed in God's name. Brother Lawrence, in a Catholic work influential on early revivalists, *The Practice of the Presence of God,* commended doing even the tedious for God and with excellence. Wesley, while rejecting Calvin's theocratic tendencies, did agree that the Christian calling went beyond church ministry. In fact, on this matter one could describe Wesley's position as pushing reform further than the Reformers. Wesley believed everyone—not just monks and nuns and priests—who followed Jesus was called to a complete and holy life. This was a duty, not a supererogatory option. The argument was influential when evangelical roots were being set during the Great Awakening in the United States and the Wesleyan Revivals in Britain.

For the Reformers and early Revivalists who laid the groundwork of evangelicalism, the believer is to at least have a sense of vocation that (1) limits which jobs are morally appropriate for the faithful and (2) requires that any job assumed must be fulfilled for the Lord. Jesus is not only the Savior, he is the Lord and that means the Lord of one's employment. Vocation is not merely employment, and not even working "as if" for the Lord, but actually is to be for the glory of God. The Christian health-care practitioner, then, is not only serving a patient, but also serving as Jesus did and is serving Jesus.

Though all parables can be understood at multiple levels, for evangelicals the parable of the Good Samaritan seems to have been told so that those who believe might simultaneously see Christ in the suffering man on the side of the road and see Christ as the example in the Samaritan. Professional skills and institutional relationships do not relieve this obligation, but rather amplify it. The service to others is a general duty for all believers, but also takes specific form. The work of anyone, but certainly of health-care professionals, is a protestantized monastic obedience and a professional vocational responsibility simultaneously. This does not occur in some idealized form, but as a particular Christian in a particular setting serving particular individuals.

All persons with higher levels of skill have higher obligations to serve those in need. For instance, firefighters have higher obligations to help those in burning houses than do those without firefighting skills, but this does not relieve nonprofessionals of their obligations. Rather, the firefighter's duties are just amplified by his or her skills. They are also amplified by relational proximity. The firefighter who is employed or is a volunteer in a given community has a greater duty to those of the community she or he serves than to those of a community she or he may be passing through. Still, if there is a need, the firefighter should offer to help by virtue of geographic proximity. Similarly, health-care professionals have a greater duty by virtue of expertise than do those of the general population in the same geographic proximity to a suffering individual, and higher still if that practitioner is in a professional relationship with the sufferer.

For Christian providers, the obligations are amplified. Assuming one does not receive a call to full-time service to the indigent or otherwise deprived, the Christian provider should volunteer for mission trips, give weekly hours at free clinics, assist with screenings through their local congregations, retire on the mission field or provide some equivalent service that is beyond the expectation of the world. The Text on healing the sick and cleansing lepers continues: "Freely you have received, freely give" (Mt 10:8). And, though elsewhere Scripture notes that the "ox should not be muzzled," which means pay and respect for vocational service, including in health care, are not inappropriate, the obligation to serve the needy neighbor should never be displaced by a desire for wealth or earthly honor.

All believing health-care professionals should understand that as Christians they accept their vocation as a calling forth of virtues and an entering into covenantal relations.[3] For Christians, the basic covenant between practitioner and patient assumes prior covenants with the "guild" and with the church. The relationship between patient and practitioner depends as much on the faithful character of the professing professional as on the level of expertise. This Christian professional behavior and character is, then, to be distinguished from both contract relationships as developed in health care in the 1980s and from early twentieth-century notions of professional virtue based solely on participation in the guild with its resulting paternalism.

The loss of the traditional close friendship of the family doctor has been in some ways good and in other ways bad, but in all senses inevitable.[4] The social structure of health care, which goes far beyond but is strongly influenced by economics, no longer makes true covenantal bonds between patient and professional likely. "Contracts are external; covenants are internal to the parties involved."[5] And, the communities that in the past shaped that internalization of virtues have been significantly changed. In particular, the guilds have been perhaps irrevocably weakened, at least in moral terms. In addition, the patient who enters care cannot be assumed to share any significant life values (beyond a desire to get better) with the practitioner. This does not relieve the Christian practitioner of the obligation to act virtuously.

> Generally in healthcare . . . more than a brief transaction is occurring. Consequently, if understood as having gradient, the model of "acquaintance" is extremely useful. Someone solicits an interaction. Both parties should be suspi-

---

[3]William May describes this in his seminal book, *The Physician's Covenant: Images of the Healer in Medical Ethics* (Philadelphia: Westminster, 1983). Another strong voice on this theme has been Edmund Pelligrino, "The Virtuous Physician and the Ethics of Medicine," in *Contemporary Issues in Bioethics,* 5th ed., ed. Tom L. Beauchamp and LeRoy Walters (Belmont, Calif.: Wadsworth Publishing, 1999). First published in Earl E. Shelp, ed., *Virtue and Medicine: Exploration in the Character of Medicine,* Philosophy and Medicine Series (New York: Springer, 1985), 17:243-55.

[4]See Kevin Wm. Wildes, *Moral Acquaintances: Methodology in Bioethics* (Notre Dame, Ind.: University of Notre Dame Press, 2000)

[5]William May, "Images of the Healer," in *Virtues and Practices in the Christian Tradition*, ed. Nancey Murphy, Brad J. Kallenberg and Mark Thiessen Nation (Harrisburg, Penn.: Trinity Press International, 1997), p. 334. The following paragraph quotations are drawn from the same article, pp. 333-37.

To use an analogy, the service of a contract relationship is like that of a waiter in a restaurant as opposed to the covenantal model of a friend offering table hospitality. The food may be good in either setting, but the experience is clearly different. May suggests that the interpretation of the relationship between the recipient and provider alters the actual care received. Further, he suggests that this interpretation changes the profession by changing the self-definition of the practitioner.

> cious (the days of simply "trusting" practitioners are gone and, I would argue, may have never existed since most practitioners were known as friends or at least trustworthy acquaintances before they performed professional services). They may agree on certain matters and must to proceed. However, the recognition of "*strangeness*" between the two cannot and should not be abandoned. This is not an evil, but is rather a respecting of difference.[6]

A deep and abiding moral friendship between caregiver and patient is not required. An acquaintanceship with common interests expressed in mutual, specific goals is what is called for in practitioner-patient relationships that are not otherwise specifically governed by a shared faith. Because of its practical orientation and the shared intention of meeting immediate goals, the Christian practitioner need not have a shared deep morality with the one served, only shared middle axioms and some specific outcome interests, and a personal commitment to excellence.

In typical settings at the end of modernity in the West, the position of the Christian provider has changed from missionary or brotherly/sisterly caregiver to employee or affiliate with privileges—as such, friendship cannot and should not be presumed. Christians should recognize the importance of autonomy and contract as correctives to the previous paternalism of health care even while asserting they are inadequate as a moral approach to caregiving. On the other hand, forced friendship is not friendship at all. The evangelical provider should be respectful, realizing that the relationship with many patients is one that is between deep friendship and the meeting of strangers. It is acquaintanceship and the believer should be a good neighbor to acquaintances. And, for Christian health-care professionals, serving an acquaintance in a neighborly manner, as did the Samaritan, is morally sufficient.

At one end, when someone is not really sick but would simply be better off with kindness, the Christian practitioner is obligated to render such care. This is more than mere civility or good manners, though politeness is not a bad place to begin. It may require a quick discharge, but always with gentleness. At the other end of the spectrum, the Christian maintains an obligation to the truly ill longer than does the world. The dying person or the person who is so severely disabled as to be defined as no longer human by some in the world does not cease to be an obligation for the virtuous Christian practi-

[6]James R. Thobaben, "Pleased to Make Your Acquaintance: A review of Kevin Wm. Wildes' *Moral Acquaintances: Methodology in Bioethics*," *Christian Bioethics* 7, no. 3 (2001): 425-39.

tioner. When the Christian character of the vocational call is manifest, then the patients will be served across the whole spectrum of physical need.

Somehow, believing practitioners must exemplify Jesus Christ and yet often must do so in a secularized setting with those of the world. In the past, the Christian vocational aspect of a believer's profession might have been readily accepted. The relationship of doctor, nurse or therapist to patient used to be accepted as quite similar to that of pastor to parishioner. The desire to serve the best interests of the patient extended beyond treating illness or injury because there was a continuing mutual commitment and often a common faith. Today, the societal demand for the Christian practitioner to continue that genuine concern for the whole person may not exist.

There cannot be true, deep friendship if there is not a common morality. This does not mean that a successful practitioner-patient relationship cannot be established. In fact, the practitioner should be honest about his or her value system and differences that may exist with the recipient of care. Acknowledgement of differences can allow the practitioner and the patient to recognize their common goals and establish a covenantal bond.

PART THREE: CHRISTIAN BIOETHICS AND THE WORLD

No one should expect Christian virtues from those of the world. While believers must view their professional life as a vocational calling, those of the world need not—they need be only skilled technicians who accept the standards of the social contract and the guild, including a willingness to fully abide by service contracts in their various forms. The Christian can and should expect those of the world to abide by the expectations of the social contract and to express in behavior the virtues of the professional guilds, even while she or he offers more. Christians cannot and should not expect practitioners of the world to act as neighbors in the sense of the Good Samaritan parable. That is a Christian moral standard.

That does not mean that medical professionals are not called to a different and in some ways higher moral standard than laypersons. Because of the difference in professional calling, the practitioner is allowed to move into a social circle called "friendly acquaintance" without the typical process of relational negotiation. This social location is maintained on the basis of demonstrated technical abilities. As noted, recently, this relationship is of a more temporary nature and more imbalanced than a true friendship. In the past, the role of health-care professional provided an even deeper access into family life. This was, after all, the man (usually) who took out the tonsils, removed the inflamed appendix and escorted a patient through the end of life right up to the moment of death. Using the language of sociology of religion, fifty years ago physicians filled priestly roles and sometimes served as prophetic guides for families. Now, they tend to have a professional character that is more a mix of managerial and pastoral.

Prior to the advent of modern medicine in the West, the family assumed caregiving responsibility.[7] Physicians and surgeons would provide treatments, often coming to the bedside in the home, but the care of the patient before and after such treatment remained the responsibility of the family. The poor, especially the dying poor, might turn to religious institutions for care (thus the creation of hospitals in Europe), but most people would remain in the care of relatives. Given the state of medical knowledge prior to the late nineteenth century, being treated by family members was often a more efficacious course than turning to professional healers anyway.

In the West, with the American Civil War and the Crimean War came the transformation of specialized caregiving. The nineteenth century also brought the development of germ theory. These changes, along with the struggles between the various schools of professional practitioners, finally led to the rise of modern, scientific medicine. The Flexner Report (1910) cemented this change. With professional differentiation, increasing urbanization, the rise of the assembly line and belief in technology, as well as the shrinking of family from extended kin group to nuclear household, health-care treatment of persons moved away from the family to the professionals. Certainly, family members have maintained some responsibilities, especially in caring for those with disabilities and in initiating entry into the health-care system, but the end result has been that caregiving is increasingly a function of caregiving specialists.

Through the twentieth century, the caregiving professionals moved from paternalism (ca. 1910–1960) to emphasis on the social contract and rights lan-

[7]See Paul Starr, *The Social Transformation of American Medicine* (New York: Basic Books, 1982). See also John Duffy, *The Healers: A History of American Medicine* (Urbana: University of Illinois Press, 1979); Nora Groce, *The U.S. Role in International Disability Activities: A History and a Look Towards the Future* (study commissioned by World Institute on Disability, the World Rehabiliation Fund and Rehabiliation International, 1992); and Michel Foucault, *The Birth of the Clinic: An Archeology of Medical Perception*, trans. A. M. Sheridan Smith (New York: Vintage Books, 1973). For two interesting discussions of the difference in the role of the family in non-Western societies, see Paul Brand and Philip Yancey, *Pain: The Gift Nobody Wants* (New York: HarperCollins, 1993); and David Werner (with Carol Thuman and Jane Maxwell), *Where There Is No Doctor: A Village Health Care Handbook*, 2nd ed. (Berkeley, Calif.: Hesperian Foundation, 1992), which bears a striking cultural similarity to Wesley's *Primitive Physik*.

guage (ca. 1960–1980) to business contract (ca. 1980–present). All of these professional self-understandings remain to some extent, tinged with "therapeutic" language. Additional models of care have been built up and appear in different institutions and in different locations within institutions.

Experts define their caregiving by assuming different models of treatment, or interpreting the patient-practitioner dyad in different ways. In order to function as friendly acquaintances with professional responsibilities, these models of practitioner, patient and institution must be acknowledged and accepted to the extent necessary to serve the common goals of treatment. All of the categories of recipients and practitioners in table 9.1 have been used during the last half of the twentieth century or the beginning of the twenty-first century to describe the relationship of the professional caregiver and his or her patient. The categories are not mutually exclusive. On some occasions and depending on the setting, one model may be preferable to another, though no single understanding of the relationship of patient-practitioner should operate to the exclusion of all others.

Table 9.1. The Language of Curing in Early Twenty-First-Century U.S.

Recipient	*Virtue/Value*	*Environment*	*Practitioner*
Child	Paternal benevolence	Home (familiar)	Parent
Battlefield	Victory	War	Soldier
Patient	Treatment	Medical system	Expert technician
Student	Knowledge	School	Teacher
Tumor in 401	Cause & effect	Laboratory	Scientist
Client	Advocacy	Adversarial society	Advocate
555-55-5555	Management	Bureaucracy	Bureaucrat
Citizen	Rights	Plurality/public square	Citizen
Partner	Cooperation	Community	Partner
Consumer	Product/service	Market	Supplier/sales

The categories are not mutually exclusive, though some practitioners do tend to identify themselves one way in particular.[8] Importantly, these understandings may come into conflict in a given institution at any particular moment. For instance, if a patient is being referred to with childish, familial language and then is confronted by an employee from finance who uses the

[8]The first four are modified from William May. The covenantal model is modified from May and appeared earlier in Paul Ramsey's *Patient as Person: Explorations in Medical Ethics* (New Haven, Conn.: Yale University Press, 1970).

language of Social Security numbers or the marketplace, there may be some hard feelings. Some of these models lead to contract thinking (e.g., the Social Security number and managed care) and some tend toward covenantal reasoning (e.g., teacher/student). All have their place and can be modified within context; for instance, while the physician is often the teacher, the patient who is dying or experiencing a disorder new to the practitioner is the teacher, such as to the intern/resident and even to the attending doctors on occasion. The Christian can use any of the models, depending on the setting, but always as a Christian who is teaching or advocating or even filling out forms.

What can and should be expected is that regardless of the professional-patient model operating, the practitioner will function civilly, like a friendly acquaintance who has the best interest of the individual at the center of decision making—that acquaintanceship being further shaped and delimited by the standards of the service contract, the social contact and the virtue standards of the guild. Any person, Christian or not, who chooses to practice as a professional health-care provider should acknowledge that she or he is professing to be part of a value system with concomitant obligations and benefits.

While civility and friendly acquaintanceship is expected morally, accountability is necessary. Perhaps in the past the professional guilds rendered that accountability, but no longer. Since individual virtue cannot be assumed and the professional-patient contract relationship is imbalanced, the practitioner's power must be limited and that currently occurs at least at six levels of accountability:

1. Laws and governmental requirements
2. Additional accrediting standards
3. Professional/guild standards
4. Institutional standards and rules
5. Widely accepted moral standards (middle axioms)
6. Personal virtuosity based on community of identity[9]

Law and government. To some degree, the society can and should demand service from health-care professionals beyond that for which they receive

[9]These "Levels of Professional Obligation" are drawn, with significant modification, from Pellegrino, "Virtuous Physician" in *Contemporary Issues in Bioethics,* ed. Beauchamp and Walters. Pellegrino develops further the role of virtue in the physician's practice of medicine in his collaborative work with David C. Thomasma, *The Virtues in Medical Practice* (New York: Oxford University Press, 1993).

compensation. The government provides education, medical research funding, health-care infrastructure and reimbursement mechanisms that make the practice of medicine far more lucrative and significantly easier than it might otherwise be. This is not to diminish the significant efforts that are put forward by nurses and doctors and allied professionals during their education, not to mention the continuous and frustrating interaction with bureaucracy and the legal system, as well as, usually, a huge educational debt. Still, the obligation remains as long as the profession—both individual professionals and their guild—receive special treatment and respect.

The state, as noted above, has made an investment in the practitioner and can make some demands on him or her by virtue of that training. In addition, and far more importantly, the state exists in order to serve as the protector of the contract makers. This includes protection from foreign enemies, but also from other contract makers who would attack the vulnerable. The extraordinary technical expertise of the provider and the neediness of the patient create such imbalance that the state legitimately intervenes to protect the vulnerable recipient of care. Patients may be free to select their practitioners and their payors/insurers, but cannot possibly be assumed competent to make critical decisions on health care without the protection of the state in assuring that the needed information is sufficiently and fairly presented, not through governmental micromanagement but through assuring individual accountability of practitioners and institutions. Often the state transfers this task, under subsidiarity, to those with more expertise and those closer to the actual practice site, namely, accrediting bodies.

Accrediting bodies. The accrediting bodies are essentially cooperatives established by professional guilds and providing organizations to prevent conflicts among themselves and to form a common front for and against the state. The individual practitioner agrees to the rules of accrediting bodies because (1) it is a surrogate for the guild, (2) it is a surrogate for the state and (3) the accrediting bodies have substantial power over the institutions in which the individual practices. Accrediting bodies provide precision, on occasion precision that is actually more precise than accurate. Reliance on numbers when the numbers themselves do not accurately measure all significant aspects of care can be problematic, even deceptive, and thereby harmful to the provider-patient relationship. Still, the accrediting bodies do allow accountability by "experts" without forcing the institutions and practitioners into governmental bureaucracies that are utterly unyielding and painfully slow in adapting to new technologies and new organizational forms.

Professing/professional guild. Guilds operate as mediating institutions between the society and the individual practitioner. They have the characteristics of labor unions, trusts, oligarchies, schools and fraternal organizations. As a union, the guilds of practitioners protect the individual from being abused, especially financially, by hiring organizations. Some guilds are hesitant to take this role, especially those made up of physicians. This is in part because traditionally physicians have been individual "companies" and their guild allegiance was more like a trust among corporations than like employees in a single industry—though this is changing. The oligarchic tendencies of guilds come through in their control of standards and of admissions into the field. The latter occurs both through limiting admissions to medical, nursing and allied health schools and through keeping marginal professions at bay—such as chiropractors. Though this is asserted as being in the public interest, it is also a way of limiting competition. The guilds are like schools through control of both initial and continuing education, setting the technical and ethical standards of practice. Finally, the guilds are like fraternal groups in that they tend to both protect the individual practitioners from outsiders, and they hold the individual practitioners accountable, to some degree, for how they practice. To not do so would diminish the guild and harm all the other members; membership would cease to be an indicator of quality, of expertise. Unfortunately, sometimes the guild is not diligent in assuring that incompetents are quickly held accountable and, given that this involves health and life itself, that is more than a mere professional turf concern. Theoretically, this is where the state and accrediting bodies step in.

The rise of modern medicine wove itself into and ultimately solidified the medical guild. Indeed, some have argued that the organization of health-care providers was as important as the technological advances. Leaders of the profession used the law, the media, the authority of universities, and shame and degradation, as well as reward and honor, to form the profession. They defined the profession in relation to other groups, institutions and patients. In doing so, ironically, they may have weakened the expectation of personal virtue, substituting guild rules. As evidence, one need only consider the typical ethics course, taught in medical or nursing school, which is far closer to the dissemination of regulatory standards than the inculcation of virtues. Regardless of the historical causes, the treatment of the sick and injured is frequently turned over to experts with defined territories of responsibility gathered together in guilds under the assumption that the "patient" generally will fare better with their care. It is usually true.

Institution. Health-care institutions are intentionally designed to meet the needs of customers, that is, patients. In other words, the provision of health care can be a product. For-profits are answerable to stockholders. Not-for-profits that are part of other not-for-profit groups are answerable to those organizations and their moral standards; for instance, a religious hospital is to serve patients to the extent that such serves the ends of the religious organization. Not-for-profits that are community-based are to satisfy the ends established by that community through the trustees of the health-care organization; such can be through an independent board or, in the case of government-owned facilities, through appointees of the state.

The practitioner must adhere to the standards of the organization to the extent agreed upon when she or he entered into a contractual employment or affiliation relationship. The trustees or directors of the institution do not set up rules that trump either the state or the accrediting bodies, but they do establish more restrictive standards within the range acceptable to those other organizations. At times the institution and guild may come into conflict, and the practitioner must decide which rules to follow, though in practice the individual institutions tend to have more power than the guild when the accreditation standards are vague or open. An example, and one that pleases evangelicals, is a hospital's refusal to demand that medial residents in obstetrics and gynecology be taught, by actual practice, how to perform elective abortions.

If a health-care facility is governmentally operated, then it tends to have less limited moral standards, though it may have substantially more in the way of bureaucratic rules than, say, a religious hospital. Community and government facilities tend to operate with the broad "middle axioms" of the social contract society and will sometimes have stricter limits depending on specific legislation. The practitioner, again, agrees to abide by the standards when she or he enters into a practice contract with the facility, even if she or he does not agree with them.

General societal values (middle axioms of social contract). All practitioners have some degree of obligation to the broader community. The support the community provides through education subsidies and the development of medical infrastructure elicits a professional duty from the practitioner to help the community, perhaps even through charity service. Primarily this should be expressed in service to individual patients but also to the broader public.

Obviously, if the obligation to the broader community becomes overwhelming, then the duty to the individual patient weakens and that would be contrary to the professional purpose of health-care practitioners.[10] A preferable model for the Christian is to see these as simultaneous obligations, with deference given to the individual being served if a conflict is discerned. One area in which conflicts arise is at the point of supposed community expectation to serve all or at least the deserving poor while not providing sufficient funding or proper distribution mechanisms. Not formally providing preventive and primary care that is reasonably accessible to the poor exacerbates funding and broader distribution problems as well as jeopardizing some individual care relationships. Christians can respond, even if laws are not changed, by providing service, perhaps a tithe of working time, to the socially marginalized. They should not expect such of those of the world unless mandated as payment for the cultural benefits of professional status.

The community values that are most often discussed center around distribution, but equally important are those values that are established by or assumed by the social contract and should be extended into practitioner-patient relations. A practitioner may not need Christian virtues, but she or he does need to be a personally reliable human being. That is a civil standard. Perhaps the central moral expectation, besides developing technical expertise, is honesty. Honesty is a virtue of the profession, a virtue of the faith and a middle axiom for behavior in the civil society. Honesty is expressed in rules of truth-telling, promise-keeping and confidentiality maintenance in health care. The patient, in spite of being in a relationship of unbalanced power with the health-care professional, is deemed a person deserving of the truth as a member of the society, unless reasonably deemed too evil or too incompetent to hear the truth.

The best way to understand the civil society's expectations of honesty for the practitioner-patient dyad and for functioning inside health-care institutions is by considering the possible violations.

---

[10]Wesley J. Smith, *Culture of Death: The Assault on Medical Ethics in America* (San Francisco: Encounter Books, 2000).

Deception comes in at least seven forms:

- Distortion: something that could mean more than one thing
- Omission: intentional concealing
- Falsification: intentional false information
- Quantity misleading: providing incomplete or excessive information for a decision
- Qualities misleading: providing altered information
- Misplaced relevance: implying greater or lesser significance of information than appropriate
- Lack of clarity: unclear representation of information[11]

Again, this is not the same as personal moral virtuosity. Honesty is a minimal standard of society that is extremely important in health care.

Personal virtuosity based on community of faith/community of values. In the United States, most practitioners might appeal to their own "conscience" for guidance if asked to do something immoral. For instance, if the rules or practices of an employer are deemed immoral or are implemented in an arbitrary manner, then the practitioner should actively protest. A practitioner, on the other hand, who insists on doing that which is contrary to the standards of the institution should be removed unless there was a prior agreement to allow such. Standing up for what one believes is not a sign of integrity if other options for employment exist and the institution's values were evident at the time of the professional affiliation (assuming those values are not illegal or utterly immoral by civil standards). Integrity, in such a case, requires keeping one's word, using appropriate mechanisms to change the organization if possible, or withdrawing.

A morally difficult situation arises when someone is hired and the policy changes or the person's values change. This creates a freedom-of-conscience conflict. If the person's values change, then she or he can seek a waiver and, if not granted, should politely leave. If the organization changes, then there should be allowance for deferring participation in what is deemed immoral. It is also possible that a higher authority (say, the state) would allow freedom of conscience that would trump the rules of the institution. For the Christian, freedom of conscience is important as the values of the Chris-

[11]Modified from R. H. Gass and J. S. Seiter, *Persuasion, Social Influence, and Compliance Gaining* (Needham Heights, Mass.: Allyn and Bacon, 1999), especially chapter 13.

tian practitioner are not exclusively those of the state, the guild or its surrogates, or the institution—they are also the values of his or her foundational communities. The Christian is first and foremost a Christian, not a doctor or nurse. Christians profess Christ, and then work out their professing in various professions.

CONCLUSION

For the Christian professional, obligations must extend beyond service contracts and even the social contract. The Christian practitioner must also demonstrate the character of one conforming his or her life to the life of Jesus Christ. The most important model for caregiving, then, is not established by the managed care organization, or the medical school, or the state, or even the Hippocratic tradition. The virtuosity of the Christian practitioner is generally Christian and then specifically applied within the field of practice. Into table 9.1, the Christian could insert Practitioner as Samaritan, Patient as immediately present person who stands in need, the Environment as the lonely byway in which other practitioners may or may not be available, and the Virtue as neighborliness that is governed not only by acquaintanceship but by *agape* love.

For the Christian, his or her virtuosity as a believer must compel adherence to the best possible professional practices. The believer must seek to exceed the acceptable and move toward the excellent. No believer should willingly function at the edge of the law, accrediting regulations or guild rules unless those standards are in direct contradiction of the gospel. In the past, physicians, surgeons and nurses were asked to function as virtuous persons as the profession defined character expectations. Those days are gone for most, with deontological reasoning governing the morality of practitioners. This is not satisfactory for believers. They must be virtuous—having virtuosity in skills whenever possible, and in morality without exception. As with other Christians who are professional (e.g., lawyers) they must extend care with at least some degree of personal sacrifice (though that may be legitimately limited by their own capacity, including impact on others to whom they have obligations and their own self-preservation).

The relationship of professional to patient is a voluntary and highly variable construct. Certainly all societies have healers and these healers have "duties" to their patients.[12] The Christian practitioner is part of at least two soci-

[12]Talcott Parsons, *The Social System* (Glencoe, Ill.: Free Press, 1951), p. 320.

eties—the late modern West and the body of believers. The believer's professional effectiveness is tied to the success of the scientific method and the technology that it has generated, and to seeking to be a healer of the kind of the Great Physician, Jesus.

10

Managing Care and Serving Needs

HUMANS AS ORGANIZERS

Organization is one of the distinct characteristics of human beings. They organize to economically produce, for education, to worship and to meet other needs. In the Scripture, the death and raising of Lazarus shows a basic organization—organization to grieve, to properly handle dead bodies for religious and sanitation reasons, and to provide care for the sick and their families. Such organization is always based on values and always must be managed. Since no society is truly a Christian society and in the United States religious pluralism is both legally and culturally endorsed, the best that can ever be achieved are organizations run by Christians under Christian values and standards or secularized institutions that respect the religious beliefs of Christian patients and practitioners.

> Now a man named Lazarus was sick. He was from Bethany, the village of Mary and her sister Martha. This Mary, whose brother Lazarus now lay sick, was the same one who poured perfume on the Lord and wiped his feet with her hair. So the sisters sent word to Jesus, "Lord, the one you love is sick."
>
> When he heard this, Jesus said, "This sickness will not end in death. No, it is for God's glory so that God's Son may be glorified through it." Jesus loved Martha and her sister and Lazarus. Yet when he heard that Lazarus was sick, he stayed where he was two more days.
>
> Then he said to his disciples, "Let us go back to Judea."
>
> "But Rabbi," they said, "a short while ago the Jews tried to stone you, and yet you are going back there?"
>
> Jesus answered, "Are there not twelve hours of daylight? A man who walks by day will not stumble, for he sees by this world's light. It is when he walks by night that he stumbles, for he has no light."
>
> After he had said this, he went on to tell them, "Our friend Lazarus has fallen asleep; but I am going there to wake him up."
>
> His disciples replied, "Lord, if he sleeps, he will get better." Jesus had been speaking of his death, but his disciples thought he meant natural sleep.

So then he told them plainly, "Lazarus is dead, and for your sake I am glad I was not there, so that you may believe. But let us go to him."

Then Thomas (called Didymus) said to the rest of the disciples, "Let us also go, that we may die with him."

On his arrival, Jesus found that Lazarus had already been in the tomb for four days. Bethany was less than two miles from Jerusalem, and many Jews had come to Martha and Mary to comfort them in the loss of their brother. When Martha heard that Jesus was coming, she went out to meet him, but Mary stayed at home.

"Lord," Martha said to Jesus, "if you had been here, my brother would not have died. But I know that even now God will give you whatever you ask."

Jesus said to her, "Your brother will rise again."

Martha answered, "I know he will rise again in the resurrection at the last day."

Jesus said to her, "I am the resurrection and the life. He who believes in me will live, even though he dies; and whoever lives and believes in me will never die. Do you believe this?"

"Yes, Lord," she told him, "I believe that you are the Christ, the Son of God, who was to come into the world."

And after she had said this, she went back and called her sister Mary aside. "The Teacher is here," she said, "and is asking for you." When Mary heard this, she got up quickly and went to him. Now Jesus had not yet entered the village, but was still at the place where Martha had met him. When the Jews who had been with Mary in the house, comforting her, noticed how quickly she got up and went out, they followed her, supposing she was going to the tomb to mourn there.

When Mary reached the place where Jesus was and saw him, she fell at his feet and said, "Lord, if you had been here, my brother would not have died."

When Jesus saw her weeping, and the Jews who had come along with her also weeping, he was deeply moved in spirit and troubled. "Where have you laid him?" he asked.

"Come and see, Lord," they replied.

Jesus wept.

Then the Jews said, "See how he loved him!"

But some of them said, "Could not he who opened the eyes of the blind man have kept this man from dying?"

Jesus, once more deeply moved, came to the tomb. It was a cave with a stone laid across the entrance. "Take away the stone," he said.

"But, Lord," said Martha, the sister of the dead man, "by this time there is a bad odor, for he has been there four days."

> Then Jesus said, "Did I not tell you that if you believed, you would see the glory of God?"
>
> So they took away the stone. Then Jesus looked up and said, "Father, I thank you that you have heard me. I knew that you always hear me, but I said this for the benefit of the people standing here, that they may believe that you sent me."
>
> When he had said this, Jesus called in a loud voice, "Lazarus, come out!" The dead man came out, his hands and feet wrapped with strips of linen, and a cloth around his face.
>
> Jesus said to them, "Take off the grave clothes and let him go."
>
> Therefore many of the Jews who had come to visit Mary, and had seen what Jesus did, put their faith in him. (Jn 11:1-45)

PART ONE: THE TEXT

Does the care of God vary? Did Jesus care for Lazarus? Did he care more or less for him than for others he met along the dusty roads of Galilee or the crowded streets of Jerusalem? Did he care for the family members who seemed to have suffered along with the dying man? Apparently, some of his contemporaries thought not, for they noted that Jesus could heal the blind but did nothing to keep Lazarus from dying. Though Jesus recognized the emotional pain of Mary and Martha and others, he apparently allowed it to be extended. He was not in the immediate area, but he could have hurried to the village. Instead, Jesus seemingly decided that his ministry elsewhere was more important than healing Lazarus, or perhaps he wanted a spectacular reclamation from death to be seen by the crowds, or perhaps he had confidence about the power of God that the others did not share.

Whatever the reason, the delay came at a price. The relatives faced additional sorrow. And this one whom Jesus loved, Lazarus, had to face the anguish of death (Jn 11:3). Further, facing death would now occur twice. Was the price worth it?

The Text implies at least five things are true. (1) Sickness and death are real and are evil, but neither is the ultimate evil. (2) Sickness and death are evils that affect us with particularity—that is, only when a particular person is sick or dies or recognizes she or he will die. (3) When someone specific is sick or dies, it impacts not only that person but also others who recognize an evil against one they love and, by extension and consequence, the evil against them. (4) This evil—sometimes by prevention, sometimes by being transformed—can be overcome. (5) Finally, this evil should be resisted when possible and mitigated when not by actions of an organized caring community.

Though later turns in philosophy have pushed Christian ethics toward descriptions of love as disinterested, that is not the biblical pattern. Love for neighbor is not abstract and certainly love of enemy requires a genuine recognition of who the person is who must be loved in spite of previous interactions. The biblical pattern is to have extraordinary concern for all persons without denying the particular responsibilities and the peculiar love one may have for given individuals. It may not be more evil for one to suffer as opposed to another, but the experience of that suffering by observers appropriately varies in accordance with relationship and obligation.

Lazarus is described as a man Jesus loves. Jesus himself asks Martha about her belief in him by asking whether she believes her brother is cared for by God. Jesus wept because of his relationship with the particular people and their particular experience. Even if the suffering of all individuals is somehow identically significant to God in his love, it is not and need not be identically significant for humans. Love of family, friend, acquaintance, stranger, sojourner and enemy differ significantly in levels and types of affection, and in moral obligation.

It is natural for people to hurt more when someone for whom they have affection suffers. But although such feelings are natural, giving up the particularity of human concern for specific people would be to either overwhelm with sorrow given the vast numbers sick and dying or push believers and those of the world alike toward an equality of callousness. For that reason, Paul tells the believers to "rejoice with those who rejoice; mourn with those who mourn" (Rom 12:15). In commending this, he does not exclude the enemy or non-Christian neighbor—quite the opposite—but he does particularize the experience of affection. Further, he uses the plural, implying that Christians are to share with one another in this responsibility of compassion.

The community in John 11 organized to support specific people (Mary and Martha), and possibly to provide assistance prior to the death with the caregiving responsibilities for Lazarus. Community care is not exclusively Christian; one can readily assume that such would happen in most, if not all, premodern social groupings. Apparently Jesus did not discourage such community care, and Paul elsewhere encourages it. Simply put, this was the way that risk could be spread and managed. Few family members could individually negotiate the various services required during a serious illness, so the community would provide some assistance, recognizing that they too would have need in the future. Mutual assistance of one sort or another is foundational for societies from so-called primitive social groups up to and through late modern societies with highly specialized insurance.

In Bethany this mutuality of care rested on mutuality of affections. One cause of moral problems in health care at the end of modernity is that affection has been severed from community obligation, with bureaucratic efficiency substituted. Sometimes high degrees of organization and clean, disinterested procedures actually serve persons well. There is no doubt that tertiary-level hospitals and economic protection from catastrophic diseases could not be readily managed in small villages. Still, when a health-care organization is only defined by procedure, then the peculiar needs of individuals are often ignored in the process of bureaucratic categorization and prioritizing. Further, the lack of affection can mean obliviousness or callousness that ultimately leads to the disregard of the individual. It is not that evil is intended, it is that the given individual in his or her particularity simply does not matter to the ones managing or giving care. The evils of sickness and death are, thereby, amplified by the evil of disregard.

Even in Jesus' time, who would do what for whom was a concern. Apparently Jesus thought the concern was one believers could organize to address. The healing of the ten lepers is an example. Another powerful example is the healing of the paralytic in Luke 9.[1] And again, when the disciples were sent out two by two "they went out and preached that people should repent. They drove out many demons and anointed many sick people with oil and healed them" (Mk 6:12-13).

The crowd organized to seek the messianic Healer for Lazarus, for the paralytic on the pallet and for all those located throughout Judea who might be seen by the dispersed apostles. Later in Acts, the deacons are organized precisely for this purpose. These actions reveal that the faithful are to organize themselves for the delivery of this care, to "drive out evil spirits and to heal every disease and sickness" (Mt 10:1). Presumably that can include organization for the use of scientific medicine and public health techniques.

PART TWO: CHRISTIAN BIOETHICS

Christian social morality has found expression in organized care for over a millennium. Without exception, a coherent Christian morality includes social

---

[1]The words *leper* and *paralytic* are used intentionally, following Paul Brand, M.D. (See chapter 4, note 16.)

expressions of caring ministry—of mutual accountability and of service. Institutional expressions of Christian morality are found in the church through organized extension ministries of health service, education and so forth. The particular organizational forms assumed reflect, formally or informally, the doctrine of the church (ecclesiology) as well as the social and cultural milieu. Care institutions are a structured declaration of belief about how Christians should live in the world.[2]

In the early twentieth century, Ernst Troeltsch described the connection between social ethics and ecclesiology by examining how Christians organized in relation to the state. Though a strong argument can be made that Troeltsch's schema is inadequate when applied to non-Christian organizations, it remains useful in understanding American Christianity, especially when supplemented with the sociological work of H. Richard Niebuhr. Troeltsch described three forms of societally based Christianity with Niebuhr adding a fourth. The terms are used here in the sociological sense, not as in common vernacular. These categories are ideal types. In other words, no single religious group fits perfectly in any category. Furthermore, religious organizations change self-understanding and relationship to the state and society over time. Still, the categories are good descriptions of tendencies.

The *state church* (called simply the "church" by Troeltsch) has a high degree of citizen-to-church-member correspondence, but with low expectations for personal religious experience. Generally, those born in a given nation-state are considered members unless they opt out. The *sect* requires voluntary affiliation and usually noteworthy religious experience, along with a high level of moral behavioral expectations. The *privatized syncretist* has a highly individualistic religion, with little ethical accountability because of low organizational affiliation, but high levels of personal religious experience (called "mystic" by Troeltsch, but his use of the term seems to disregard the strong connection of traditional Christian mystics—at least those prior to the Reformation—with the institutional church, so *privatized syncretist* is substituted). Privatized syncretists do sometimes form groups, though with loose affiliation and with some other characteristic, often social issues, serving to hold them together (e.g., contemporary Unitarians).

[2]This paragraph modified from James R. Thobaben, "Ecclesiology and Covenant: Christian Social Institutions in a Pluralistic Society," in *Living Responsibly in Community: Essays in Honor of E. Clinton Gardner*, ed. Fredrick E. Glennon, Gary S. Hauk and Darryl M.Trimiew (Lanham, Md.: University Press of America, 1997).

> history, it reached its apex in nineteenth-century America when sectarian fervor combined with voluntarism. Typically, these institutions (hospitals, retirement homes, colleges, etc.) were begun to meet specific needs as an expression of Christian concern and ministry. Increasingly, however, these institutions have little (if any) religious accountability or sensibility.[4]

Methodism, for instance, was a sect within the state church in England and upon its introduction to what became the United States functioned as a sectarian movement. Ironically, then, many of the health-care institutions that now remain may be Methodist, but are not Christian.[5] Methodist splinter groups, the best example being the Salvation Army, attempted into and through the twentieth century to maintain evangelical, sectarian distinctives in their service.

In the meantime, other evangelicals in the early twentieth century—of holiness, fundamentalist or Pentecostal varieties—did not usually develop public institutions, except doctrinally-specific colleges. Basically from the period of the Scopes trial until the election of Jimmy Carter, evangelicals stayed on the side of the public square. The rise of the Religious Right followed, and then the increased political diversity among evangelicals today. What has not occurred with the return of evangelicals to public life is a significant return to building institutions, other than educational.

The extent of this mix of desire and disdain conditions the degree of participation in the world and the shape of institutions. Recently, evangelicals have tended to create K–12 schools and colleges as places for Christian education but have not similarly built health-care facilities (except pregnancy centers)—at least not in the Western world. The lack of focus on domestic health care is partially due to the prioritizing. The need for distinctive educational alternatives is felt more strongly than the need for an explicit evangelical Christian presence in health care. Even more, the cost of building and maintaining health-care facilities or organizations and the general satisfaction of evangelicals with available facilities and organizations pushes developing new facilities or services down on the ministry priority list. While these points are reasonable, they should not eliminate organized evangelical health-care outreach.

Organizations are necessary. Reticence about participation because of the dirty hands one might get in the process is not a sufficient excuse for limiting

---

[4]Thobaben, "Ecclesiology and Covenant," p. 134.

[5]Ibid., p. 145.

serving ministries. Just as the church has organized to meet the spiritual needs of people throughout the world (Lk 24:47), so also the obligation of caring for physical needs has expanded and requires the coordinated use of resources. Consequently, there is moral demand to provide organizations, or to participate in organizations, that through economy of scale and division of labor can provide better health care and more health care.

Admittedly, claiming there is a moral demand for organized care should be concluded from the Scripture only with some hesitancy. The healings of Jesus and the apostles were, after all, miracles. Though interventions using technologies and bureaucracies delivered through group effort can sometimes appear miraculous, they are a blessing from God but are not miraculous in the usual sense of the word. The conclusion that organized care is acceptable, and sometimes mandated for believers, can be drawn (with great caution) from passages like the sending of the disciples two-by-two. In particular, evangelicals should be wary of the utility and power necessary for the functioning of any institution. Still, if believers do think that any participation in the public arena is warranted, then it should include cooperative participation in forming health-care institutions that are distinctly Christian or by participating in existing institutions without embarrassment for being Christian. These are the ways those in need can be served.

The expectations are high for Christian practitioners and organizations because "[f]rom everyone who has been given much, much will be demanded; and from the one who has been entrusted with much, much more will be asked" (Lk 12:48). Something is woefully inconsistent with paying executives huge amounts of money, building aesthetically stunning facilities, ignoring the indigent or downplaying the need for all to hear the gospel and then claiming to be Christian. It dishonors the name of Jesus. So does paternalistic "charity" given at a powerholder's whim, rather than *agape/caritas* given as an expression of the institutional Christian character.

What is not needed are more in-name-only Christian health-care institutions. If they look like all other health-care centers, then they have no reason to exist as a Christian institution. A desire to reassert Christian character must be evident. Christian character in a health-care institution is, minimally, evidenced by care for the forgotten poor, socially dismissed and inconvenient (such as persons with significant disabilities or the unborn), and the historically disregarded (especially persons of minority groups).

Practically speaking, establishing new hospitals in the United States is all but outside of reasonable consideration for economic reasons and, further, is unnecessary given the number of available hospital beds.[6] Likewise, Christians do not need to build more nursing homes for the middle and upper middle classes as persons in those groups can generally fend for themselves, or have family members who should assume more obligations. Evangelicals should develop facilities that meet needs at the margins of health care. These should include, but not be limited to, hospice facilities; housing alternatives for the impoverished or otherwise marginalized chronically ill; transitional living facilities for persons following physical rehabilitation; residential facilities for persons with mental illness and for persons with developmental disabilities; primary care missions into impoverished areas, especially by cooperating with congregations already present in poor urban and rural areas; formalized respite care programs; and additional refuge pregnancy centers.[7]

Believers should develop the organizations in such a way as to maintain the peculiar values of evangelicalism. Complete control over the values will not be possible with any health-care institution, especially when outside accrediting bodies (such as the The Joint Commission on the Accreditation of Healthcare Organizations with hospitals) wield considerable authority. To put it another way, Christian care facilities should be hospitable in the historical sense while offering services at the highest standards. Christian caregiving facilities should mix the virtue of hospitality with technical expertise and organizational savvy. In organizing or working in health-care organizations, believers should be as shrewd as serpents and as innocent as doves (Mt 10:16). The roots of Christian institutions go back to Christian providers developing habits of service—for instance, the outreach of monks and nuns in hostels—and, even further, back to Jesus healing his friend Lazarus out of concern for him and the community. Christian health-care providers and institutions should be true to this heritage.

---

[6]Political factors can also play a part. The Oral Roberts Hospital that was supposed to bring together medical education with a treatment approach that yoked traditional medicine, pastoral care and psychological support was a victim of financial over-extension, a lack of understanding about Certificate of Need, political pressure from those who disliked the project and overconfidence.

[7]A similar argument is in Erwin W. Lutzer, *Why the Cross Can Do What Politics Can't: When They See You, Do They See Jesus?* (Eugene, Ore.: Harvest House, 1999). This is from the evangelical literature, usually sold through Christian bookstores, that is commonly ignored by mainline/old-line churches and by secularists.

PART THREE: CHRISTIAN BIOETHICS AND THE WORLD

Health care institutions in the world operate as contract-oriented institutions composed of various professionals and support employees with widely varying value systems. Certainly, some of these institutions were and continue to be focused primarily on providing health care in the sense of caring for the individuals served. For most, caring is strongly limited by demands of various constituencies and individuals for money, prestige and so forth. This is not necessarily wrong, unless unchecked.

In the distant past, health-care institutions were good only for care in the narrowest sense, as the medical or surgical treatment was of dubious quality. Most in the West were monastically supported hospices or, eventually, state-supported once urbanization accelerated. People who were sick and indigent did find compassion in the best of the hospitals, near-imprisonment in the worst and iatrogenic infections in all of them. Truly significant improvements did not really come until the nineteenth century and, then, genuinely improved care with the increasingly availability of antibiotics in the mid-twentieth century.

After World War II, with antibiotics available and soldiers returning home with high expectations, along with the rise of the suburban middle class, standards for hospitals went up quickly. Hospital buildings went up quickly, as well. The Hill-Burton Act and other government and charitable initiatives led to rapid expansion of in-patient beds. In the 1960s hospitals began to become medical centers. They were funded by fee-for-service charges paid by Medicare and Medicaid, and by the insurance employers offered at the demand of the workforce. During this time the traditional language of professional virtue and leadership of the hospital by a physician gave way to the rights language of the social contract and leadership by professional administrators. To no little extent, this was spearheaded by the patient's right movement at the end of the 1960s and in the early 1970s. The moral reasoning was deontological and sometimes became legalistic. The social contract rules were boiled down to the principlism of the Belmont Report.

Principlism is useful in that it brings the categories of the U.S. social contract into a highly pluralistic setting, thus providing some basis for discussion. Unfortunately, the words were and are often tossed about without genuine consideration of what they mean or, worse, with people meaning quite different things while using the same words. When discussing a bioethical concern, one could hardly avoid hearing *autonomy, nonmaleficence, beneficence* and *justice* offered as if speaking them had the power of an incantation. The principles were helpful in breaking patterns of paternalism and maternalism, but became formulaic.

A leading defender of principlism says that the principles of "respect for autonomy, justice, nonmaleficence, and beneficence (including utility and proportionality)—along with such derivative rules as telling the truth, keeping promises, not violating privacy and maintaining confidentiality—are only prima facie binding . . . binding at first impression and . . . sufficient to establish rightness or wrongness of an act unless they are outweighed or overridden."[8] This is a bit of an exaggeration, as some of those "rules" existed long before principlism and the rest could be derived from other approaches to bioethics concerns. Still, there is significant value in the principlist approach as it provides a basic language for initiating conversation among strangers, and, as such, can be used by those who hold minority views, including (quite often) evangelicals, to receive a legitimate hearing in a bioethical discussion in a secular institution.

Principlism is, basically, an incomplete version of just war theory. When modified to include the remaining criteria (noted in parentheses in italics), the principalist approach facilitates genuine discourse. Decisions should be made

- seeking the best for the patient first, but also for the community *(just cause);*
- not to facilitate unrelated goals of practitioners or family members *(right intention);*
- so that interventions, costs and possible suffering are commensurate to the treatment goal (*proportionality*; this is similar to "do no harm" or nonmaleficence);
- because circumstances indicate that the status quo is problematic *(last resort);*
- on the basis of a probability analysis that this treatment is superior to alternatives *(reasonable chance of success);*
- by the patient or the person selected by the patient or a person having a sustained relationship with the patient, though others may provide nonpaternalistic, nonmaternalistic professional guidance (*legitimate authority;*

[8]James F. Childress, "A Principle-Based Approach," in *A Companion to Bioethics*, ed. Helga Kuhse and Peter Singer (Oxford: Blackwell, 1998), pp. 66-67.

this is the principle of autonomy for both the patient and freedom of conscience for the practitioner);

- so as to not adversely affect others directly or through the setting of precedent *(discrimination).*

The main disadvantage of an excessive emphasis on principlism in practice has been that autonomy becomes the dominant value and, in turn, is used to justify two major bioethical immoralities—the euthanizing of those with disabilities and elective abortion.

Many other bioethical concerns, however, arise in health-care institutions because of an emphasis on an entirely different form of moral reasoning—utilitarianism. In the 1990s rights contractualism, while not disappearing entirely, gave up moral territory to managed care. Though frequently attacked as evil opportunism foisted by greedy corporations, there are good reasons why managed care appeared and why some form of managed care is good for the recipients of medical care. However, in excess it can lead to significant moral concerns.

What is managed care?[9] It is the coordination of patient care through the health-care system, usually by an agent of the payor. Managed care at its best facilitates care from prevention through rehabilitation and lowers costs to the individual and society. At its worst, it is costly to the patient, callous and leads to the further marginalization of the disabled and chronically ill. The dominant moral language of managed care is utilitarianism, the business contract rather than the social contract.

Utilitarianism is a useful (this term selected intentionally) tool at a secondary level of analysis. Indeed, it would be irresponsible to not take into account the costs and benefits of given actions. Members of the social contract should favor the organizational use of utilitarianism, but in a restricted manner that allows certain socially shared values to trump utility.[10]

Utilitarianism is extraordinarily susceptible to abuse. First, utilitarianism assumes a decision made prior to calculation in which the guiding value is determined. Whether it is interests, pleasure or anything else, there must be some basis for deciding such will be the value maximized. Abuse arises when

---

[9]Much of the following is modified from James R. Thobaben, "The Impact of Managed Care on the Moral Character of Rehabilitation Institutions," *Journal of Head Trauma Rehabilitation* 12, no. 1 (1997): 10-20.

[10]Allen E. Buchanan, "The Right to a Decent Minimum of Health Care," *Philosophy and Public Affairs* 13, no. 1 (winter 1984): 55-78.

the powerful determine the value to be counted in such a way that they benefit. People with power tend to intentionally or unintentionally validate their own social positions and support their own desires in the selection of values and measuring of utility. Second, the calculations are extraordinarily difficult to make. After all, what constitutes a unit of happiness or pleasure or interest? Utilitarianism works when money is what counts precisely because money can be counted. Third, anything not easily measured tends to not be measured and, therefore, disregarded. This is particularly important to Christians, as it is hard to count the worth of salvation or the units of mercy or the score for healing a soul. It may be that such things should not be funded in secular health care, but they should not be demeaned nor should the opportunity of patients and providers to offer such for themselves and others be denied. Utilitarian-dominant organizations tend to be intolerant of what cannot be counted or what their leaders think should not be counted. Fourth, outlying individuals, those defined as not fitting the usual treatment protocols or who are defined as having a quality of life that makes living not worth it (note the near-economic utilitarian language) are threatened with service withdrawal or simply ignored.

Managed care is not brand new. It has been the organizational pattern for years in the Veterans Affairs system, in the military, for rehabilitation, in some nursing homes and in some psychiatric institutions. Why, then, is there such high visibility now? Most importantly, because it now affects the middle-class and the United States is a middle-class nation. Managed care has moved from governmental systems and facilities treating the marginalized to the broader population. Also, not-for-profits have adopted the management approach. Some factors pushing managed care are the trends of the business world. Among those are

- increasing emphasis on information management;
- downsizing as a means of saving money;
- downgrading (hiring at lower levels of professional competence) to save money;
- corporation buyouts (seen as consolidation in health care);
- for-profits, not-for-profits and government adopting sales and marketing strategies;
- rise of marketable product lines;

- appropriation of continuous quality improvement in business, education and health care;
- growth of self-insurance (combining funding mechanisms with other functions of insurance and health care).

But the change to managed care also occurred because employers in other sectors of the American economy have raised the issue of health-care costs to the point that it has become a political topic. Employers, the primary purchasers of health-care services after the government, want to purchase a package with a continuum of care that lowers costs—not only the costs of the actual treatment, but also of the managing of the health insurance benefit. Or they want the government to assume all the responsibility.

Managed care is based on certain assumptions about health-care delivery. First, continuity of treatment leads to higher quality of care. The absence of coherent treatment programs from prevention through acute care and into rehabilitation and reentry was one of the primary weaknesses of the fee-for-service approach. Another weakness of fee-for-service was the excessive expenditures associated with doctors and hospitals being paid for doing as many expensive procedures as possible. Second, continuity of treatment under managed care can provide equal or higher quality at lower costs. Third, this can be assured if the process is overseen by the payor or the payor's agent, not users or practitioners. The employers who pushed for managed care argued not only was this a matter of efficiency in health care, it was also their market right as the real purchasers of the services. (This market right would be assumed by the nation-state under a single-payer/single-provider system; in turn, this would mean using constraint in the form of explicit rationing.) Fourth, continuity, quality and cost are quantifiable, and therefore measurable for purposes of evaluation.

Currently in the United States, there is significant disagreement over the best way to perform this management task of maximizing utility in the distribution of health-care resources while protecting a basic minimum of services for all who are covered, helping to provide for those who are not covered, and protecting everyone's social contract rights. Moral problems with managed care tend to arise when utilitarianism and deontological reasoning, as well as the virtue claims of professional guilds and the demands of individuals that their values and virtuosity be protected, come into conflict.

Moral reasoning can be divided into four basic categories. Deontological thinking is category-based reasoning. The most famous philosophical example is Immanuel Kant. It is the primary language of the U.S. social contract. Utilitarianism is the end justifying the means. This form of reasoning philosophically arose at the end of the eighteenth and beginning of the nineteenth centuries, being most clearly stated by Jeremy Bentham and John Stuart Mill. Utilitarianism is teleological in that it is end- or goal-oriented (there is a *telos*—the maximization of "utility"—which is usually happiness or profit or interests). It is the primary moral reasoning method of the market and of conversations about pleasure and pain. When this same approach is applied with only consideration of one's personal experience of pain/pleasure it can be called *hedonism*. Another form of teleological thinking is virtue reasoning. In this the end conditions the means. The most famous philosophical examples are probably Thomas Aquinas and Aristotle. It is the traditional language of professional guilds and the typical language of families and religious communities. Finally, a form of moral reasoning that is often ignored is analogical thinking in which the moral appropriateness of an action is based on correspondence with other actions already deemed acceptable or unacceptable. The Christian philosopher Søren Kierkegaard exemplifies this in his extensive use of stories and Jesus used this in the telling of parables. This kind of language gets used to explain new concerns.[11]

Ideally, health-care institutions combine the various forms of moral reasoning, using values that find general agreement in the culture (middle axioms) or represent a specific community (e.g., a Catholic or evangelical institution), making those values clear before persons use services provided by the institution. This means the moral health-care institution at the end of modernity in the West will

[11]To further explain these forms of reasoning, one can turn to biblical examples. The Ten Commandments (though actually expressions of the covenant) are often thought of as rules and used deontologically. Caiaphas's decision is an example of utilitarianism. Paul's commendation to "have the attitude of Christ" in Philippians 2 is an example of virtue teleology. The call to imitate Christ is a call to virtuosity. The use of Israel as an analog for the church is analogical reasoning, as would be the warning to come away from a life of sin as Israel left Egypt in the exodus.

Consider a nonbioethical example: adultery. Christians should not commit adultery. Why? Some might assert that they should not because it is against the direct command of God (deontological reasoning). Some might say the moment of pleasure is severely outweighed by the eternal suffering, not to mention the personal anguish and social condemnation that might occur on earth (utilitarian teleological reasoning). Others might say they should not because to do so would push one off the path toward Christlikeness (virtue reasoning). Still others might conclude that the Scripture compares adultery frequently to idolatry and it must be considered similarly despicable by God (analogical reasoning). Indeed, the Christian might legitimately use all these forms of reasoning to conclude that the act is immoral.

- have leaders who can explain the basic purpose (telos) in morally coherent language compatible with the social contract and/or the values of the originating organization;
- hire virtuous individuals as providers (virtuosity as technical skills and virtuosity of personal character);
- enforce specific minimum expectations in behavior and skills for patients and staff;
- measure quality of care/practice (including "soft" aspects of care) in order to evaluate outcomes;
- intentionally involve payors;
- protect outliers as rights-holders;
- protect the institution through efficiencies that do not violate other expectations (accept the reality of the market while realizing health care is never a completely open exchange among equally knowledgeable participants);
- view contract participants, family members, practitioners, administrators and suppliers as members of a community in which their individual interests must be considered while recognizing the value of the whole and, in so doing, promoting institutional values;
- recognize individuals are members of other communities of value.

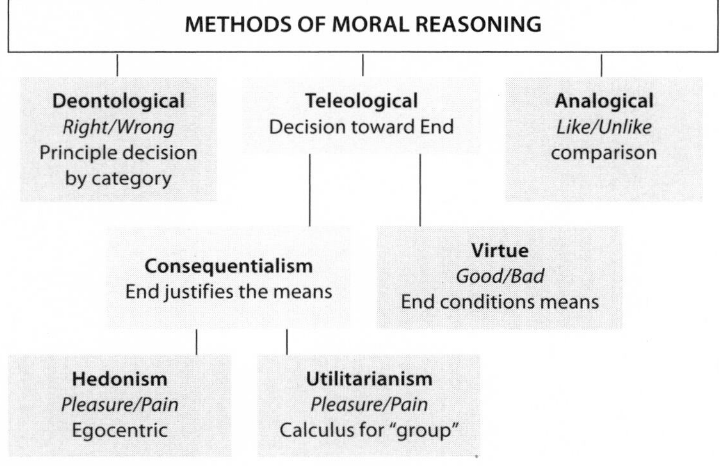

Figure 10.2.

CONCLUSION

Christians should recognize the need to develop and maintain health-care institutions. To do so, the institution must not operate at a loss or must depend on contributions to make up the difference in expenditures and income. Given the changes in technology and the growing disconnection (breakdown in kinship obligation) in society, such organizations are necessary. Especially in the West, given the strong power of market forces, utilitarianism tends to rise in significance as an ethical reasoning method in health-care organizations. There is nothing wrong with this. But utilitarianism should never be the primary means of moral evaluation for health-care organizations. Certainly, the market can function in health care, either in the future patient selecting a managed care provider or insurance companies determining which providers to use or in the government or corporations deciding on insurers, and so forth. What is not necessary is for utilitarianism to become the dominant form of moral reasoning in such institutions.

Secular institutions should operate with the basic standards of the social contract as the foundation. Currently, this means respecting basic negative rights (rights of noninterference). If health care is defined as an entitlement, then the right to the basic minimum must also be foundational. The institution must also use utilitarianism. Even a not-for-profit must operate in the black—if not directly through operations, then from charitable giving or governmental supplement. Just as importantly, the institution must be organizationally tolerant, leaving room for virtuosity. Practitioners can legitimately appeal to the moral standards of their various guilds, but also the institution should be structured to leave room for the values and virtues of the individual patient's and practitioner's community of value.

When Christians and nonbelievers have established some shared goals for the broader community, they can and should work together to accomplish them. In health care this means developing and maintaining more and more diverse health-care settings. When Christians cannot participate in such joint efforts or when such cannot or will not be initiated by others, then the faithful are obligated to serve the broader community in the name of Jesus Christ by facilitating the provision of high quality health care through new organizational efforts. In particular, evangelicals should establish institutions that fill the gaps of the health-care system, especially for the poor and otherwise marginalized. Such institutions should be explicitly and unapologetically Christian.

When Jesus sent out the disciples two-by-two to heal, he did so with the full expectation that the organized effort to end physical suffering would be more successful, in part, because it was organized. Yet such efforts will never be entirely adequate. Those who banded together to care for Lazarus and then his grieving sisters could not keep him alive and could not provide them with complete comfort. Only Christ could do this. That did not relieve them of the duty to do all they could.

11

Societal Membership and Rights

HUMANS AS CITIZENS

Justice is the ordering of creation as intended by God. Though believers may seek to express the deeper justice of that intention in their relationships with each other, in the broken world the original justice can only be approximated. Relationships, especially among moral acquaintances, strangers and enemies, are best managed with procedures and rules derived from social contracts under which key aspects of the original justice are maintained. These contracts are built on the assumption that individuals have intrinsic worth expressed morally by forming political entities specifically to protect those rights in a fallen world. Importantly for bioethics, negative rights (or rights of noninterference) are prior to and foundational for the social contract. Positive rights or rights of entitlement, while not natural in the sense of existing before the contract, can be established by the agreement of the contact makers. One such right would be a right to health care. These positive rights cannot be instituted in a fallen world except in given places under given agreements and with given resources. Regardless, Christians should do all they can to meet health-care needs in every society. Negative rights, on the other hand, should apply everywhere whether or not the social contractors have agreed on such.

> But some of them went to the Pharisees and told them what Jesus had done. Then the chief priests and the Pharisees called a meeting of the Sanhedrin.
>
> "What are we accomplishing?" they asked. "Here is this man performing many miraculous signs. If we let him go on like this, everyone will believe in him, and then the Romans will come and take away both our place and our nation."
>
> Then one of them, named Caiaphas, who was high priest that year, spoke up, "You know nothing at all! You do not realize that it is better for you that one man die for the people than that the whole nation perish."
>
> He did not say this on his own, but as high priest that year he prophesied that Jesus would die for the Jewish nation, and not only for that nation but also

> for the scattered children of God, to bring them together and make them one. So from that day on they plotted to take his life. (Jn 11:46-53)

PART ONE: THE TEXT

During Jesus' trial, Pontius Pilate recognized that killing Jesus was unjust. He rhetorically asked, "What crime has the man committed?" (Mk 15:14). None. Jesus was being deprived of his rights (though the language of rights was not developed in the contemporary sense of the term). Jesus' rights were abrogated and he was executed. For Pilate, the killing of Jesus prevented a riot and satisfied some local officials. He had no standard against which such an injustice itself could ultimately be judged; after all, "what is truth?" (Jn 18:38). This sounds more like nihilism than belief in any moral standard. Simply, he did not want the irritation of dealing any longer with the Christ and his followers.

For Caiaphas, the high priest, the death of Jesus was justified with more subtle reasoning. Using what is now called utilitarianism, the priest argued that it was better that the one should die, that the nation might live. As with all pure utilitarian reasoning, rights were meaningless—Jesus' rights under Jewish law were dismissed with superficial adherence to procedures. Even while condemning the high priest's character, ironically, the Text declares that Caiaphas's calculus was faulty morally but not finally incorrect—ultimately God would use Caiaphas's decision.

The dialogue between Pilate and Christ at his so-called trial and the conversation of Caiaphas with the rest of the Sanhedrin the night before reveal two truths for Christians about social justice. The first is that justice requires a standard for judgment, a truth. Justice requires that individuals be judged as intrinsically of value. Individuals do have basic rights, or ways they should be justly treated. The fact that Caiaphas's staged religious trial appears so unjust demonstrates there is a minimal standard. Even those who think Jesus was a false Messiah must acknowledge the trial was immoral. An innocent man was killed. Pilate's wife acknowledged such, saying, "Don't have anything to do with that innocent man, for I have suffered a great deal today in a dream because of him" (Mt 27:19). Second, justice requires consideration of what is good for the group, as well as how the group and others treat the given individual. Evangelicals, out of justice and love, must care for each person and for the group of persons in their "calculus" of morality. No individual can be forgotten or deemed insignificant for the sake of the total happiness or the overall minimization of pain. And yet, the group should not be destroyed for a disproportionate individual want or even need.

Drawing from its Reform stream, which in turn was reaching back to the arguments of Augustine, evangelical theology often includes the assertion that Jesus' death satisfied the demands of justice—divine justice, not human justice. Additionally, debates using various theories of the atonement center on how the standard of justice relates to the omnipotent God who is subject to no morality, but himself generates morality. Regardless, there is no disagreement that Jesus was completely deprived of earthly justice. As the prophecy traditionally applied to this event from Isaiah, in one of the Servant Songs, states:

> He was despised and rejected by men,
> a man of sorrows, and familiar with suffering.
> Like one from whom men hide their faces
> he was despised, and we esteemed him not.
> Surely he took up our infirmities
> and carried our sorrows,
> yet we considered him stricken by God,
> smitten by him, and afflicted.
> But he was pierced for our transgressions,
> he was crushed for our iniquities;
> the punishment that brought us peace was upon him,
> and by his wounds we are healed. . . .
> By oppression and judgment he was taken away.
> And who can speak of his descendants?
> For he was cut off from the land of the living;
> for the transgression of my people he was stricken.
> He was assigned a grave with the wicked,
> and with the rich in his death,
> though he had done no violence,
> nor was any deceit in his mouth. (Is 53:3-6, 8-9)

The reality of this earthly injustice, even though it served the purpose of eternal justice, compels Christians to act against the kind of behaviors that were exemplified in the treatment of the Lord. The social activity of Christians must be opposite that of Pilate and Caiaphas. There is a standard of truth and that truth guides believers in knowing that individuals have rights and the community has value.

The demand for justice arising out of the Christ's egregious mistreatment amplifies Jesus' stated concern for the poor, the sick, the broken and the lost. Christians are required to exhibit a similar attitude and corresponding behavior. Depending on the circumstances of one's civic location, including whether or not one is subject to genuine persecution for being a Christian, this concern may be expressed in political engagement. This does not necessarily mean staging protests to get other people to adhere to a particular Christian moral position, but it may include efforts to create a more just society for all, including for Christians. While living in a social contract state, proper procedures and reasonable protections of justice are a legitimate, albeit small, expression of divine righteousness, and believers can legitimately advocate for them.

In the case of Jesus bar Joseph the Nazarene, the rights of which he was deprived were negative rights, that is, rights to noninterference. In the broadest form, negative rights protect the individual from unwarranted intrusion from the state and from other individuals. Negative rights include the right to free speech, religious association and so on. When the Sanhedrin and Roman authorities arrested, abused and finally killed Jesus, they abrogated his right to not be imprisoned and deprived of life. Those rights, from an evangelical point of view, are based on the identity of every human being as a bearer of the image of God. Rights are evident in the underlying values of the Text, even if not in the specific language later developed by eighteenth-century political philosophers. Again, using the example of the killing of Jesus, Jesus' betrayal by Judas is often thought of in personal terms, of a friend turning on a friend; but as is clear from Judas's words, there was also a sense that the action violated rights.

> When Judas, who had betrayed him, saw that Jesus was condemned, he was seized with remorse and returned the thirty silver coins to the chief priests and the elders. "I have sinned," he said, "for I have betrayed innocent blood."
>
> "What is that to us?" they replied. "That's your responsibility."
>
> So Judas threw the money into the temple and left. Then he went away and hanged himself. (Mt 27:3-5)

The limit to the notion of rights at that time and in that place, and the critique of that limit by the Scriptures' authors, is also evidenced in the description of the beheading of John the Baptist. Another clear example of negative rights is Paul's appeal to Caesar, though in that case the plea is not based on negative rights existing prior to the state, but on a citizenship-based claim (Acts 25:11). Underlying the scriptural presentation of the stories of Jesus' crucifixion, of John the Baptist's execution, and even of Paul's failed appeal is that these were just men who did not deserve to die according to a reasonable standard evident to all, a standard that today might be called negative rights.

While this is the assumption made in the Text, it was certainly not the claim of the Roman Empire or the Herodians. Likewise, even today, in various places in the world, core rights are not properly acknowledged. Notably or notoriously, depending on one's interpretation, some philosophers at the end of modernity are asserting that the notion of rights posited by a Creator on every human being is preposterous. At best, they claim, rights are a useful social construction. At worst, the entire notion of rights should be abandoned, they assert, for the purpose of the masses (or the greater interests of this or that individual) so that inevitably the weak are crushed. Evangelicals should and must disagree.

The starting assumption of the American social contract upon which the whole civil structure is based is that some core negative rights belong to each person prior to being part of any state. Negative rights are intrinsic to human nature, or at least everyone should act as if they are. And the United States, and much of the West as well as international organizations like the United Nations, claim that rights are inherent or natural (even if they do not act on that assumption).

Positive rights are the right *to* interference from the state or some other authority in order to obtain some highly valued (and limited) good. In less complicated and more affirming language, a positive right is a right of entitlement. Some lists of positive rights include the right to education, to health care and so on. The New Testament does not seem endorse or deny positive rights. This makes sense given that the New Testament church is a community of the culturally marginal and often socially marginal, not engaged in political change per se. Earlier models of civil responsibility requiring provision for other tribal members and for sojourners under chieftains or Old Testament regents come closer to the concept of positive rights than anything presented in the New Testament.

Mark's description of the healing of the woman with the flow of blood makes no comment about who should have paid for the services she received. He does include (while Matthew does not) that she suffered under the failed treatments of doctors. Being sick had been costly for this woman, both physically and economically. For what it is worth, the physician-author Luke does not include this incident in his Gospel, though he does note elsewhere that people were healed by touching the edge of Jesus' garments. Still, there is no condemnation of doctors nor is there a statement that everyone has a right to access medical care. She is coming to Jesus simultaneously out of poverty and in the hope of the near desperate. No right to care is asserted in the report of the incident.

> A large crowd followed and pressed around him. And a woman was there who had been subject to bleeding for twelve years. She had suffered a great deal under the care of many doctors and had spent all she had, yet instead of getting better she grew worse. When she heard about Jesus, she came up behind him in the crowd and touched his cloak, because she thought, "If I just touch his clothes, I will be healed." Immediately her bleeding stopped and she felt in her body that she was freed from her suffering.
>
> At once Jesus realized that power had gone out from him. He turned around in the crowd and asked, "Who touched my clothes?"
>
> "You see the people crowding against you," his disciples answered, "and yet you can ask, 'Who touched me?'"
>
> But Jesus kept looking around to see who had done it. Then the woman, knowing what had happened to her, came and fell at his feet and, trembling with fear, told him the whole truth. He said to her, "Daughter, your faith has healed you. Go in peace and be freed from your suffering." (Mk 5:24-34)

While the New Testament writings have little anticipation that the state will provide entitlements, there is a powerful expectation that those within the body are to care for one another and should expect care from one another. In another healing miracle, this one recorded by Mark and Luke, friends fulfill their duty to serve one another in a time of sickness by carrying the paralytic to the healer, Jesus (Lk 5:17-26). Their duty to do so was based on the *phileo*, familial or fellowship love, and perhaps on the *agape*, self-sacrificing love. The Christian is obligated to care for his or her own biological family and those of the fellowship (the "brothers and sisters") and, though apparently in a lesser degree, to render care to the acquaintance and the stranger. This care included then and includes now health care. It was not based so much on the existence of a positive right held by all humans as on the moral character of the provider—caritas in its truest sense.

Though the foundations for negative rights can be readily derived from the New Testament, such is not a primary moral language in the Text. Still, it is certain that the reasoning of Caiaphas is not acceptable to believers precisely because of its injustice. That leaves natural rights the best alternative for a society not governed with Christian values. The lack of specific rights language in the New Testament is not particularly problematic for the evangelical. As to whether the ready acceptance of negative rights translates into the acceptance of any or all positive rights currently being discussed in the United States—education from preschool through college, welfare assistance and health care—is another question.

PART TWO: CHRISTIAN BIOETHICS

It is not true that one's duties inevitably generate rights for another. The believer has a duty to serve the poor, but that does not mean that a particular poor person can demand particular social goods from a particular believer. The inverse, though, is true. One's rights generate at least some duties for others.

In the case of what are often called negative rights, the primary duty generated is simply to not impede someone in his or her practice of religion, speech and so on. The cost is relatively low—leave other people alone. Also, under the social contract, there is an additional duty to pay taxes and generally facilitate the protection of everyone from external or internal threats to those rights. The duty of noninterference is a duty that exists prior to the social contract, but is enforceable only by the contract or by what the earliest contract theorists called a war of all against all. The former is far more efficient, and cooperation is the shared risk and cost to protect everyone in the contract. The duty is double-layered: do not interfere with other's rights and sacrifice enough to protect the contract as a whole. Negative rights are a remnant of the original justice of God. They are an expression of his will for the relationships of persons with each other. In the broken world, these rights can only be maintained by banding together against those who would threaten them. The primary reason for a state existing is protection of the negative rights. However, people who have banded together can expand their rights.

Positive rights do not exist outside of the contract. As an expression of the community, the members of a social contract (in the case at hand that would be those under the U.S. Constitution) may assign rights of entitlement. These must be distributed justly, which means fairly and with disinterested procedures. The costs, too, must be justly distributed. This usually means fair taxation to pay for the provisions such as the right to education or right to basic welfare or, arguably, the right to health care. Positive rights or rights of entitlement are not rights of noninterference, but essentially rights to interference in the form of some social good. Obviously disagreements arise over whether an entitlement does or should exist, how it is distributed, and how the burden of providing it (primarily through taxation) is distributed.

Positive rights are always contingent on negative rights. In other words, under the contract one cannot be entitled to a given social good in a manner that would create a greater injustice (especially of negative rights) for others. Positive rights require fair distribution of benefits and burdens, though that does not always mean identical or equal distribution. This is unlike negative rights which everyone should have in equal proportion. In some situations, rights are balanced, but positive rights should never take priority over negative rights except in the most dire of circumstances, and then only temporarily.

The difficulty of balancing rights is obvious. For example, some would claim that everyone should have an equal opportunity to a given job on the basis of qualifications with no secondary characteristics considered. Others might say affirmative action is appropriate to redress past wrongs, but only to correct the lack of reasonably equal opportunity. Still others might argue that quotas should be put in place temporarily to force a justice order. It, however, would always be unjust to have quotas, "cronyism," nepotism or racism as the basis for determining who obtained employment or a position in a school. Procedures of distribution must be fair, which means that the principle of individual liberty and the principle of equality among individuals constrain each other under the social contract.

The balancing of entitlement with freedom means the positive right must always be limited. The educational right, for instance, does not include any nursery school the parents prefer nor the college of one's choice. Some argue that the education entitlement should be expanded to cover preschool and after-school with the debate taking shape around the social function of parenting and economic opportunity for parents. While that may be a legitimate argument, it is not appropriate to assume that entitlement rights can be expanded ad infinitum. Resources limit entitlements, but even more so, liberty limits entitlement.

In practice, it seems that basic housing and food, through various welfare programs, are entitlements as well. Though these are not so outlined in the U.S. social contract, they would generally be accepted as such by most Americans. This does not mean one is entitled to the most expensive food or a house in a gated community with satellite television. This entitlement has always been restricted, as any positive right must be. For both education and welfare, the main debate is about which limits should exist and to what extent.[1] One side claims that without proper entitlement, other rights—even negative rights—will be effectively curtailed. The other side declares that the "pursuit of happiness," not "happiness" itself, is a basic right.

Entitlement, or not, to health care is even more complex ethically, including for Christians. Given the lack of direct biblical guidance about health-care services that did not even exist in the time of the writing of the Scrip-

---

[1]Since the Personal Responsibility and Work Opportunity Reconciliation Act of 1996 was enacted, certain expressions of this entitlement have a time limit.

tures, it is most appropriate to consider historical Christian sources for some kind of moral instruction. Such sources must be evaluated on the basis of general compatibility with the core doctrinal and moral assertions of the faith that can be verified by the Text. Also, as historical sources, they can and must be evaluated by the outcome of the moral choices over time. In addition, when using any extrabiblical sources, believers must clearly test whether their decisions are simply reflections of the values of the culture in which they live.

Prior to the church being formally accepted within the Roman Empire, Christians were distinguished by the care they gave one another and strangers, especially the sick and desperately needy. Soon after Constantine's edict, Basil of Caesarea in the fourth century founded a facility for treating the sick. Throughout the Middle Ages, churches in the West were sites for much of the medical care. By the 1200s churches and monasteries had assumed the social responsibility for providing hospitality in primitive forms of what are now called hospices and hospitals. In the English-speaking world, the most famous prior to the Reformation was St. Mary of Bethlehem, which eventually became an asylum for the mentally ill known by the shortened name Bedlam.

After the turmoil of the Reformation, the Protestants reexamined how health care was rendered. In Britain, Guy's Hospital and Thomas' Hospital were developed for serving the sick, with special provision for those injured in war. Most famously, Puritan Thomas Sydenham changed how medical care was provided in the English-speaking world, emphasizing the need for the empirical verification of treatments. In addition, he was a friend of Boyle's and extraordinarily influential on his apprentice, John Locke. Sydenham promoted care for the suffering, including those suffering during the 1665 plague. Still, at that time, except for those who had been injured while serving in war, there did not seem to be an assumed right to health care. Care and public health interventions were provided, including by the civil government—not as a right but as a duty for civil well-being or as charity.[2]

In the preevangelical Protestant tradition, Calvinists and, to a lesser extent, Pietists sought social change. Jonathan Edwards, who laid much of the intellectual foundation for the Great Awakening, strongly believed in the political protection of Native Americans. John Wesley, in his time, declared the legitimacy of political activism in the matter of slavery, not only activities like Wilberforce's but going so far as to assert the acceptability of violent rebellion

---

[2]Daniel Defoe, *A Journal of the Plague Year*, originally published in 1722. See Project Gutenberg, <www.gutenberg.org/etext/376>.

by those in bondage.[3] He also made strong appeals to the personal moral obligations of those who might have held slaves, prohibiting the ownership of slaves among the Methodists. With slavery, as with so many other justice issues, Wesley called for personal reform, for care of those hurt by the social sin, and for societal reorganization. The Wesleys also asserted that society should protect the freedom and life of all, claiming that the state under certain circumstances should control prices, use rent control, offer opportunities for education and so on. Both Edwards and Wesley asked for some health interventions by the state.

Through the first half of the nineteenth century in the United States, when evangelicals—at least those in the north—did participate in political activism, it was usually focused on obtaining respect for the negative rights of an oppressed people (the enslaved population of the southern United States). Finney and others used the New Testament endorsement of negative rights, the Christian notion of *caritas*, and combined the parable of the city on the hill with Old Testament theocratic obligations for the just distribution of social goods. Especially after the Civil War they even made claims about everyone having access to health care. In practice, there was little political activism for such, which makes sense given the technological limits of the medicine of the day. Health care was usually only given charitably to those defined as the deserving poor (e.g., widows, orphans), not as a right to which all could make appeal. As part of the broader Protestant triumphalism of that period, evangelicals supported the building of hospitals and sometimes medical and nursing schools.

At the end of the nineteenth and especially the beginning of the twentieth century, for reasons previously outlined, evangelicals began to sever relations with mainline Protestantism and withdraw from most political discourse at the national level. Certainly, local organized efforts and face-to-face support of the poor and sick continued, but rarely at society-wide levels. Engagement with the issue of abortion and the resurgence of evangelical political presence in the 1970s and 1980s began to change that. Contrary to the nineteenth century, there was much more ambivalence about the possibility of the state making society morally good, and most rights arguments were about restraining the government rather than about expanding entitlements.

[3]John Wesley, "Thoughts Upon Slavery," 1774 <http://gbgm-umc.org/umw/wesley/thoughtsuponslavery.stm>. See also John Wesley, "Letter to William Wilberforce," 1791 <http://new.gbgm-umc.org/umhistory/wesley/wilberforce/>. Both of these are published on the General Board for Global Ministries website of the United Methodist Church.

Generally, evangelicals at the beginning of the twenty-first century continue to emphasize the right to life and the liberty to proclaim the gospel much more than call for positive rights to education, welfare or health care. Without displacing concern for protecting negative rights, including the expectation that evangelicals will be tolerated by the broader society, a renewed look at the possibility of supporting some entitlement rights should occur in the church.

To state the obvious, health care has significantly changed from the early days of evangelicalism. The knowledge of how to prevent and treat disease has grown phenomenally. The ability to provide services and "empower" persons with chronic and disabling conditions so that they can "function" in society has been equally impressive. Though the moral obligation of Christians to take care of themselves and to provide care to others in difficult situations has not changed, the capacity for successfully treating disease and injury now makes possible more efficacious responses to the needs of others. Christians should consider the possibility of an entitlement right for those residing in the United States because health care has improved and the society has the economic capacity to fund it. While such a positive right is not intrinsic to human nature or constitutionally mandated, it is compatible with the gospel and may be a more effective means of meeting ongoing individual and social needs. In other words, evangelicals can support a right to health care if (1) it works, (2) it does not become an excuse to significantly impede other rights and (3) it does not corrupt the church.

There are three great risks in all this. First, it might not work. Entitlements tend to generate bureaucracies and bureaucracies are not well known for innovation or for compassion, both of which are desirable characteristics for health care. On the other hand, any provision of entitlement services will require large scale management and accountability. The price is worth it, if the price is not too great. The right to health care is similar to the positive right for education. It must take a particular form in the United States because this is a particular society. For education, that means an assurance of schooling through the secondary level, though in other nations apprenticeships might be the best expression of such an entitlement and it might be best managed by the family, not the state. Similarly, health care must be tailored to U.S. circumstances. The notion of entitlement, as opposed to precontract negative rights, is dependent on whether or not the entitlement makes sense for the society at the given time.

Second, as with any positive right, the more implementation demanded, the greater the risk for the loss of freedoms. Whenever someone has an entitlement, someone else has not only a duty to pay more in taxes but also to place less value on other things that might have been financed with that money. There is a lost opportunity cost, and though a right to health care is not illogical for evangelicals, it should be asserted only with every effort to not diminish other freedoms. Not only does this mean there should be limits on taking money through taxation, but also individuals should have maximum freedom even if that freedom means being free to do stupid things with their own health. For that reason, this right to health care, if implemented, should be some kind of voucher-mandated insurance or cooperatives system that would assure a minimum level of care along with maximum individual choice.

Third, Christian duty does not lessen if the entitlement is implemented. Believers remain personally responsible with a Christian duty to care for those in immediate need. Believers are supposed to take care of themselves, help others and work toward a just social order. It would be simple to deny, if health-care treatment is a right, any sense of obligation to take care of oneself or, conversely, take orders from government bureaucrats setting standards for healthy behavior. Likewise, it would be easy to fall again into the trap of believing that Christians have ministered if this or that political candidate or referendum is supported. People can vote all they want for the correct causes, but if they do not assume an obligation for their own well-being or if they fail to minister personally to the sick, injured and dying when called by God to do so, then they are in sin.

Indeed, the greatest condemnation of evangelicals today is that so few recognize their responsibility to provide personal care, either in their homes or through the giving of their time and money, to the socially marginalized or even to their own families. Further, some do not even take care of themselves. Given the tendencies in American Protestantism, it would be easy for the Religious Right to place all the blame on the victims and for the Left to seek health-care salvation through the state. The Right should know that whether or not someone "caused" his or her illness does not change the believer's requirement to minister, including through changes in society to maximize the life and liberty of all. Likewise, the Left should not delude itself into believing that lobbying is a substitute for caring for individuals or respecting the temple of the Holy Spirit through reasonable discipline and personal purity (1 Cor 6:19).

All believers must assert a biblically-validated moral obligation to care for the Christian brother and sister and to care for the neighbor. This does not imply a right in the legal sense. For instance, the good Samaritan saw injustice and acted out of charity in the moral sense of *agape/caritas*. His actions did not arise from a legal obligation (legal in our twenty-first-century U.S. sense—it was a legal responsibility in accordance with the Pentateuch). It was not a duty to someone generated by that person's rights. It was not a duty derived from his social position in the civil society, neither a *noblise oblige* manifest in paternalistic/materialistic notions of charity nor the duty of the lesser to render services to a social superior. The Samaritan had a duty, but the injured man had no legal claim on that specific Samaritan. Rather, it arose from the character of the Samaritan, who had given himself over to the way of God.

Laws can be better or worse, but even the best are never more than partial goods. Committed Christians should never think they will have less to do in serving the disenfranchised (in this case, by illness or injury) by virtue of some law. A legal right always implies a duty for others, but all moral duties do not arise from legal rights and Christians have higher moral duties. If a neighbor is in need, then the believer is compelled to help, given resources and abilities, in a manner that will meet that need. A believer can legitimately advocate for a neighbor's right to health care, but never at the expense of losing accountability for his or her own behavior or diminishing the obligation to care for familial needs, nor at the cost of lost religious liberty.

The society has a duty to its citizens that might include some health care, given the changes in society's capacity to provide and the importance of health for functioning in a late-modern society. Also, Christians have a duty to care for those who are sick that arises from the general Christian obligation to those who suffer. The question for believers is to what extent do these two duties (that of the state for citizens and of Christians for people who suffer) correspond? Or, to consider a specific implication, should the believer go beyond his or her understanding of his or her own duty to the sick to advocate for the legal right to health care and, hence, to argue for the duty of society and all its members (including nonbelievers) to provide for it?

There is no clear biblical requirement to support a positive right to health care. There is, likewise, no clear biblical argument against such an entitlement. A Christian "yes" to a health-care entitlement is based on the current possibilities of Western societies. Further, there is no coherent argument that such a positive right is intrinsic in a social contract society. Christian support arises out of the functions of citizenship as they work out in this specific society. In the case of the United States, entitlements can be justified only as they directly or indirectly support the pursuit of happiness or the individual *telos*. Evangelicals, then, must decide about a right to health care on the basis of their being both citizens of an earthly land and citizens of a heavenly kingdom.

PART THREE: CHRISTIAN BIOETHICS AND THE WORLD

Americans generally do not die of malnutrition, usually do not drink their own sewage, and are inoculated against childhood diseases. The risk of early death is significantly lower than during the nineteenth century or first half of the twentieth century for virtually the entire population of the nation. Unfortunately, while the public health in the United States is generally good, and though acute care has astoundingly improved over the past fifty years, the treatment and prevention of individual disorders is nowhere near as well managed as it could be. For a significant portion of the population, health care is poorly or sporadically delivered through emergency rooms, public health clinics and church charities. Health care is not formally, but is in practice, a right in the United States—but one poorly distributed.

Currently, there are distribution problems with health care—both of macroallocation and microallocation. A limited resource is distributed among those with competing claims. At one level, the resource of concern is the services and supplies for individual treatment—medical equipment, drugs and so on—but given that the United States and most of the world operates on an intermediated exchange system—that is, not bartering, but using money—the resource of immediate concern is usually money. This can be quickly resolved by shifting funding away from other socially valued efforts to health care. That, though, would reveal macroallocation problems—questions about from where or from whom the money will come and what will be sacrificed in the process.

Regardless of how and who directly pays, positive rights or entitlements always involve cost to someone because limited resources always have value. This reality is what prevents the broader assignment of entitlements. For instance, there are significant arguments over whether or not the application of public moneys to education, accrued through taxation, are worth the cost—the cost to taxpayers and the lost opportunity cost of not having that tax money for other governmental purposes or for personal use by the taxpayer.

To put it simply, there are doubts the society is getting its money's worth.

Arguably, higher taxation or shifting funds from other federal and state programs would lead to a healthier population that would then produce more goods and services. This is an argument used for public education. It is a "trickle-down" theory of funding. But instead of running from large corporations, it runs from large government entities. The claim in the case of health care is that putting the money into the treatment of individuals means they will get healthier and they will use that health to produce more, which in turn will provide more funding to pay for more health care as well as other social goods. Of course, that is by no means assured. Perhaps healthier people, especially the many aging people in the United States, will simply extend retirement or the many immigrants will simply go back or send funds home. And soon the health-care right will look like a failed Ponzi scheme. Or perhaps the system would hold together but get increasingly expensive. Opportunities would be lost because of expenditures with the whole nation losing competitive advantage as do some U.S. corporations now.

Whenever considering entitlements, a starting point must be the recognition that the positive right must be limited by economics. While true that health care will generate money as new technologies are developed and sold, such society-wide profits are not significant compared to the cost. Also, it is true that a healthier population can work better than a sick one and the improvement in the overall economy will tend to help raise funds for the government. And, perhaps, some companies will become more competitive in some markets as their health care costs are spread across the society. Yet another truth is that paying for health care will require drawing resources or effort from other sectors of society to resolve even the most basic concerns of prevention, acute treatment and rehabilitation. Individuals who could use that money in other ways will have to provide it via taxation for those who cannot pay.

An entitlement, then, is an intrusion on the liberty of others. The only way such can be justified is if that infringement is relatively minimal and leads to significant benefit not only for other individuals but for the society as a whole, including those who disproportionately pay. In other words, while negative rights are evaluated on the basis of a deontological appeal to the intrinsic character of humans, entitlement rights must satisfy an additional standard of utility. Entitlement rights have to work at making society better by strengthening the capacity of marginal individuals to "pursue happiness" within the limits of the social contract, which in turn, strengthens that contract. Positive rights or entitlements are always conditioned by input and output, by the availability of resources, and by the effective use of those resources. They are conditional. They are conditioned by the emerging capacity of the society.

This can be understood most simply by considering that freedom of speech or of religion should look similar, whether in the United States or any place else in the world. To the contrary, health care as a right varies significantly through place and time—more can and should be expected in the U.S. at the beginning of the twenty-first century than in a rural area of a developing country in the nineteenth century. This is not to excuse inadequate health care elsewhere, but to acknowledge that since it is a positive distribution, it is necessarily shaped by circumstances. Emergent rights are based on the social capacity to provide and the improved possibility of fulfilling the individual *telos* (pursue happiness, in the sense offered in the U.S. Declaration of Independence). Negative rights are intrinsic to the human condition, foundational for the social contract, and nonnegotiable.

> In making the claim that health care should be a right, it is important to understand two things: (1) a right to health care may not functionally exist in other nations and still be appropriate for the United States, and (2) though not formal, health care is already distributed to most people in the United States, but very inefficiently. Additionally, though not readily demonstrable, I would argue that the legal formalization of the right to health care would, if properly administered, actually maximize the efficiency of health-care dollars already spent. If the emergency room is no longer a primary care center and persons are compelled to assume more responsibility for themselves earlier in disease processes, money in health care will be saved and health-related social losses will decrease.[4]

Unfortunately, distributing a limited social good is always complicated. First, the question of whether the right should exist at all must be legally resolved. Then come questions of efficiency, the maintenance of quality, the possibility of diminished innovation, ongoing costs (direct and indirect), and the curtailment of liberty through both taxation and the restriction of health-care choice. Three approaches offered to address these problems are libertarian, egalitarian and utilitarian. The citizenry should evaluate each, recognizing that all vested interests will not have the same interpretation of expectations nor the same evaluation of the costs, quality and so forth.

---

[4]James R. Thobaben, "A Wesleyan Argument for Responding to Real Needs: The Case for Action in Health Care," *Christian Social Action* (June/July 2001), pp. 3-6.

Libertarian arguments center around opening the market, assuming that competition will generate higher quality, and on freedom from the paternalistic/maternalistic intervention of the state. If disease treatments and disability assistance are fully subsidized, then there will be increasing numbers of persons with those difficulties—not that more may actually be sick, but more will assume sick roles because of various cultural and economic benefits. On the other hand, if (using the most extreme arguments) everything is deregulated—from credentialing through pharmaceuticals to insurance—then the market will create higher quality at cheaper rates, though certainly some outliers will fall to the side.[5] This will, most libertarians acknowledge, create a two-tier or multiple-tier system of care. Equality, according to libertarians, is best understood in ethical terms as equality of opportunity, with liberty the central societal value.

Libertarianism not only protects the individual as a decision-maker, it generally protects the family as a site for decisions. If the family can provide care, it should. As costs and competence make familial, fellowship and neighborly care impossible or ineffective, others could step in to assist; then and then only, a libertarian would claim, should society enter to provide—and that as charity, not as an entitlement.

Most libertarian arguments strongly assert the need for freedom and the beneficial character of freedom for the development of both technology and distribution. The great flaw in the libertarian argument is that just participation in the selection of actual health-care services is impossible for the vast majority as they cannot have true market knowledge about each and every practitioner they may need, let alone each and every treatment that might be required. Generally, most patients cannot fully understand their health-care needs or the competency of the seller of services. This could be addressed by having persons buy expertise instead of treatments—in other words, selected insurers or managed care providers would screen the competence of providers. That is not unlike using a stockbroker or financial manager—and the incumbent problems are similar (excessive fees, corrupt alliances, etc.). Further, this may push the problem back, as the individual might not have the proper knowledge to select a health services manager. The market is often the best way to distribute goods for their true worth when real incentives come into play. However, knowledge and competence

---

[5]Hans-Hermann Hoppe, "A Four-Step Health Care Solution," *The Free Market* 11, no. 4 (1993) <http://www.mises.org/freemarket_detail.asp?control=279&sortorder=authorlast>.

restrict the ability to judge properly and, thereby, skew the market.

Another factor that twists how a market works is desperation. Even those who were previously healthy will not be able to enter the marketplace as equals if they are desperate or, at least, under duress. Arguably, according to strict libertarians, when a disaster strikes, bottled water should be worth more because the supply is limited and someone was smart enough to have extra. Even if that were true in disasters, it is a problematic argument when applied to individuals, and the sellers of products are not equally vulnerable.

The most significant concern with libertarian arguments is the undeniable fact that there are and will be losers of both natural and social lotteries. More extreme libertarian positions do not protect the innocent victims of such. Even if one wanted to assert that such was acceptable for adults, it surely is not for children who cannot make choices. It is neither logical nor consistent with U.S. social contract theory to assume that impoverished children should be free to pay for health care. They do not have the competence necessary, the physical access to providers, nor the money to purchase the product. A libertarian might argue that is the responsibility of the parent, and it may be a legitimate use of subsidiarity. Yet, though the parent is one of the responsible parties (the most significant one) she or he is not the party of last resort. Subsidiarity requires moving up levels of accountability to protect the weak and highly vulnerable. The child within the social contract is not just a family member of some adult who is a rights holder but is a rights holder of his or her own. This leads to the conclusion that at least a moderate libertarian should allow that the weak and deserving poor, especially children, ought to receive some health-care coverage.

An additional but equally important limit on libertarianism is the protection of the public health. As with liberty claims about the environment, there must always be a limit created by externalities. Externalities are costs that are not taken into account by those who generate the cost and, subsequently, pass them on to those in social or physical commons. The problem or tragedy of the commons occurs when persons own something corporately and can draw from that good disproportionately in their favor, while paying back only partially or not at all, and do not fear punishment for doing so. Some will intentionally take advantage and they will increase in number as others recognize that the good is being distributed unjustly. For instance, a person's right to dump something on his or her land is always restricted by the dangers presented to other individuals through the spreading of pollutants into the air and water used by others. Liberty in health care should not be the freedom to destroy herd immunity through refusal to accept inoculations, poison through the creation of water or air pollution hazards, and so forth.

The second major position on health care as a right is the egalitarian. Egalitarian arguments assume that all human beings are equal, not simply in opportunity, but in what they receive, or should receive, from the state and perhaps from others in meeting basic needs. This argument is framed, especially in the United States, with the claim that all persons are "created equal" not only "endowed by their Creator with certain unalienable rights among which are life, liberty, and the pursuit of happiness." At first glance, it might seem that a right to health care requires that health care be equally distributed. In the strictest sense this is useless. Men do not need obstetricians and gynecologists and children do not need gerontologists. So the idea of equality must give way to equivalence and a debate over what actually constitutes fairness when different uses and resources are being measured.

The most popular recent version of the egalitarian argument is based on the assumption that justice requires that rules of government and the market be constructed without knowing who would be peculiarly benefited or be injured by those rules, that is, constructed from behind a "veil of ignorance."[6] The closest everyday example is when two children are told they must share a piece of cake and one slices the cake and then the other gets to choose. This method, and generally all egalitarian approaches, promote the maximization of care for those at the minimum level. Egalitarian arguments, by their nature, assume preference for a one-tier medical system, which would necessitate strong regulatory control or outright service provision by the state. Some egalitarians call for an entirely socialized system, with all persons having exactly the same access to all services, including the type of room and food offered during hospitalization. A more common, and more moderated version is found in the call for a basic minimum. Arguably this is already done to a limited degree with public health clinics and emergency rooms.

More efficiently, the society could fund a basic minimum. The minimum would be defined relative to the society's values and capacities; the minimum is different in the United States than in a developing country. However, it should not vary significantly within the United States, which would mean there would have to be compensatory efforts for regions like the Appalachian

[6]John Rawls, *A Theory of Justice* (Cambridge, Mass.: Belknap Press, 1971). Also, see The National Commission for the Protection of Human Subjects of Biomedical and Behavior Research, *The Belmont Report: Ethical Principles and Guidelines for the Protection of Human Subjects of Research* (April 18, 1979) <www.nihtraining.com/ohsrsite/guidelines/belmont.html>.

spine, the Mississippi Delta, the Rio Grande Valley and so on. The basic minimum approach allows individuals, rather than society, to pay for special desires. The minimum health-care services would include at least basic preventative care, basic primary care, readily available surgical and pharmaceutical interventions for life threatening or debilitating conditions, and basic rehabilitative care.[7] Also, a reinsurance that protected individuals against the costs of catastrophic disorders may be needed. The basic minimum model is egalitarian with a bit of libertarianism placed on top.

It is by no means assured, but it would appear that egalitarian approaches would not allow the trading of long-term needs for short-term efficiencies. Certainly, if a unified, one-tiered system developed, there would be continuity of care between practitioners because there would be only one system. The services would be generally available because the government could build facilities and mandate that practitioners serve in previously underserved communities. One of the biggest advantages of egalitarian models is that the public health could be readily protected, as persons with contagious disorders and information about disease would be easily tracked.

Serious problems, however, would likely arise. Persons with orphan disorders or serious disabilities might fall out of the system as too expensive. Egalitarianism would likely be window dressing for the exclusion of persons on utilitarian grounds. As the population aged, assuming some degree of a correlation of increased illness with increased survival as one ages, then ever greater demand on the system should be expected. The only ways around that are improved health until the moment of death (perhaps through new technologies or through allowing people to die faster) and/or increased economic input through more taxpayers or higher taxes or both. Even if full coverage were denied to those with expensive disorders, the system would likely require a significant elevation in taxes. Additionally, in a government-run system, the risk to confidentiality, long time delays and so on would mean less acceptability for the vast majority of users. There is a risk that the most extreme egalitarian version—a government-run system—would be, as one bumper sticker puts it: "Government Healthcare—Post Office Quality with IRS Service, All at Pentagon Prices."

The third major set of arguments is the utilitarian. Utilitarianism is a form

[7]Based on Allen E. Buchanan, "The Right to a Decent Minimum of Health Care" in *Contemporary Issues in Bioethics*, 5th ed., ed. Tom L. Beauchamp and LeRoy Walters (Belmont, Calif.: Wadsworth Publishing, 1999).

of moral reasoning, but is also a philosophical approach to social problems. Most strictly it is a method of calculating applied in political analysis or in economics. In this case, it would take shape along the line of maximizing health care outcomes and minimizing cost. Utilitarian arguments depend on the maximization of a good and minimization of a bad for a group of interest-bearers. A utilitarian system could be one using the market or one operated by the government or something in between—whatever worked. There would be an emphasis on the use of preventative care and a movement away from high technology and expensive drug expenditures.

The cheapest insured persons are the very healthy or very dead, so those managing the system would emphasize making people healthy as fast as possible or, conversely, having them die as soon as possible. Expensive ICU and ER care would be discouraged. Essentially, proprietary managed care narrowly understood is a utilitarian system, but with the benefits accruing disproportionately to the stockholders of the providing organization. However, utilitarian distribution of health care could just as easily be a government program.

Public health requirements and continuity likely would be properly addressed using utilitarianism. The distinct advantage of a utilitarian model is that costs could be controlled relative to benefits gained. However, availability, access, appropriateness and acceptability would not necessarily be achieved for many potential users. In the most extreme form, persons with disabilities or those living in rural areas would be systematically excluded from the system as outliers, too expensive to warrant care.

Essentially, utilitarians would turn health care into a closely managed market with some excluded as natural or social lottery losers because they were too costly. Under the U.S. social contract this would be problematic. Health care would not be a right, and often utilitarians avoid the language of rights for this reason, because some would be systematically excluded. Of course, such people could be defined out of the system as no longer interest-bearers and therefore no longer persons and therefore no longer under the social contract. This would be a fundamental violation of the United States understanding of the function of the state. The state should not be able to buy housing, education and so forth by intentionally excluding persons at the margins from receiving health care; such should be blocked exchanges, that is, deals that cannot be made by the government.[8] Rights language, by its nature, limits the

[8]Michael Walzer, *Spheres of Justice: A Defense of Pluralism and Equality* (New York: Basic Books, 1983).

power to use utility in directing final, social decision making.

A combination of these three approaches is necessary for just distribution of health care. If health care is a right (a positive right), then all persons within the nation are entitled to it, though accessing services in a way that provides the least restriction on choice and that, given that criterion, must be cost-effective relative to the other needs of society. Criteria by which various proposed programs for implementing a right to health care could be evaluated include, but are not limited to, the following:

- *Availability/existence of services.* Available services means there should be practitioners, equipment, facilities and so on in the area. In the case of approaches requiring the market, the availability must include more than one option.
- *Appropriable services at existing sites.* Appropriable services refers to the capacity of the individual to obtain what is available. This includes physical accessibility to the site and a manageable bureaucracy.
- *Acceptability.* Acceptability includes the provision of services that are culturally and morally tolerable to the consumers of the services, both the payors and the patients, and to the providers. This includes satisfying basic concerns of confidentiality, quality of medical and nursing care, and basic "hotel amenities" (comfort during hospitalization). It also includes reasonable freedom of conscience for providers.
- *Affordability.* Affordability means having the money and/or insurance necessary to be served. Affordability is a concern of the service user, the one who facilitates the funding (e.g., government, employer) and the providers. Affordability requires efficiency.
- *Continuity.* Continuity has three components:
  1. *Continuity between practitioners:* This includes the ability to transfer when necessary, share information among practitioners as needed to prevent treatment errors and protect the public health.
  2. *Portability:* Patients must have the ability to continue care for a pre-existing condition when the user changes employers, insurers and so forth.
  3. *Catastrophic Protection:* Patients must maintain continuity in non-futile care even after the costs to the funder have become significant (possibly by reinsurance beyond the contracted cap).

- *Applicability.* The services provided must work given the diagnosis.
- *Protection.* Protection of the public health is necessary no matter what the need of the individual.

Needless to say, no real-life program can perfectly satisfy all the demands for the expansion of health-care coverage in the United States. Most tend to be too libertarian or ignore liberty all but entirely (any of the centralized distribution plans). The two delivery models that seem the most likely to satisfy all three criteria to some reasonable extent are health-care vouchers and mandated insurance. Vouchers would be funded by taxation and distributed to all persons, perhaps in the form of a tax credit, allowing the purchase of a health-care service contract; this contract, in turn, would have certain services guaranteed while additional services could be purchased. The primary way in which these vouchers would be provided is through taxation. Mandated insurance does not provide funding, but rather requires purchase (as car insurance is required of anyone driving). The health-care service contracts purchased, as with vouchers, would have to have certain basic services required with vouchers provided to those justifiably unable to afford their own mandated coverage. The primary way mandated insurance is paid is from the paycheck of the individual or family, as with automobile insurance. If health care is a right, someone has to pay and the cost will be significant and will not be made back in improved health in every case.

As crass as it may seem, when the calculations of cost are made, it appears that a healthier population lives longer than one that is not healthy and unless there are significant changes in retirement expectations, that means a lot more cost to the society as a whole. Technology, too, drives up cost frequently, but is demanded nonetheless. Still, higher cost does not mean it is not socially warranted.

The following are a few advantages of vouchers and mandated insurance:

1. allow the user to remain free to select services on the basis of perceived quality, thus allowing market competition to drive higher quality;
2. minimize the risk of expansive rationing of health care since the patient/user would pay for add-ons to the minimum;
3. promote innovation through competition (users could choose management groups or cooperatives);
4. allow maintenance of a basic minimum without determining all aspects of care;

5. create an opportunity for strong, but not overbearing, oversight.

On the other hand, vouchers and mandated insurance could mean:

1. persons unqualified to actually define quality (the patients/users) would push the market the "wrong" direction by valuing relatively unimportant characteristics (e.g., no copays over $25, cable television in physician's waiting rooms, aroma therapy in dental treatment rooms).
2. decisions might be made in vulnerable periods and unnecessary or inadequate service may be selected;
3. multiple services may not be available in rural and impoverished areas, thus negating the possibility of competition;
4. competition may threaten professional collegiality;
5. the vulnerable/"outliers" (persons with severe disabilities, etc.) may not have sufficient coverage without substantial supplementation.

Each issue would have to be addressed. Still the advantages of vouchers or mandated insurance, especially if outliers are protected, seem to strongly outweigh the disadvantages. Both provide freedom of market, while recognizing that the individual is not knowledgeable enough to select specific treatments in specific situations. They, generally, protect the vulnerable, whether they are vulnerable due to lack of funding or lack of knowledge or from the onset of a disorder. They also minimize the risk of harm from incompetent bureaucracies. At the macroallocation level, they provide equity, but allow at the personal level individual choice. If properly monitored, they will also provide utility.

Indeed, no right to health care exists in the formal statement of the U.S. social contract (i.e., the Constitution), yet the expanded capacity in treatments and greater recognition of the consequences of poor health care provide a basis for claiming this expansion of rights should occur. Ideally, the "emergence" of the health-care entitlement or positive right should not cost the society any more than it already does as a portion of the gross domestic product. Using the market whenever possible can help control cost, but additional, initial governmental costs (likely paid through taxation) should be expected with the possibility of "reimbursment" by improved workforce production.

CONCLUSION

A secular argument for the right to health care rests on the idea that the primary function of the social contract is the protection of the rights of its members (at least in the Lockean-Jeffersonian version), and health care would allow citizens to more fully pursue happiness or the fulfillment of their personal *telos*. To put this another way, health care has improved to the point that it is actually effective in changing the quality of an individual's life. It is not the function of the state to eliminate all barriers to achieving life purpose, but it is the state's responsibility to facilitate the minimization of inequity arising for those who are losers of the natural lottery, and arguably the losers of the social lottery as well. As such, it is a matter of justice.

Of necessity, if there is a right to health care, it

> should be limited, but then every right has some limit (the classic example is that free speech does not mean someone can yell "Fire!" in a crowded theater). Still, people in the United States should have a minimum level of health care available regardless of personal financial resources.
>
> This right is new. It has emerged from improvements in health technologies, from development in health care organization, and from the increasing recognition that when one "loses the natural lottery" by being sicker or more vulnerable than others there is often a corresponding loss of fundamental freedoms. Of course, everyone gets sick eventually and everyone dies. However, those who get sicker or get sick earlier lose relatively more freedom and lose it sooner. This matters because the purpose of the State, as understood historically in the United States, is to protect life and maximize freedom.[9]

Having said this, it would be inaccurate to the point of falsehood to claim that such a right is explicit or implicit in the founding documents. Indeed, health care at the time those documents were written was so abysmal that to have received certain treatments would have been more of a punishment than entitlement. It is possible, though, to make an argument that the fundamental values of the founding documents call forth from the broader society new entitlements. But this creates genuine dangers such as abuse of the commons. Any positive right must be limited by cost capacity and, most importantly, by liberty.

Evangelicals in the United States could legitimately hold three basic positions: (1) Since there is no positive right to health care even suggested in the New Testament, and given that such is not intrinsic to the U.S. political order, health care should remain the obligation of the individual. (2) Given the parables of the Good Samaritan and the Sheep and the Goats, there is an obligation to render care and when the mechanisms of the state can facilitate that

[9]Thobaben, "Wesleyan Argument for Responding to Real Needs."

without impinging on negative rights by controlling all distribution nor diminishing the quality of health-care services available, they should be used. (3) Given those same arguments about care and the assumption that the state exists as an agent of God, a governmentally controlled system for distribution is best.

The second position is the most morally consistent with evangelical history over the past two hundred years. The libertarians are correct in asserting that freedom genuinely matters, including freedoms of the market and of professional activity. Further, the libertarians are correct in asserting that the market tends to raise quality and lower costs as services develop. The egalitarians are correct in claiming that the society should not allow the magnification of the impact of social and natural losses, especially those beyond the control of the individual. The utilitarians are correct in noting that there is a macroallocation limit to the expansion of the health-care right. The second option comes closest to satisfying all three.

12

The Body of Believers and the Public's Health

HUMANS AS PUBLIC

Evangelicals, as opposed to some other subsets of the Reformation stream and both Catholicism and Orthodoxy, have generally supported the idea of the strong separation of church and state. While there have certainly been exceptions, the argument is made that what belongs to God is God's and what belongs to Caesar is Caesar's. What happens, though, when Caesar makes a demand on the Christian as citizen? This is especially important to consider in paying taxes, serving in the military and participation in the protection of public health.

> Keeping a close watch on him, they sent spies, who pretended to be honest. They hoped to catch Jesus in something he said so that they might hand him over to the power and authority of the governor. So the spies questioned him: "Teacher, we know that you speak and teach what is right, and that you do not show partiality but teach the way of God in accordance with the truth. Is it right for us to pay taxes to Caesar or not?"
>
> He saw through their duplicity and said to them, "Show me a denarius. Whose portrait and inscription are on it?"
>
> "Caesar's," they replied. He said to them, "Then give to Caesar what is Caesar's, and to God what is God's."
>
> They were unable to trap him in what he had said there in public. And astonished by his answer, they became silent. (Lk 20:20-26)

PART ONE: THE TEXT

What belongs to Caesar? This has been one of the central questions in Christian social ethics over the past two thousand years. There is no debate that the religious life does not. But that assertion only raises more questions for a Christian. Can the spiritual life be rent from the work life, the family life or even the political life? Can the faithful split their existence into spheres with varying sets of rules or is Christianity a comprehensive worldview that demands of the believer that all things are defined by the relationship with God? It seems that both must be answered with a yes. Christians must differentiate the spheres of social existence in such a way that institutional boundaries and authority are distinguished, even while believing that Jesus is Lord of all.

The denarius was the largest denomination of coinage commonly available in Jesus' day. It was silver, while coins of higher value were gold and not usually in general circulation. Presumably, the coin Jesus looked at bore the image of Tiberius on the obverse. Perhaps the denarius he pointed to had an enthroned woman on the reverse with scepter and branch, possibly Tiberius's wife, Livia. While the image of the Julio-Claudian Dynasty that had been initiated with Caesar Augustus and would end with Nero was on the coin, that specific piece did not belong to the Caesar except in the most formal terms. Rather, it was the possession of the holder. Nonetheless, Jesus declared that the coin could finally be claimed by the emperor. He then implies that as the image of a Caesar was on the coin, the image of God is on each human being, so, each human could finally be claimed by God.

The use of the metaphor leaves open the question, what claims can Caesar or any state make on citizens? What claims of the state should the Christian community accept? Do individuals residing in a given land owe resources to the state? Yes, according to Christ. Money is a resource and is owed in the form of taxes. Does the individual also owe other resources, such as time, to the state, perhaps in the form of military or alternative service? Does the person owe obedience to the state? Yes, in the Christian tradition, unless there is a good reason for disobedience. Jesus does not imply in any way that this payment or obedience is conditioned by affection or admiration. Tiberius had, after all, expelled Jews along with Egyptians from Rome several decades earlier, allowed corrupt Jewish surrogates and Roman authorities to rule the Holy Land, and was more than willing to use armies as policing forces. Not surprisingly the Romans were hardly considered close friends by most of the people of Israel. Still, Christ called the coin the possession of the emperor.

Obedience to the state, then, is the *prima facie* moral obligation of believers. They obey the state, not because the state necessarily deserves it, but out of obedience to God. The passages in Romans 13 and Acts 4–5, when combined, describe both the extent and the limit of this obedience. The state, minimally, restrains some forms of evil and Christians should support such as long as the state does not become too evil itself. In particular, Christians may disobey the authorities over genuine religious matters. This pushes one back to the start: for the believer, is not everything religious? For instance, should the believer obey when drafted into the military or even alternative service? Some Christians (the radical Anabaptists) argue no and consistently live out their separation. Some say yes, but cautiously, and attempt to carefully keep their obedience to the state subject to their obedience to Christ. Others are inconsistent. Some assert believers cannot support the military and that they will not participate in such, but then willingly vote and run for offices that include authority over policing functions. Some, likewise ethically inconstant with the gospel, will serve in the military and take orders without reservation, including obeying immoral commands on the grounds that the leader bears the final responsibility.

Another example is schooling. School is mandatory, but some public schools use material that is actually anti-Christian. Should believers keep their children out? Only if they can still accomplish the purposes of education that the state can legitimately expect to be satisfied. Or, they can stay in the schools and attempt to influence them. On the one hand, it is not acceptable to turn public schools into Christian schools. On the other, it is irresponsible to allow Christian children to undiscerningly accept everything taught in public schools.

An example pertinent to bioethics is Christian participation in the public health efforts. Arguably more intrusive than taxes, compulsory education is action of the state to assure the public health. When public health interventions are attempted that seem of limited value and appear to be serving non-public health agendas, Christians can legitimately resist. When useful, Christians can and should participate. When a need is recognized but not addressed, Christians can legitimately speak up to encourage public health interventions. The ethical questions for believers center around how the level of Christian participation in such state efforts is to be determined.

These questions that arise can be answered only hesitatingly. In some sense, Christians must live paradoxically as citizens of both the world and the kingdom to come. Or, using another model from the New Testament, they must live as sojourners in a foreign land, functioning as ambassadors of the gospel, yet also as the salt of society. To the extent that the state acts in a manner consistent with God's will or at least not blatantly contrary to it, the believer as either a dual citizen or alien sojourner should accede to its commands. When there are direct conflicts, then the level of resistance should correspond to the degree of violation of the gospel. When believers recognize something without specific religious content that could help the society, they can and should speak "prophetically" in favor of such to the leadership of the state.

In response to the increasing prominence of National Socialism (Nazism) in the 1930s, the Confessing Church Movement in Germany described the permeable boundary between the church and state:

> The various offices (official positions) of the church establish no lordship of one over another; instead, these practices are entrusted and commanded for the service of the entire community.
>
> We reject the false teaching (doctrine)—as if the State should and could, above its specific (special) assignment (commission)—[that the State ought to] become the sole and total order (ordering authority) of human life and thus also fulfill the Church's destiny.
>
> We reject the false teaching (doctrine)—as if the Church should and could, above its specific (special) assignment (commission)—[that the Church ought to] assume the state-like manners (behaviors), state-like jobs (responsibilities), and state-like rank (propriety), thus becoming itself an organ of the State.
>
> We reject the false teaching (doctrine)—as if the Church could [appropriately act] in self-lordship—of the placing of the Word and work of the Lord into the service of any unauthoritatively selected (inappropriately chosen) desires (wishes), ends (purposes/designs), and plans.[1]

The Barmen document appropriately describes the limits on state authority. It also declares the limits of church engagement in state functions. And, by its structure and presentation in defiance of the Nazis, it also commends "prophetic" proclamations by the church to correct and protect the society.

In the past, evangelicals have on occasion cooperated closely with the state or even tried to push the state to accomplish some otherwise-ignored but worthy end. For example, Charles Finney, in antebellum America, considered it a Christian duty to change the government in order to have the government change the society.

---

[1]Selections from Karl Barth et al., "The Barmen Declaration of the Confessing Church," trans. James Thobaben (1996). German text from "Die Sechs Sätze der Barmer Theologische Erklärung, vom 31 Mai 1934," *Barmer Theologische Erklärung 1934–1984: Geschichte, Wirkung, Defizite*, ed. Wilhelm Hüffmeier and Martin Stöhr (Bielefeld: Luther-Verlag, 1984). Consulted translation: Arthur C. Cochrane, "Text of the Barmen Declaration," in *The Church Confronts the Nazis: Barmen Then and Now*, ed. Hubert G. Locke (New York: Edwin Mellen Press, 1984).

> The very profession of Christianity implies the profession and virtually an oath to do all that can be done for the universal reformation of the world. . . .
>
> The church with a great many ministers have resorted to the plea of using moral suasion as the means of ridding the world of intemperance, licentiousness, slavery and every other legalized abomination; but pray what can be meant by moral suasion? Moral Government surely is a system of moral suasion. Moral suasion includes whatever is designed and adapted to influence the will of a moral agent.
>
> Laws, rewards, and punishments—these things and such as these are the very heart of moral suasion . . . they are afraid to employ government lest it could be a departure from the system of moral suasion. . . . the great sin and utter shame of the Church and of so many of the ministry in neglecting or refusing to speak out and act promptly and efficiently on the great questions of reform. How could they more directly grieve and quench the Spirit of God than by such a course? . . . no wonder that such a ministry should look coldly on revivals.[2]

This seems a long step away from rendering to Caesar what is Caesar's. But is it a step that must, nonetheless, be taken? The difficulty lies in the fact that the instruction from Christ was given when the possibility of Christians directly influencing or serving in government was remote. That is not the case today. Besides abolition, the great social issue of nineteenth-century evangelicalism was temperance. The Prohibition effort at the end of the nineteenth century and in the early twentieth century drew evangelicals together in a way that virtually no other issue ever has, excepting perhaps abortion at the end of the twentieth century. Pulled together as a social force, they entered into the political process. The Women's Christian Temperance Union and similar groups used arguments much like public health protestations against smoking and transfats today. To many of the world (and probably a substantial number of today's evangelicals) looking back, those sound more prudish than prophetic, more intrusive than instructive. At the time, the efforts were considered a Christian duty. Was the problem that the church was imposing its moral teaching or was the problem the overdrawn analysis of the alcohol problem, especially compared to other social ills of the day? Put another way, was the church usurping state authority or was the analysis of alcohol consumption as a social crisis a misreading or, at least, an exaggeration? If the former, then the church was blatantly immoral; if the latter, then the

---

[2]Charles G. Finney, Letter #23, *Letters on Revival* (originally presented in 1846) <http://gospeltruth.net/1846OE/46_lets_art/460121_let_on_revival_23.htm>.

church was mistaken. Or, the evangelicals of the late nineteenth and early twentieth centuries may have been completely correct and the society may have suffered for lifting the ban in 1933 that had been imposed in 1920.

What is clear is that the state and church should remain distinct. Christian theocracy is immoral. It is counterproductive for society and spiritually corrupting for the faithful. Even so, complete separation is not possible in this life. The closest believers can come to that position is that assumed by the Hutterites and the Amish, though even they participate in the marketplace and pay taxes for infrastructure. The question for evangelicals is where between these two extreme positions, theocracy and complete separation, should they stand? Even if believers should participate in politics and social change, should it only be as individuals? Does the church ever have a responsibility for speaking authoritatively on nonreligious issues? Should Christians try to change institutions or use non-Christian institutions to effect social and cultural transformation? Arguably, the answer is yes when the issue is significant enough or, to use language more fitting for bioethics, when there is a great enough risk. And that leads to another question: how does one decide what is risky?

PART TWO: CHRISTIAN BIOETHICS

When Christians work with the state or encourage major shifts in approaches to public health concerns they are, almost inevitably, participating in the state's intrusion into the lives of its citizens. To legitimately warrant government intervention, some danger must be risky enough to enough people who have no other means of addressing the concern. Risk can be calculated:

Risk = Expected Frequency of an Event

Of course, the risk of something bad occurring is never completely known, but is always a matter of probabilities. Therefore, an event always has the range of possibly happening of 0 to 1.0, or if one prefers percentages, 0 percent probability of occurring to 100 percent probability of occurring.

Still, knowing this, even to a high level of confidence, is not sufficient to estimate the implications of a risk and, subsequently, drive public health or moral decision making. Risk is always conditioned by the severity of the hazard.

Risk = Expected Frequency x Severity of Hazard

Even this is not enough information to make a decision. After all, some truly dreadful or truly wonderful things might happen, but for them to occur something else would have to not occur. To use economics language, all choices have lost opportunity costs.

Risk = Expected Frequency x (Severity of Hazard – Benefit from the Choice)

One more important fact about risk must be included in any consideration of public health dangers, that is, the comparison of the risk with other risks of other options, including the option of doing nothing. Risk is always comparative.

$Risk_A : Risk_B$

Jesus suggested using risk assessment in ethical analysis.

> Therefore keep watch, because you do not know on what day your Lord will come. But understand this: If the owner of the house had known at what time of night the thief was coming, he would have kept watch and would not have let his house be broken into. So you also must be ready, because the Son of Man will come at an hour when you do not expect him. (Mt 24:42-44)

As an example, what is called Pascal's Wager is a risk assessment for one's soul. Pascal asks how one can decide for or against a personal relationship with God through Jesus Christ when one simply cannot know every fact and every possible outcome of the choice to believe or not believe. He suggests that the probability cannot be known—that believing and not believing are equally rational (or, perhaps, arational, which is not irrational, but beyond rationality). So, assuming these are the only two options, one could estimate the probability of one or the other occurring as .5 (50 percent). Since the probabilities of occurrences are assumed to be equal, one must differentiate between the choices by considering the danger or consequences of each decision, that is, the severity of the hazards.

The weakness of the wager argument, when simplistically presented, lies in the problem of discerning if all reasonably possible choices and their consequences are considered. To complete the wager, then, one needs to assert that if one chooses believing over atheism that, in the next analytical step, believing in the Christian God is more rational than any other option. This, evangelicals are more than willing to claim—believers assert that enough information is available to compare religious systems, even if there is not undeniable scientific proof there is or is not a God. This finally, then, leads to a decision to accept Jesus as Lord, to trust in the relationship one can have through Jesus

Christ, because it is far more probably true than other religions and equally probable and vastly less severe than not believing in any religion at all.

Not all evangelicals would agree with nor use the wager argument evangelistically. Some might think it is too calculating. Others think there is, after all, clear scientific evidence for the Christian God. Regardless, this kind of risk assessment occurs in decisions all people make every day. Even when they do not consciously think through the numbers, people use risk assessment in countless decisions every waking hour. Sometimes they misjudge the probability. Sometimes they misunderstand the danger of a given outcome. And, sometimes, they are manipulated when others use misinformation or political power to compel a given course of action when the risk is weak or the threat is minimal. Still, "assess" is something all people do, and something governments must do well to fulfill its purpose.

The use of power, not the risk assessment per se, is what makes public health interventions problematic. They are intrusive and the justification for that intrusion is not always clear. Yet, epidemiological uncertainty should not necessarily lead to moral uncertainty. Some interventions are worth the risk because the alternatives are so egregious or because the interventions are fairly minimal. For instance, there is a risk to treating water with fluoride, but it is minimal relative to the notable minimization of dental cavities. As evidence, the current increase in bottled water and fruit juice consumption by children whose parents want what is "natural" for their offspring is associated with a rise in cavities. The risk for those children goes up, and it is not clear whether or not other risks go down because of a supposed reduction in carcinogenic pollutants, and so on. For this reason the state should (1) continue to fluoridate water and (2) encourage sufficient fluoride intake for children. The state, however, should not intrude on parental care, defining bottled water or fruit juice as child abuse. Christians can and should encourage those in their own communities to follow such reasonable and fairly unobtrusive public health guidelines.

Another example is keeping sewage out of water supplies and making sure food is generally pure. The state can and should limit the freedom of anyone who wants to dump pollutants into sinkholes or sell prepared foods canned in unsanitary facilities. For the state to do this, it must intrude. Christians should allow such intrusion. A specific case would be limiting raw milk sales from organic farms, and even requiring pasteurization. The believer who lives on such a farm may not like this rule and may actively try to get it changed, but should abide by it while it is the law. That does not mean all such intrusions make sense, as some risk has to be accepted in order to avoid extremely high lost opportunity costs. In other words, there are trade-offs.

Roughly speaking, believers should speak and act in such a way that they could, on matters of public health, be guides, examples, challengers and partners. First, the guide instructs, but as a knowledgeable peer or equal on the public square. Analogically this like a school teacher, not a spiritual mentor. Unfortunately, in terms of public health, individuals in the evangelical community are often too uninformed on the science to offer instruction. To guide others one must first be willing to be taught. Evangelicals have a lot to learn about disease and disability in populations and about public health regulation.

Second, evangelicals should set examples by the way they live. Often American Christians are poor models given the notable presence of obesity and lack of exercise among them. They may not be significantly worse than the general population, but are surely not significantly better. Christians should hold one another accountable. In the past, gluttony was considered one of the seven deadly sins, but is now ignored or laughed at. Christians are called to exceed the standards of the world, not acquiesce because marketers create new and tastier snack foods. Still, alcohol abstinence or temperate consumption, defense of heterosexual monogamy, and disdain for tobacco use seem to promote good public health. Religious people, defined by participation rather than intellectual affirmation of a belief system, do tend to be a bit healthier insofar as that is defined by longevity.

Third, believers may question the worldly when the behaviors of the world lead to diminished public health. It is right to challenge persons to live monogamous lives, for instance. It is right to challenge those who drink excessively or drive at twenty miles over the speed limit day in and day out. However, the first challenges must be to other believers in the form of mutual accountability. All must be done with humility, as this exemplifies Jesus and helps avoid the accusation of hypocrisy, which would allow others to dismiss the concern of the faithful.

Fourth, partnering is necessary. No believer, even the most sectarian, does not have to interact with those of the world. While there may be many points of disagreement, cooperation on social actions based on shared middle axioms (even when the fundamental reasons for those moral positions differ significantly) is preferable to not helping those who stand in need. For instance, churches that might be used as public health satellite clinic sites (that might provide instruction to ethnic or economically marginal groups, that could assist in gathering people for blood pressure and other kinds of screenings and so on) should willingly open their doors.

Perhaps the best example when determining how Christians do and should consider the issue of public health is HIV/AIDS. AIDS is primarily a sexually transmitted disease. In the United States in 2007, the reported estimated total number of cases with method of transmission was as listed below:

Adult males:	male-to-male sexual contact	487,695
	injection drug use	175,704
	both	71,242
	high-risk heterosexual contact	63,927
	other	12,108
Adult females:	injection drug use	80,155
	high-risk heterosexual contact	112,230
	other	6,158
Children (< 13)	perinatal	8,434
	other	775[3]

So, in the case of males, only about 23 percent of the infections were not tied directly to sexual behavior (and only 1.5 percent were not attributable to sexual behavior or intravenous drug abuse). In the case of women, the rate due to high-risk sexual behavior is 56.5 percent. High risk heterosexual behavior is engaging in sexual relations or similar behaviors with a person known to be infected or known to participate in high risk behaviors himself or herself. The rates of infection vary with income and ethnicity, but the causal relation is to the behavior.[4] The general pattern of the physiological and anatomical infection mechanism is the same across ethnic and economic lines. The disorder has both behavioral and cultural category implication.

AIDS is not just an individual's disease; it truly is a disorder of society. First, non-risk-taking persons are put at risk. Though the numbers are pro-

[3]Table 4. "Estimated numbers of AIDS cases, by year of diagnosis and selected characteristics, 2003-2007 cumulative—United States and dependent areas," U.S. Department of Health and Human Services HIV/AIDS Surveillance Report, 2009, vol. 19 (Atlanta: Centers for Disease Control) <www.cdc.gov/hiv/topics/surveillance/resources/reports/2007report/default.htm>.
[4]Ibid.

portionately small, some who could not have controlled their situation are put at high risk (notably, spouses and partners and newborns). Second, the long latency means persons may be vulnerable who are unaware of or naive about the risk. Third, the treatment is expensive and society is bearing much of the cost. Fourth, those most likely to get infected are of the age group that is most important to the long-term maintenance of society. There is a lost opportunity cost, as well as a treatment cost. Fifth, the groups that do seem to get the most infections are marginalized for other reasons completely unassociated with the disorder and the disease may increase that marginalization (this is not a reference to practicing homosexual men whose behavior is causally associated with disease, but blacks and Hispanics whose ethnicity is clearly not). "In the modern world, particularly in industrial societies, inequalities in morbidity and mortality are often more social than biological phenomena."[5]

Social inequality is a factor in iatrogenic spreading of HIV. For instance, transmission by improper blood transfusion in the United States seems to have been properly managed. This, however, is clearly not true in the developing world. As part of missionary outreach, Christians who believe in participating in politics should encourage improvement in health care that would minimize HIV transmission risk. Further, Christians should encourage making reasonably priced antiretroviral drugs available.

Still, AIDS is basically a sexually transmitted disease, and secondarily a disease of blood transmission through intravenous substance abuse. The term "venereal disease" is no longer commonly used in public health and that change is appropriate, for the term is derived from the name of the Greek goddess of love, Venus. There is nothing loving about spreading this infection. Of course, the English word *love* is a more inclusive term than the word used in Greek. Venus was deemed the goddess of erotic love, not *agape,* and AIDS is clearly associated with erotic behaviors.

Ideally, from a Christian viewpoint, sexual intercourse occurs only when love as *agape* and *phileos* are present and endorsed in heterosexual monogamous marriage. The ultimate physical expression between man and woman is woven together with the ultimate legal, spiritual and emotional expression. While this is the morally desirable condition, evangelicals are not naive about sexual behavior in the general population nor among some of their own. Yet the primary mech-

[5]National Research Council, *The Social Impact of AIDS in the United States,* ed. Albert R. Jonsen and Jeff Stryker (Washington, D.C.: National Academy Press, 1993), p. 9 <www.nap.edu/openbook.php?record_id=1881>.

anism and epidemiological pattern being essentially one of promiscuity cannot become an excuse for ignoring persons who suffer. Christians must do what they can to alleviate suffering in the United States where the disease is disproportionately homosexual as well as in the other regions of the world where the disorder is primarily heterosexually transmitted and large numbers of monogamous wives and children become infected.

By Christian standards, there is not any moral legitimation of sexual intercourse or equivalent behaviors outside of heterosexual, monogamous marriage. Certainly no honest reading of the New Testament can be used to endorse such. Still, the moral concern for those with or who could potentially get an STD, including HIV/AIDS, should be as significant as the moral concern for protecting sexual purity. Indeed, to set these up as if they are in moral conflict is itself morally suspect. Some evangelicals have implied that one legitimate moral concern, the human family as endorsed by the creative and prevenient grace of God the Father, should be prioritized over another—in this case, helping persons avoid sickness. That is a false dichotomy.

On the other hand, those who trivialize the family are more than willing to legitimate their own sexual agendas using fear of disease or social dislocation. They attempt to use the coercive power of public health authorities to achieve their sociopolitical ends. It appears, for instance, that Planned Parenthood did this, using unintended pregnancy and the danger of STDs to assert a political agenda only tangentially related to public health. Similarly, various homosexuality advocacy groups have done so with fear of HIV/AIDS more specifically. These groups have asserted that rejecting the inevitability of promiscuity and the legitimacy of homosexual behaviors are putting people at health risk, and hence people who do so are either morally reprehensible (prejudiced) or have a psychological disorder (homophobia). This, in spite of the fact that everyone in the general U.S. population is clearly not equally at risk to contract STDs, including HIV. In fact, it would seem dangerous to the public health to expend public or private funds on the basis of such reasoning. To the contrary of that argument, subsets of the population should be targeted for prevention and treatment corresponding to the risk behaviors in which they engage, and behaviors that put people at risk should be discouraged. Christians should be willing to be challengers on this matter, even while they partner to provide care.

While perhaps understandable, the initial response of U.S. evangelicals to AIDS included too much condemnation. Indeed, immorality did and does lead to the majority of U.S. infections but that did not and does not excuse the duty as Christians to care and as citizens to minimize threats to the public health. The lack of immediate concern for the suffering actually became an opportunity for politicizing the disease in a manner that worked contrary to Christian values. In other words, the slow response was both a moral failure and a strategic one.

In the United States now, for believers and for those in the high-risk pools, the availability of the drugs seems to have lowered the fervor of calls for prevention. Christians should insist, having learned from their mistake two decades earlier, that such an attitude is not for the public's good. Prevention is accomplished best by monogamous sexual relations with a monogamous person or by complete abstinence. From a public health viewpoint, this could include both hetero- and homosexual monogamy. Christians must oppose the legitimacy of homosexual partnering, but may need to tolerate public health instruction to those of the world who choose to do so.

Christians can tolerate, though not endorse, monogamous homosexual behaviors as preferable for the public health (this need not mean the endorsement of homosexual marriage). This toleration should not be offered inside the church where appropriate morality can and should be expected, at least among leaders. Toleration is a social attitude located between affirmation and rejection. When appropriate, it is a moral good that allows for the functioning of society, in this case by protecting the public health.

A good public-health model, and one that evangelicals can readily support, is used in sub-Saharan Africa by some Pentecostal groups. It initially appears that persons active in those groups do have a lower probability of contracting AIDS, which is not true of all other Christians in the region. Reportedly, these Pentecostals tend to

1. strongly indoctrinate on sexual morality;
2. have their religious experiences confirmed by the group which, in turn, confirms the veracity of moral claims associated with the group;
3. have behaviors socialized by the whole, not merely taught to the individual;
4. expect persons violating the standards to be excluded (or, to use the Anabaptist term, shunned).[6]

Other possible factors, such as the association (or lack thereof) of circumcision with Pentecostal belief or prior commitment to communities that have

---

[6]Robert C. Garner, "Safe Sects? Dynamic Religion and AIDS in South Africa," *The Journal of Modern African Studies* 38, no. 1 (2000): 43-69.

stricter sexual mores, may or may not play a role.[7] So, if those other factors do not impede the gospel nor create major risks, then they should be practiced. This would include circumcision, for though the gospel does not encourage such for spiritual reasons, there is no prohibition for other reasons.

Whether inoculations or controlling sexual behaviors that spread HIV or the fluoridation of water or the control of pollutants or inspection of food-processing facilities, the public health requires some limits on individual freedom. There can be no free riders on the public health train. Rendering to Caesar does not mean agreeing with him on everything. It does mean that, given the necessity for social order, Christians should not attempt to stop reasonable efforts by the state to facilitate orderly function. Indeed, sometimes Christians should participate in those efforts and even encourage them as guides, examples, challengers and partners.

PART THREE: CHRISTIAN BIOETHICS AND THE WORLD

Among the shared values, or values that are expected to be shared, under the U.S. social contract is the value of human life. The state's duty to defend individual human lives gives rise to police powers for the public health. This means that some choices—personal and social choices—cannot be tolerated when they are a significant risk to others. Other choices, even if morally objectionable, should not generally be prohibited by the social contract state.

The police authority of the state should not be extended to use for the public health unless there is a significant and likely threat to others. Thus quarantines are appropriate for contagious diseases that are contractible by casual contact, though not for diseases that are clearly not, such as AIDS in the case of an infectious disease and lung cancer in the case of a noncontagious disorder—even if the cause is a possibly objectionable behavior like homosexual promiscuity or a two-pack-a-day cigarette habit.

Once risk evaluations have been made, the question arises as to how much power the state should use in promoting the potential improvement of health. This is not a black-and-white decision. Some marginal improvement might be

[7]Stefan Lovgren, "Circumcision Can Reduce AIDS Risk, Study Says," *National Geographic News*, July 27, 2005 <http://news.nationalgeographic.com/news/2005/07/0726_050726_circumcision.html>; "WHO and UNAIDS Announce Recommendations from Expert Meeting on Male Circumcision for HIV Prevention," UNAIDS Press Release, World Health Organization <http://data.unaids.org/pub/PressRelease/2007/20070328_pr_mc_recommendations_en.pdf>. See also "Adult Male Circumcision Significantly Reduces Risk of Acquiring HIV: Trials in Kenya and Uganda Stopped Early," *NIH News*, December 13, 2006 <www.nih.gov/news/pr/dec2006/niaid-13.htm>.

had at the cost of draconian control over individuals' lives. It is not worth the trade-off. On the other hand, some minor interventions significantly improve health and help not just a given individual but also the society by lowering health-care costs.

Christians using just war or just coercion criteria have traditionally evaluated the legitimacy of a state intervention and Christian participation. It remains one of the best analytical tools available. Bioethicists working in secular settings have advocated the same method.[8] The actions of public health need this kind of justification because they involve coercion, or the loss of liberty, and may involve a risk for loss of health or life for given individuals for the sake of the pool of individuals. In other words, there is always a cost to someone and the question must be asked before hand, Is that cost justifiable? Should the risk be taken?

Just coercion theory, though sometimes listed in slightly different ways, usually includes seven criteria: just cause, right intention, legitimate authority, reasonable chance of success, last resort, proportionality and discrimination. In the case of public health, the *just cause* is always the health of the public. In the United States the general assumption is that public health measures are intended to improve the physical well-being of individuals by improving the health of the population as a whole.

Right intention can be defined as the matching of motive with just cause. In other words, does the moral agent's action coincide with what she or he says is the reason for coercing? The public health response to AIDS provides examples from each side of the sociopolitical spectrum. It would be immoral, in that it lacked proper intention, for evangelicals to try to control homosexuality as an immoral act, but under the guise of public health—even though the two are associated. Likewise, it would be immoral for Planned Parenthood to advocate for condoms or certain forms of "sex education" on the grounds of public health when the real agenda is to promote a promiscuous lifestyle.

Legitimate authority is defined legally, at least in a Lockean-Jeffersonian social contract state such as the United States, as the agreed upon social authority. This does not always mean the federal government. Following subsidiarity, it can mean that the family (as with fluoridated water consumption), the county or state (as with fluoridation of water supplies), or the federal gov-

[8]For instance, see Lawrence Gostin, Benjamin Berkman and Members of Working Group Two; "Project on Addressing Ethical Issues in Pandemic Influenza Planning: Draft paper for Working Group Two," October 6, 2006 <http://www.who.int/eth/ethics/PI_Ethics_draft_paper_WG2_6_Oct_06.pdf>.

ernment (as with funding of fluoridation research) is the locus of decision making. The idea of subsidiarity is in the U.S. Constitution as the Tenth Amendment: "The powers not delegated to the United States by the Constitution, nor prohibited by it to the States, are reserved for the States respectively, or to the people." Obviously how this is interpreted for public health is open to debate.

Legitimate authority can extend to controlling persons who are not legally guilty, but legally threatening. For the public health a person's liberty can be restricted even if she or he does not deserve, on the basis of criminality, a limit on his or her freedom in the form of quarantine or compelled inoculation. Besides quarantining persons with an infectious disease, the police power of the state may legitimately be used to directly quarantine or constrain the infectious agent. Mandated inoculations do this. The goal is to achieve "herd immunity" by providing the antibodies necessary to prevent the infection from gaining a foothold in the individual and, thereby, the population. If enough people are inoculated, then the "herd" blocks exponential expansion of the disease, critical mass is not reached, and epidemic is averted (it may continue at a low endemic level).

The protorevivalist movement in its earliest days strongly supported such interventions under leaders such as Lady Mary Montague, Cotton Mather, Jonathan Edwards and Edward Jenner—even with some lay and physician opposition. Ironically, Edwards actually died after receiving a small pox inoculation meant to demonstrate to the students of the school where he presided (King's College, eventually to become Princeton) that the treatment was both safe and efficacious. The sad outcome of Edwards's efforts points to an important reality of public health measures. They frequently limit the freedom and/or put at risk a small number of persons for the sake of the general well-being of the state and its citizens.[9] In the United States, the state uses a utility calculation to protect the rights to life, liberty (in the long run) and the pursuit of happiness.

---

[9]Jenner was a believing Anglican, from a family of clergy and missionaries. He observed that milkmaids who had been infected with cowpox were far less likely to come down with small pox. Jenner intentionally vaccinated and then attempted to infect with small pox a youth named James Phipps. This would be a problematic protocol today. Jenner, though, was not inclined to abuse the vulnerable. He was also strongly opposed to slavery. Before Jenner, Lady Mary Montague had reported on variolation as practiced successfully in the Ottoman Empire, and which had centuries earlier been practiced in China and India. Records exist of variolation by a slave, perhaps named Onesimus, in the American colonies, and Benjamin Jesty in England vaccinated his own family, prior to Jenner's work. Still, Jenner verified scientifically the efficacy, provided a mechanism and published the work allowing its dissemination.

Traditionally, to allow state compulsion there must be a strong benefit measured against the relatively smaller risk to liberty. For instance, in order to protect the public health, a vaccination against a communicable disease can be mandated. The legal precedent was set in the United States with *Massachusetts v. Jacobson* (1908), in which the U.S. Supreme Court declared as fundamental that

> real liberty for all could not exist under the operation of a principle which recognizes the right of each individual person to use his own, whether in respect of his person or his property, regardless of the injury that may be done to others. This court has more than once recognized it as a fundamental principle that "persons and property are subjected to all kinds of restraints and burdens in order to secure the general comfort, health, and prosperity of the state; of the perfect right of the legislature to do which no question ever was, or upon acknowledged general principles ever can be, made, so far as natural persons are concerned."[10]

To justify any coercive act in the name of justice, including in the name of the justice of saving the public from health crises, that intervention must have a genuine probability of succeeding in comparison to the status quo and other alternatives. In just coercion theory, this is called a *reasonable chance of success.* Ideally, this is something that can be determined scientifically. Often, though, *reasonable* must be defined as "more likely to limit or minimize the risk than maintaining the status quo or other alternatives." In other words, the intervention should lead to the lowest possible "incidence" of new cases and the best chance of lowering "prevalence" (Prevalence = New Cases + Existing Cases). This assumes that an epidemic can be restrained, that an endemic can be lowered in prevalence or that a pandemic can be restricted in geographical distribution.

---

[10]The *Jacobson v. Massachusetts* case was the culmination before the U.S Supreme Court of an ongoing argument in the country and particularly in Massachusetts (e.g., *Commonwealth v. Pear, Commonwealth v. Jacobson,* 67 L.R.A. 935, 183 Massachusetts 242, 66 N.E. 719 [Massachusetts 1903]). Pear refused to pay a $5 fine for not getting the smallpox inoculation. The state courts recognized the police powers of the commonwealth took precedence over Mr. Pear's liberty when a true and significant threat to public health and safety existed. In *Jacobson v. Commonwealth of Massachusetts,* 197 U.S. 11 (1905), Jacobson's argument hinged on his claim that the science was inadequate and that, to the contrary, the science demonstrated a genuine risk to his well-being and that there is an "'inherent right of every freeman to care for his own body and health in such way as seems to him best." An earlier Massachusetts case, *O'Brien v. Cunard S.S. Co., Ltd.,* 154 Mass. 272, 28 N.E. 266 (Mass. Sep. 01, 1891), had resulted in Cunard being held clear of any liability for battery when it required a passenger to be vaccinated prior to traveling on their steamship; her standing in line and accepting the shot demonstrated that she had given permission to the doctor to vaccinate her.

Police power should be used for public health only as a *last resort.* For instance, instruction may be preferable, through public service announcements or through physicians. Some argue that health education in schools is a last resort, arising because of the failure of parents to properly guide their own children. A better example is compelled quarantine after education and voluntary self-restriction have failed.

The *proportionality* of a response to any risk is dependent on the availability of a range of responses. In public health, the evaluation of a hazard is properly yoked to a risk-benefit analysis of the possible responses, their efficacy and costs. "The U.S. Preventive Services Task Force (USPSTF) grades its recommendations according to one of five classifications (A, B, C, D, I) reflecting the strength of evidence and magnitude of net benefit (benefits minus harms)" and this model is quite useful for making decisions in light of partial certainty/uncertainty.[11] The USPSTF Model, with the language significantly modified to include decisions beyond individual treatments/screenings, is

A. Action strongly recommended because good evidence that the choice will improve important health outcomes and apparent measurements leads to the conclusion that benefits substantially outweigh harms.

B. Action recommended because good evidence that the choice will improve important health outcomes and apparent measurements leads to the conclusion that benefits outweigh harms.

C. Action neither recommended nor not recommended because though some evidence that the choice will improve important health outcomes exists, measurements cannot be used to determine if benefits outweigh harms for a general decision (each must be made individually, not as a group or for the public at large).

D. Action is not recommended, especially routinely (in asymptomatic situations), for fair evidence indicates the choice would lead to ineffective outcomes or that harms outweigh benefits.

I. Action cannot be recommended as the evidence is insufficient because it is lacking, of poor quality or conflicting to recommend for or against routine

[11]"U.S. Preventive Services Task Force Ratings: Strength of Recommendations and Quality of Evidence," *Guide to Clinical Preventive Services, Third Edition: Periodic Updates,* 2000–2003. Agency for Healthcare Research and Quality, Rockville, Md. <http://www.ahrq.gov/clinic/3rduspstf/ratings.htm>. See also "Grade Definitions" for differences before and after May 2007 <http://www.ahrq.gov/clinic/uspstf/grades.htm>.

action or the balance of benefits and hazard is virtually indiscernible.

Proportionality and last resort are linked to the efficacy of the various possible interventions (including the status quo) as well as the comparability of the risk of the disease and the benefit of the treatment (to the individual or to the public). For a significant, but not immediately life threatening disease, this might mean that first physicians are asked to instruct their patients. Then, public service announcements are used. The next step might be optional screenings. This could be followed by mandated screenings, but only if the health threat was high or if the cost of treatment for the disorder to the state was significant. If the health risk was high, then quarantine might be instituted.

Discrimination is not a negative term under just coercion theory. To the contrary, it is a good thing to discriminate between combatants and noncombatants, those who must be coerced and those who need not be. So, if a person is not infected with a disease and another person is carelessly serving as the vector for that disease, then the state—assuming it is a debilitating or life-threatening illness—might intervene to protect the vulnerable and unwary. In public health coercion, however, as in war, there may sometimes be innocent bystanders who get coerced. For instance, the relative of a sick person may not have caused his or her illness in any way, nor have the disorder but may still need to be quarantined for the sake of the population.

Evangelicals should have no problem with quarantine and other coercive public health actions when appropriate, though must insist on clear, even if not absolute, scientific evidence of a risk and of the efficacy of the means for abatement. Just coercion criteria should be satisfied. An example would be favoring the state over religious liberty when the physical life of the child is threatened, including not only cases when there is an immediate threat such as with the refusal to allow a blood transfusion by Jehovah's Witnesses parents, but also requiring reasonable inoculations/vaccinations as an appropriate preventative for the individual child and means to develop herd immunity, regardless of religious belief, and then returning the child to the care of parents. A simplistic utilitarian calculation should not be used to abrogate the rights of those holding minority opinions, only significant problems with just interventions.

It is not necessary for evangelicals, or anyone else, to accept the use of public health power to accomplish other social or political ends. Assertions for moral positions that are not strongly needed for the public health but are masked underneath the label of health concern should be exposed. Sometimes this happens when neopuritans insist that persons be held legally responsible for their cigarette smoking or consumption of fatty foods. Such self-destructive behaviors clearly do not warrant approval and may even call for moral condemnation, but not rigorous use of police power by the state. The state should not be given the power to arrest gluttons. While this sounds silly, it is not different from arresting smokers. Second-hand smoke is a relatively minor but real health risk; it certainly may be argued that children should not be exposed or even that places of employment be smoke-free, but not that persons should not be permitted to smoke in their own cars, homes, and so on in which they expose only themselves and those who voluntarily choose to be present.

Responses to smoking and, to a lesser degree, obesity have been harsh—using shame and legal enforcement to culturally degrade the smoker and, increasingly, the overeater. On the other hand, the response to potentially deadly infectious diseases has been quite confused and often legally inconsistent. For instance, some favor or tolerate inoculating underage girls for human papillomavirus (HPV) against their parents' wishes, using public school enrollment as leverage. This is inconsistent to the point of hypocrisy when the same public figures refuse to compel or at least strongly encourage behavior alterations of those who might casually pass HIV/AIDS. Further, such efforts are problematic not only because they seemingly ignore other reasonable public health controls (education about behaviors—after all, HPV is not going to casually pass but needs intimate contact) but also because the use of the public schools for this is an extraordinary expansion of the police power of the state through the education sector. An institution may have legitimate authority for some social purposes and not for others.

This raises a specific question: Is AIDS exceptional, or are sexually transmitted diseases treated differently than other public health concerns? Why have public health methods used successfully in the past not been used in the same way or not used at all with HIV/AIDS and now with HPV? The answer is fourfold: (1) the belief in magic-bullet medicine; (2) a political agenda of groups denying primary legitimacy for heterosexual, monogamous marriage; (3) the assertion, made by various organizations and prevalent in the popular media, that individuals, especially young individuals, cannot restrain their sexual behaviors, and (4) freedom/liberty.

First, Americans specifically, but increasingly persons throughout the world, tend to "believe" in technological progress to such an extent that they will not alter personal health behaviors if there is the slightest possibility that a magic bullet treatment can be found. Even those protesting against pharmaceutical companies want pills that cure so they do not have to change what they do. Perhaps such is innate to human beings as much as cultural. The HIV magic bullet has never materialized, at least not one that inoculates. The initial insistence on mandating the HPV vaccination did, to some extent, reflect this belief. This type of belief, when generalized, is a genuine threat to the long-term public health. Precaution in personal behavior is most often useful.

Second, there was a political agenda. AIDS has served in the West—though certainly not in the same way in the rest of the world—to achieve institutional and civic power for persons favoring the lowering of sexual behavior barriers. HPV education and advertising may be used in the same way. While almost everyone agrees that persons who intentionally pass these diseases are prosecutable (and some have been), there seems little desire to hold the careless accountable. In the United States there is often a legal distinction between criminal intent and negligence. The spreading of HIV has often been through behaviors that, in other types of legal cases, would be clearly deemed gross negligence. An intoxicated individual does not "intend" to get into a car, careen down a road at 90 miles per hour and kill someone. To the contrary of what should be expected using public health reasoning, there has been extreme reticence to use strong cautionary or critical language about high-risk sexual behaviors by too many public health officials and politicians. Evangelicals, obviously, have not been as hesitant to complain about such carelessness, though unfortunately, too often tinging it with self-righteousness.

Third, the claim is made and asserted to be scientific—though suspicion about social research on such matters is quite appropriate—that individuals cannot restrain their sexual behaviors. Usually this is made on the basis of some unverifiable assertion about human nature. Presumably for those making this claim, there is a genetic encoding for promiscuity or, at least, experimentation that cannot be overcome. Ethically, this is an intentional indulgence in the naturalistic fallacy—that what is is what ought to be. Further, even given some of the assumptions, the evidence does not seem to support the conclusion.[12] The argument, then, is fallacious on two counts: this is not

[12]"Positive Trends Recorded in U.S. Data on Teenagers" *New York Times*, July 13, 2007. See <http://childstats.gov>.

an inevitable natural behavior pattern and even if the tendency toward such carelessness were, it would not thereby be morally/socially preferable or worthy of encouragement. Needless to say, evangelicals disagree with assertions about the inevitability of promiscuity.

Indeed, the same argument has resurfaced in justifications for the HPV vaccination. Teenagers will act promiscuously; therefore, they should be inoculated. And, so the argument goes, the school system is an important agent of the state public health machinery and should be used to compel submission to vaccination. The difficulty for evangelicals should not be the vaccination per se—assuming it is not high risk. The use of such magic bullets is fine if the parents are intentional in telling their children its use is for minimizing a risk that they, the children, can even more significantly lower by their careful behavior as they grow older.

The faithful should not be naive—innocence is a virtue, naiveté is not. A higher incidence of sexual promiscuity exists among church-going teenagers and young adults than many would like to believe. The real problems with the way the HPV vaccination is being promoted is (1) pharmaceutical companies appearing to have used state power or at least connections to maximize sales and (2) the state using the schools as a vehicle for policing public health when there is no immediate threat, thus violating one of the core social contract assumptions about limits on the police powers of the state.[13]

Does this mean no STD or HIV/AIDS education should be directed at evangelical teenagers, operating on the assumption that they are not at risk? Absolutely not, for it is clearly verifiable that some are. Still, it may mean that public health efforts take into account both the risk to the evangelical population subgroup and the cost to family and values that might occur. The family matters, not only to Christians but to the state as a mediating institution that far more efficiently addresses most societal needs than does a centralized bureaucracy and, if for no other reason, should be supported and not attacked.

Fourth, freedom. There is an inconsistency, bordering on self-contradiction, when an argument for freedom in sexual behavior is made at the same time that it is asserted that people have no choice but to participate in such behaviors. One is not free if compelled—by genetics or by police power of the state. Nonetheless, liberty matters so much for the strength of the social con-

[13]Glenn McGee and Summer Johnson, "Has the Spread of HPV Vaccine Marketing Conveyed Immunity to Common Sense?" *The American Journal of Bioethics* 7, no. 7 (July 2007) <www.bioethics.net/journal/j_articles.php?aid=1288>.

tract that the freedom to engage in high-risk behaviors that do not directly harm others should not be constrained unless indirect risk is demonstrated to create extraordinarily high cost for society generally and other means of assigning that cost specifically to the risk takers cannot be found. Freedom is the most compelling argument against quarantine and lesser uses of police power in the case of HIV/AIDS. The just coercion criterion of proportionality requires that the cure is not worse than the disease (this shows how important freedom actually is because this is a truly dread disease). What remains unclear is why persons advocating for such freedom in this case do not advocate for freedom from unneeded police power in other less dangerous public health cases such as overeating and smoking.

Some less controversial cases can serve as illustrations. Children playing sports should be compelled to have physicals as the cost is low and it protects the otherwise legally vulnerable sponsoring agency; the state does not need to mandate this, but the organizations should be free to require it. Seat belts and helmets should only be mandated if the costs to the state are so significant and the cost (loss of freedom) to the driver/rider so low as to warrant the inconvenience; and, such seems to be true for drivers and motorcycle riders and so can be mandated unless persons waive all societal obligation to provide health care. Similarly, kayakers wanting to use flooded creeks, climbers wanting to ascend difficult routes and people wanting to enjoy snuff should be free to do so, if

1. others who are asked to tolerate the behavior are likewise free to note their disapproval of the same behavior;
2. the kayakers, mountain climbers and snuff-users put no one else at risk to a degree higher than is within the range of normal daily risks;
3. those engaging in the voluntary higher risk behaviors agree individually or within an insurance pool to pay for injuries or illness consequent to said risky behavior (this would require finding the difference between the expected survival for the "normal" person and the one participating in that specific behavior, and finding that it differed from generally accepted high risk behaviors, like driving ten miles over the speed limit);
4. comparable risks are addressed by police power in equitable ways.

All of this leads back to AIDS and ways for Christians and those of the world to morally respond in a civil society that practices separation of church and state. The disorder is a threat to the public health. The best way, if rights are of no concern, to control AIDS would be to immediately quarantine all persons infected. A drastic limit on freedom might make sense if the disease were *not* a venereal disease but spread through casual contact. Since that is not true, no other restrictions on the behavior of the disease carrier should be mandated. Freedom matters that much. Still, the state should encourage public health honesty.

CONCLUSION: SOCIAL ENGAGEMENT FOR THE PUBLIC HEALTH

The moral complexity for society (not just for Christians) of public health interventions can be bewildering. The inconsistencies make moral conversation difficult. For instance, is the ready availability of condoms any different from making clean needles available for addicts? Is education emphasizing the safety of sexual abstinence different from teaching people not to smoke? Guilt and shame have been used successfully with smoking. Should the same be done with promiscuous sexual behavior?

No Christian can actually avoid interacting with the broader culture, the state at its various levels, nor nonbelieving individuals. Still, believers must make a choice as to whether the health of the population is one of the values that warrants full political engagement, by individual believers and by the organized body of believers. Without asserting that every so-called public health issue really is one, it is apparent that any Christian that agrees with the legitimacy of believers participating on the public square should support the state to the extent that it reasonably promotes the public health.

There is one caveat. Risk can be used to justify intrusive governmental actions that are only tangentially related to the public health or that do not properly take into account legitimate individual choices because they violate some nonhealth value. This may be accomplished by declarations of perceived risk as if it is real risk, and is often done with the shrillest voice. Of course, believers occasionally do the same.

Still, there is a serious risk (and the use of the risk language is quite intentional) that public health constructs will be used to intrude into the Christian community. For instance, if believing in a God who is simultaneously judging and gracious is deemed psychologically damaging by a public health bureaucrat, then for the supposed well-being of a segment of the population (children) parental rights could be challenged for believers. This is not as fantastic as it may sound. Public health law is the most intrusive subset of U.S. law, with the possible exception of the tax code. No one needs to be found guilty to have behavior restricted. This risk does not allow Christians an excuse to not support legitimate public health services of the state, nor to not provide their own public health outreach when possible—even cooperating with the state to do so. The Christian obligation to render to Caesar may, at least on some occasions, mean instructing Caesar about how to best accomplish a common task and to serve as an example to others.

13

Moral Agency and End-of-Life Decisions

HUMANS AS FREE

Freedom as a right is not the same as having the capacity to make any and every decision. The capacity to choose is limited by natural abilities (including developmental stage, psychological history, cultural location and, of course, sinfulness). The state should not restrain freedom, given those limitations, unless a choice is a direct threat to another's life, liberty or property. Freedom is a moral good that can be used for bad moral ends. Free choice can be evaluated by (1) the process of calculating outcomes and (2) consistency with the character of the moral agent. Believers can and should expect other believers to make personal choices in accordance with the gospel. They should expect those of the world to make choices minimally in accordance with the rights protections of the social contract. This means evangelicals must tolerate some immoral decisions and actively oppose others. In bioethics, the concept of free choice comes up most often in end-of-life decisions, specifically passive and active euthanasia.

> Suppose one of you wants to build a tower. Will he not first sit down and estimate the cost to see if he has enough money to complete it? For if he lays the foundation and is not able to finish it, everyone who sees it will ridicule him, saying, "This fellow began to build and was not able to finish."
>
> Or suppose a king is about to go to war against another king. Will he not first sit down and consider whether he is able with ten thousand men to oppose the one coming against him with twenty thousand? If he is not able, he will send a delegation while the other is still a long way off and will ask for terms of peace. In the same way, any of you who does not give up everything he has cannot be my disciple. (Lk 14:28-33)

PART ONE: THE TEXT

To become a Christian, one must make a decision.[1] At least in the Protestant

---

[1]This chapter was developed on the basis of presentations developed with Bruns Myers, former chaplain and ethicist at Methodist Rehabilitation Center in Jackson, Mississippi. Any errors remain mine.

traditions, the assumption is made that one chooses to be a follower of the Christ. The best known and dominant model is Paul's conversion. Jesus refers to the decision as a matter of calculation (Lk 14:28-33). The term *calculation* usually brings to mind utilitarian methods of reasoning, but the reasoning Jesus proposes is of a different kind. It is closer to what traditional Catholic and ancient Greek philosophers refer to as prudence. This type of prudential calculation may take a mathematical form, such as in Pascal's Wager, or as more of a sense of correctness, such as in Wesley and Whitefield.[2] The decision is not right and good solely by its consequences, but by the consequences as an expression of the character of the decision-maker and what that character is meant to be.

While not utilitarian in the true sense, this kind of decision making is clearly teleological (end-oriented). Though utilitarian philosophers often consider such a description simplistic, utilitarianism is essentially an argument that the ends justify the means. The kind of prudent calculating Christ asks is a matter of the end conditioning the means. To be his follower mandates certain means to the end and eliminates others.

The prudent believer recognizes personal understanding of pertinent subjects, proper consideration of the time allowed to make a decision, an awareness of the impact of decisions on others, and how the communities involved shape decision making. The prudent believer realizes when she or he does not know enough to make a decision completely free of ambiguity, but recognizes that making a decision may be compelled and the choices may be limited. For the

---

[2]There is certainly a point of overlap between evangelical notions of prudential reasoning and American civil concepts. See Daniel Walker Howe, *Making the American Self: Jonathan Edwards to Abraham Lincoln*, Studies in Cultural History (Cambridge, Mass.: Harvard University Press, 1997). According to Howe, the "self" as expressed is the capacity of reason engaging the passions as prudence. For a specific protoevangelical example, see discussion about Whitefield on page 45. Prudence is understood as reasonable self-interest, but with self often recognized in communal as well as individual terms. See the review of the Howe work by Kyle P. Farley (University of Pennsylvania) on H-SHEAR, H-Net Discussion Network for the Scholars of the History of the Early American Republic, November, 1997 <http://www.h-net.org/reviews/showrev.cgi?path=1071882897360>.

How passion and reason were understood in the decades before the American establishment period is discussed in Albert O. Hirschman, *The Passions and the Interests: Political Arguments for Capitalism Before Its Triumph* (Princeton, N.J.: Princeton University Press, 1977).

What is not sufficiently addressed in these excellent descriptions, though, is the moral epistemology, especially as developed in light of Newtonian physics. Frequently, the protoevangelicals as well as the nonreligious humanists emphasized the sense of morality. See James R. Thobaben, "Holy Knowing: A Wesleyan Epistemology," *The Death of Metaphysics, The Death of Culture*, Philosophical Studies in Contemporary Culture (Springer Netherlands, 2006), 12:99-132.

prudent believer, all choices should move one toward Christlikeness, or be intended to do so.

In this parable, Jesus asserts that following him is prudent, even though costly. Proper decisions are not those that are problem free, but those that are the best given the situation, needs of the participants and the final outcome. This means in any and every situation, some choice can be right and good. Some may assert that the decision for the "lesser of two evils" is morally wrong, but preferable to greater moral wrongs. Generally evangelicals would not accept such a description. If a choice is truly right given the options, it is the good choice. Bad consequences may follow, but those are due to the broken moral nature of existence or to prior decisions that created the circumstances, not to the choice of the decision-maker.

Still, the decision-maker is responsible for addressing consequences. Not being responsible for the conditions in which a decision is made does not mean that one is not responsible for the outcomes of a decision. She or he cannot simply claim that bad side-effects were not his or her intention and therefore not his or her fault. To the contrary, even in a good decision, the bad consequences are also the responsibility of the decision-maker to address. Such is the case with accepting Christ. There is a cost and the cost must be borne, even though the actual culpability for at least some of those negative costs belongs to evil persons who may strike out at believers.

To not choose the good is to choose the evil. To not choose heaven is to choose hell. So then, it is necessary to count the cost to the best of one's abilities, considering all alternatives and the effect on the character of all participants as well as immediate implications. In the case of choosing Christ, the cost for alternative decisions is infinitely bad, while the cost for choosing him is only proximately negative and well worth the eternal joy as well as earthly improvement in character.[3]

The choice for Christ is yes or no, and prudence calls for the extreme decision of accepting Christ as Lord. Such is not the case with many moral decisions. There can be degrees of relative goodness or degrees of evil that make choosing the right difficult. The ambiguity of the temporal world makes choices, on many occasions, less than obvious. The nature of a given evil or good may be such as to compel a decision, or there may be

[3]This is a version of argumentation that has become known as Pascal's Wager. Pascal lived at the beginning of modernity, anticipating the problems of reductionism, and his thought returns again at the end of modernity in the use of probability for moral analysis.

several choices with varying degrees of the preferable and the undesirable. In the parable of the three servants, two acted wisely with the same rate of return but had different actual outcomes. The possibility of the right choice, even with different particular outcomes, is more evident when considering the failed servant whose master tells him that he could have at least invested the money for interest. There was a right choice, and he did not make it.

With the parable of the tower, the choice of the virtuous was not simply whether or not to build the tower, but also to prudently determine how tall and how wide given the limits of skill and funding, as well as the needs of the location. If every moral choice is a small reiteration of accepting Jesus in that it is accepting his Lordship in the moments of life, then the difficult moral question is not whether or not to build our lives for him, but how.

The prudent decision to accept Christ calls forth prudence as a virtue in making moral decisions, including those in bioethics. Given that most so-called bioethical dilemmas cannot be resolved by appealing to direct scriptural references, the virtuosity of the decision-maker(s) is especially important. Simple answers are rarely available to moral questions arising with new technologies and new organizational forms. Even when direct references can be used to address specific bioethical concerns, prudence should shape the Christian's orientation. Discerning the right and the good may sometimes depend on an accurate exegesis of a difficult scriptural passage, but even that finally depends on the virtue of the decision-maker and true familiarity with the story and the values of the story as empowered by the Spirit.

Christians should always seek to be wise as a matter of character; then so-called dilemmas will be less frequent, and when they do arise, the believer will be able to respond appropriately. The training of the believer in prudence or wisdom comes through the individual study of Scripture and through accountability to the church. The latter includes reliance on saints above (the example of Christians who have gone before) and on saints on earth (it is simply not possible for a person to be a mature and wise Christian without being accountable to other believers).

In bioethics, as in all moral consideration, the prudent or wise person is the one who can take into account the values of the past, the virtues of the present and the outcomes anticipated for the future—for individuals and for communities. The prudent person is not only smart but also good to the extent that she or he allows God's grace to function and seeks the good.

PART TWO: CHRISTIAN BIOETHICS

Saul was the first king of the united kingdom of the twelve tribes of Israel. Some have claimed he was less a king than a transitional figure who was partially a federation military leader and partially a monarch, but who fully succeeded in neither role. At the end of a battle, he chose to end his life either out of dread over possible torture, shame over defeat, a desire to deprive enemies of the opportunity to kill him, an effort to maintain kingly control to the smallest extent possible, or out of emotional and/or spiritual weakness in the face of personal failure.[4] Analogically, his choice is like those who choose to actively terminate their own or another's life.

> Now the Philistines fought against Israel; the Israelites fled before them, and many fell slain on Mount Gilboa. The Philistines pressed hard after Saul and his sons, and they killed his sons Jonathan, Abinadab and Malki-Shua. The fighting grew fierce around Saul, and when the archers overtook him, they wounded him critically.
>
> Saul said to his armor-bearer, "Draw your sword and run me through, or these uncircumcised fellows will come and run me through and abuse me."
>
> But his armor-bearer was terrified and would not do it; so Saul took his own sword and fell on it. When the armor-bearer saw that Saul was dead, he too fell on his sword and died with him. So Saul and his three sons and his armor-bearer and all his men died together that same day.
>
> When the Israelites along the valley and those across the Jordan saw that the Israelite army had fled and that Saul and his sons had died, they abandoned their towns and fled. And the Philistines came and occupied them. (1 Sam 31:1-7)

The Scripture is replete with reports of moral decisions and consequences. With most of those reported, the decision has dramatic implications (that is why they are included in the Text). These implications are usually commu-

---

[4]Another, similar suicide occurred earlier when Abimelech, the first person to declare himself king of Israel, was killed at his own request by his armor-bearer after he had been injured by a woman dropping a millstone; he did not want it said that his life had been taken by a woman. Abimelech was the devious son of Gideon. He had killed off most of his family and hired mercenaries in order to establish his rule. He apparently encouraged Baal worship. The Text avoids actually saying he was a judge, as if to deprive him of the honor, though he was the authority figure for a period. A parable that Jotham told is recorded in which Abimelech is compared to a thornbush. Abimelech's death is deemed "repayment" from God (Judg 9).

nitywide, yet individuals often make the decisions themselves. In the case of Saul's suicide, the decision is his and those he tries to compel to assist, yet he is aware (and so are those around him) that it has broader implications. While he is injured, the suicide seems to be primarily based on his unwillingness to be taken prisoner to his shame or to Israel's or both. His armor-bearer, interestingly, refuses to "euthanize" or to "assist in the suicide," yet is willing to kill himself soon after Saul.[5]

Essentially, Saul was abdicating, which could be most readily accomplished by death. Suicide was an efficient means of ending his temporal experience of his problems, though not necessarily for others who continued living with the consequences of his choice. As noted, he might have been doing this for a number of reasons. In Christian terms, his suicide might be viewed as something like an inverted baptism in that it was the conscious withdrawal from the community. In 1 Chronicles 10, Saul's decision to commit suicide seems to be simultaneously added to the list of his dishonorable decisions indicative of his failures as a leader and a consequence administered by God's will for the previous immoralities. He abdicated his kingship, withdrew from the community of Israel and resigned from the human race.

For Christians reading this story and considering the implications of decision making in bioethics, the responses of David and of Jabesh Gilead are important. David inquired of soldiers from the field as to what had happened. A soldier of non-Israelite origins reported that he saw Saul dying and at the request of Saul, after he had impaled himself, had finished the task. The soldier justified his action by saying, "I stood over him and killed him, because I knew that after he had fallen he could not survive. And I took the crown that was on his head and the band on his arm and have brought them here to my lord [David]" (2 Sam 1:10). Immediately David had the man killed because he had struck down "the LORD's anointed." The harshest judgment seems to be against the man who claimed to have assisted, not against the suicide victim himself—though Saul is dead by the time David exacts punishment and so condemnation of him would be both pointless pragmatically and disrespectful.[6]

---

[5]Perhaps the unwillingness to kill Saul was due to the latter's royal status and the possible consequences for the armor-bearer and his family. David's later action indicates that this would not have been an unwarranted fear.

[6]From the text in 1 and 2 Samuel, it appears that the man was claiming he had assisted so as to gain David's favor, but likely did not facilitate the suicide and certainly did not gain David's favor.

Apparently, David did not demonize Saul for his action, either because the new king considered it understandable emotionally or disrespectful or he did not want to undermine kingly authority. Saul's status as the Lord's anointed, his past acts of kindness, the emotional vulnerability and culturally demanded shame he had experienced and even the physical pain following the self-inflicted wound seem to allow an appreciation for the good he represented in spite of this ethical error. David certainly insisted that he remain honored even though the death is represented as the will of Yahweh. Also, the people of a village Saul had helped in the past remembered his kindness and grieved for him without allowing this decision for suicide and his numerous other failures to negate all good memories of him. It seems that though an immoral effort to avoid consequences, Saul's action is condemned without his being deemed an "excommunicant" or apostate of Israel.

> When all the inhabitants of Jabesh Gilead heard of everything the Philistines had done to Saul, all their valiant men went and took the bodies of Saul and his sons and brought them to Jabesh. Then they buried their bones under the great tree in Jabesh, and they fasted seven days.
>
> Saul died because he was unfaithful to the LORD; he did not keep the word of the LORD and even consulted a medium for guidance, and did not inquire of the LORD. So the LORD put him to death and turned the kingdom over to David son of Jesse. (1 Chron 10:11-14)

People have choices, but all options are not equally valid morally. Saul, his armor-bearer and the Amalekite-Israelite soldier failed in varying degrees to act morally. The choice to kill oneself or to facilitate such remains immoral today, though immoral in varying degrees. The desperate individual is not morally culpable to the same extent as the facilitator who benefits from the self-killing. Further differentiation can be made between those who assist a suicide out of their own sorrow and those who do so in an effort to improve their own social status or push forward a political agenda. The possibility of such distinctions has been graphically demonstrated, quite vividly, in the tragico-comical actions of Jack Kevorkian. The pathologist's so-called patients were predominantly people with chronic disorders and/or disabilities, not people with terminal (in the sense of immediately dying) conditions.[7] The choice of the person with the disability would be deemed

---

[7]For a discussion on the intersection of Christian belief and the political and legal activities of Jack Kevorkian, see James R. Thobaben, "A United Methodist Approach to End-of-Life:

immoral by believers and should be actively discouraged and prevented to the extent reasonably possible by the state. The actions of those facilitating the self-killing, which is not an individual, but communal act, should be actively punished. David did not approve of the killing of a king, and the state today should not tolerate the unnecessary killing of contract makers, even when they are desperate.

This does not mean there will never be circumstances in which one accepts his or her own dying without aggressive treatment or allows another to die. Certainly, the prudent decision-maker takes into account the possibilities of improvement and/or recovery. Further, allowing the sick who are in the process of dying to go ahead and die is recognizing that physical existence is a high good, but not the ultimate good. Extending the dying process is not necessary and often not warranted.

Still, biological life is a good and the default should be on the side of preservation, both for eternal reasons and temporal. Most obviously, defaulting toward the preservation of life protects the well-being of the marginalized of society who will suffer if definitions of *unworthy* or *unnecessary* are expanded and the killing of such is defined as merciful—to the killed individual and to the family and to the society—or even obligatory on the part of the vulnerable and costly individual. While the concern of Saul's armor-bearer may have been that he would be accused of killing a member of the royalty and, thereby, acting above his station, it also appears that the taking of a human life, when not as a matter of civil justice, was not acceptable. Within Christianity, the taking of life for justice may be, according to some theories, morally acceptable under extreme circumstances, but it is never acceptable to take life as an act of mercy.

For Christians, the life does not belong to the individual, contrary to what is asserted by those enamored with Western hyperindividualism. The life belongs to God. If the sick or injured person decides from a perspective of hyperindividualism, then that is a choice made in pathetic isolation that may even reveal sociopathology or psychopathology. If the community makes the decision considering only its own well-being (including economic, the avoid-

---

Intentional Ambiguity or Ambiguous Intentions," *Christian Bioethics* 3, no. 3 (1977): 222-48; Amy M Burdette, Terrence D. Hill and Benjamin E. Moulton, "Religion and Attitudes Toward Physician-Assisted Suicide and Terminal Palliative Care," *Journal for the Scientific Study of Religion* 44, no. 1 (2005): 79-93. Aside from the legitimation of the killing of persons with disabilities, the reasoning offered by some of those defending Kevorkian from a supposedly Christian perspective was embarrassing.

ance of community shame and so forth), then it is domineering or even oppressive. From a Christian point of view, all moral decisions, but especially those having to do with life and death, must balance individuality with community obligations. Having said this is true, however, may not mean the Christian should insist that the secular culture endorse such a view. Christians must oppose decisions to euthanize and work against those who would attempt to "assist" in the death of others, when it appears that the consequences of the decision could harm others, especially the socially weak (the poor, etc.). Still, the role the state should take in preventing such decisions and actions is another question. While the state should not allow but actively discourage such, there is not a clear Christian justification for treating persons who attempt such as criminals. Those willing to assist can readily be deemed such.

Further, every person in the United States—and that includes Christians—should recognize that the social contract requires protection of every person, including himself or herself. Opting out of the contract must occur by emigration simply because there is too great a risk in allowing the state the authority to *not* act when people seek to opt out through suicide. The state must protect the lives of each individual from imminent threat; that is its primary reason for the state existing under the social contract. While some might assert that utility directs the society to kill off the costly or to equate the suicide or involuntary killing of persons with putting down horses with broken legs and cats that get decrepitly old, the right to life takes priority over utility.

Suicides are immoral, but they may not always be the actions of irrational or mentally ill persons. The crisis faced may be primarily spiritual—a sort of existential depression—rather than a psychological one. If the rational, competent decision is for suicide, and there do not seem to be any direct consequences for others, it would not be illogical for a Christian to morally oppose the action, but without additional legal penalty advocated. In reality, though, the legal line of rationality in the midst of any such circumstances that might call for suicide is quite difficult to draw. As rational as a decision may appear, suicidal efforts are all but inevitably elicited with a mixture of motives. Not the least important factor is often pressure from others or a lack of reasonable support in the midst of a difficult situation. Believers must err on the side of protecting persons and act against any laws legalizing active euthanasia. Certainly, there is absolutely no reason to encourage any legal mechanism that would facilitate self-destruction. Christians could well advocate for the provision of counseling and support against suicide funded by the state on the basis that human life is an intrinsic good.

In a similar way, many other bioethical decisions are limited by the prudential consideration of the divine purposes for each person's life. While humans may be free to make choices about biotechnologies that alter the human genome for enhancement; about periodically remaking their bodies and faces with expensive cosmetic surgery; about refusing cochlear implants for their children, it does not mean they should (or even be allowed to) do any of these things.

Evangelicals ought to make distinctions not only about the morality of a decision, but also about the morality of interfering with another's decision. So it is completely reasonable to work toward legislation that will prevent the killing off of those with disabilities, and it would be correct to support legislative action against positive eugenics through genetic engineering. It would be appropriate to raise public questions about the parent who refuses a cochlear implant in order to maintain his or her own social network's membership. It would be wrong to legally interfere with (though there is no reason to fund through insurance pools or governmental programs) persons choosing excessive cosmetic surgeries (this does not include dire cases; e.g., restoration following severe facial injury).

These examples illuminate the different degrees of restraint on choice. It is reasonable to interfere with parental control when the parent seeks to prevent a treatment that is highly likely to assist the child in moving toward functional normality[8] such as with cochlear implants or, to use an even clearer example, with blood transfusions for the young children of Jehovah's Witnesses. This kind of interference must be approached with full consideration of the implications and reasons why persons might desire to act in such a way. Persons with hearing impairments have faced discrimination and some do have a distinct subculture with a distinct language. Jehovah's Witnesses do have a distinct religion, which they take quite seriously, and there is not evidence, excepting on blood transfusions, that their children are at greater risk than the average Americans'. Cosmetic surgery in the

[8]The concept of "functional normality" developed by Norman Daniels and others is useful but open to abuse if "normal" as biological and statistical is confused with normal as the moral norm. For another critique of the language, see Anita Silvers, "No Basis for Justice: Equal Opportunity, Normal Functioning and the Distribution of Health Care," *The American Journal of Bioethics* 1, no. 2 (spring 2001): 35-36.

United States often seems frivolous, and it is more than reasonable for Christians to question the morality of such a choice. Yet such decisions do not directly threaten another individual or put a category of persons at risk, and so even excessive cosmetic surgery that puts the person at some notable risk needs to be tolerated as a bad, but permissible, moral choice—unless funded by group insurance or the state.

All moral choices by believers are simultaneously individual and communal, as Saul's, the armor-bearer's and the Amalekite-Isrealite soldier's indicate. Patients' decisions are rarely made in isolation. In the case of euthanasia, there is almost always someone facilitating. The choice to or not to participate in such activities is as important as the decision of the patient to follow a particular course of action. This not only applies to family members or professionals in cases of euthanizing, it also includes other actions of conscience. For moral consistency, then, evangelicals tend to actively support freedom-of-conscience provisions for providers, including pharmacists, when the service or dispensed drug would function inevitably as an abortifacient, that is, a pharmaceutical meant to kill what believers consider and can reasonably argue to be a member of the social contract.

The rights of persons to make choices are limited by the obligation of the state to protect persons. For evangelicals, the rights of persons to make choices are further limited when those persons choose to become Christian. There is a cost to be borne for faithfulness. Part of that cost is a restriction on options. Part of that cost is tolerating the decisions of others under certain circumstances. Sometimes the cost is working to limit the choices of others when they significantly threaten the life or liberty or property (in that order) of another.

PART THREE: CHRISTIAN BIOETHICS AND THE WORLD

At this point in U.S. health care, autonomy in decision making all but trumps all other considerations. Even the most cautious diagnosis and treatment protocol is subject to acceptance by the patient or his or her agent. This may be best. In the arena of health-care delivery, given the numerous differences on values, the moral acceptability of many decisions tends not to hinge on either the rightness or wrongness of the choice, nor goodness or wrongness of the character-shaping event. Rather, the acceptability depends on the enactment of what is considered a just procedure under the social contract: namely, that an individual makes an autonomous decision.

This would seem to represent the triumph in the health-care setting of the political concept of liberty. Yet autonomy cannot be an absolute value. Freedom is always limited; the practical question is how. In health-care decisions, one significant limit is accountability for the effect of decisions on others.

Ironically, some in medicine deny the reality of autonomy altogether. Though the terms vary, the secular argument about autonomy, freedom and choice tends to take shape around the familiar nature/nurture polarity. Strong psychoanalytic theorists and strong social constructionists assert that nurture is all that matters, with one tending to claim that morality is written on the blank slate of the human mind by family and the other by the societal order. Sociobiologists argue for the commonality of human traits on the basis of genetic mutation and natural selection, though for the group as opposed to the individual. Behavioral geneticists assume the blank slate is shaped in a particular way and that it will allow only certain kinds of writing upon it, with human difference being the compelled effect of genetics, environment and environment-genetic interaction. Freedom (the political parallel of the ethical term *autonomy*) tends to be understood as an evolutionarily selected self-deception.

Evangelicals do not dispute that persons can learn from all of these schools of thought, but they consider them woefully inadequate as worldviews. In particular, they consider the explanatory power of these theories to be particularly inadequate to explain (1) the actual human experience as decision-makers and (2) the moral order that is conditioned by the moral choices of participants. Evangelicals would agree with the claim that persons are shaped by both nature and nurture. But that dichotomy is not a sufficient description of the components of moral decision—also significant are *chance* and individual *choice*. Chance is a statistical term that has a rough equivalent in the term *chaos* as borrowed from contemporary scientific literature with modifications from physics. Chaos is that which is unpredictable at the micro-level while tending to appear in statistically predictable patterns at the macro-level and sometimes assumed to be determined entirely by highly sensitive initial states. This is definitely not what is meant in popular uses of the word *chaos* nor how the word is used in Scripture (e.g., Gen 1). Evangelicals claim that "chance" is sometimes, though not always, a miraculous expression of God's will and is always a reflection of his penultimate will.

Rather than simply nature and nurture, the capacity for choice should be

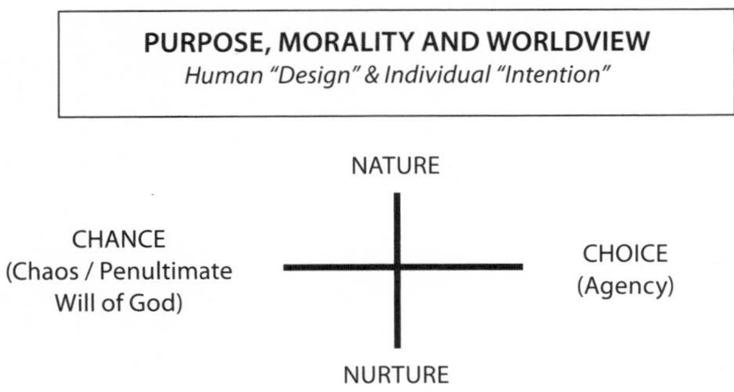

Figure 13.1.

placed on a grid with nature, nurture and chance (fig. 13.1). The responsibility of the decision-maker is indicated by the parabola on the x-y continuum (fig. 13.2). Persons who have capacity must seek to control their biology and their social location to the extent possible. Persons are also obligated to prepare to meet contingencies (chance/chaos). Control of all the various aspects of daily existence, however, can be quite limited. The greatest responsibility is for those aspects of life over which they have—or are perceived to have—the greatest choice. Moral dysfunction arises when one tries to control that beyond which one has control or, through the abdication of responsibility, avoids making a decision when one should.

Various understandings can be located on this x-y continuum. One of the most popular in the United States at the end of modernity seems to be some version of shallow existentialism in the form of subjectivism. The only concern is one's own choices without considerations of nature, nurture and chance that have shaped those options. It was described by Kierkegaard as the life of the aesthetic and is marked by shallow, egoist calculating. Such subjectivists who are personally failing at one thing or another may seek to shed blame—either attributing choices to their own genetics or blaming someone they dislike. They believe they are entirely positively shaped by decisions, while negative aspects are due to someone else. Autonomy is not a means to an end, but an end in itself. Perhaps they think that God can advise, but he cannot and should not demand; God can suggest but not set standards. Those functioning with such an operational model tend to deny there are common experiences by which everyone is shaped or they claim that these are experienced in such unique ways as to not really create commonality of understanding or values. This is moral autonomy misunderstood, for such people think they really are "an order

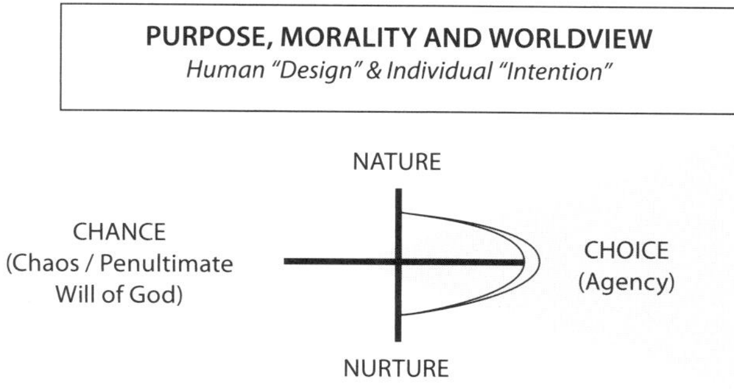

Figure 13.2.

unto themselves," which is demonstrably not the case.

The most common version of moral dysfunction is the emotive individualism that quickly developed in the 1960s and 1970s, with its strong subjectivist claims.[9] These persons strongly emphasize their own autonomy, borrowing political vocabulary from libertarianism and philosophical liberalism, but in practice tend to favor a paternal/maternal state at the same time that they try to satisfy immediate desires through excessive material consumption. Opponents are accused of being unjust, with shame and embarrassment. In bioethical terms, the immoral paternalism of pre-1960s health care is completely inverted into immoral subjectivist autonomy.

The argumentation is much like the complaining of a U.S. adolescent who wants unfettered use of the family car and tuition for college but is angered by the expectation that his or her parents may set a curfew or require the taking out of the trash. Eventually the "trash," or consequences of bad moral choices, must be taken out. This is the proverbial spoiled brat as citizen.

The philosophical argument for this moral position runs along the following lines. Everyone is supposedly equal biologically (nature). Problems must be due to bad experiences or rearing (nurture), for there is no other way to explain inequality. The possibility of unpredictable events or what might be called bad or good luck is generally denied, thus allowing credit for victories to be claimed, while personal failures are to be denied or blamed on others.

[9]See Robert Bellah et al., *Habits of the Heart: Individualism and Commitment in American Life*, updated ed. (Berkeley: University of California Press, 1996). See also Charles Taylor, *Sources of the Self: The Making of Modern Identity* (Cambridge, Mass.: Harvard University Press, 1989). A fine exposition of various philosophical and theological arguments analyzed from a Christian Catholic position applied to bioethics is John F. Kavanaugh, *Who Count as Persons? Human Identity and the Ethics of Killing* (Washington, D.C.: Georgetown University Press, 2001).

Demands on physical resources or on practitioners are made to obtain freedom of choice. The individual asserts a right to demand of others the provision of resources or particular services to increase his or her potential for achieving his or her individual *telos* while ignoring the right of others to work toward their own *teloi*.

Paradoxically, this argument, over time, leads to lessened choice. If and when the state is compelled to protect an opportunity for an individual to choose by providing options, (1) those options of necessity will be more limited than might be developed by individuals themselves as the cost of resources to the state rises and (2) they will limit the freedom of others and, as others make demands, limit the freedom of the prior decision-maker. This is especially hypocritical in bioethics when demands for freedom of choice are used to deny freedom of choice to practitioners who want to withdraw from participation in certain treatments for reasonable moral reasons. The claim is made that they should be compelled, while the service user should be free to do the compelling.

Though this subjectivism is the dominant popular argument in the world at the end of modernity, in its most extreme form becoming postmodern deconstruction, another approach dominates a large segment of the academy and cultured elite—that is physical reductionism with its denial of freedom. Sometimes the argument takes shape around individual psychological determinism or evolutionary determinism. The moral impact, somewhat contradictorily, is the condemnation of all who make "bad" choices, though not as sinners but as dismissed inferiors. More complex philosophical versions of the same can be found, ironically, in modified Nietzschian *Übermensch* (superman) arguments that take shape in both leftist (as the ideal political leader) and rightist (as the self-made capitalist) forms—both sometimes make arguments to eliminate the "weak," or at least allow them to die off.

Regardless of what secularists may claim about the ontological condition of persons, the state should act as if each competent individual can make choices, including about health care—even while realizing human decisions are constrained by nature, nurture, the choices of others and unpredictable circumstances. For instance, one can choose to accept or decline an offered treatment. The patient's choice to accept a treatment option assumes that the treatment is not considered futile by experts or legitimately cost-prohibitive, as no one is entitled to demand inappropriate services. Also, generally favoring liberty does not mean that the choice of the patient inevitably trumps the freedom of conscience of the practitioner. Still, the Christian should strongly endorse the liberty to choose and should reject paternalism/maternalism in health care.

The autonomy of an individual is also limited by the cost of health care. While sometimes choices have been immorally restricted for financial reasons, all financial constraints are not thereby immoral. Someone's choice might be undue taking from others and would, therefore, be immoral. In the case of taxation for health care, the system to be developed should be demonstrably superior or equal to what currently exists and, then, provide increased freedom for a substantial number of individuals seeking to fulfill their individual *telos*.

Liberty can also be limited by the capacity of the decision-maker—both the internal capacity to make rational decisions and the externally generated capacity. If a person has received (1) an appropriate level of information (practitioners have a duty to remedy deficiencies in information), (2) has the mental capacity to understand the information, (3) is not unduly pressured into making a particular decision by caregivers or others with a vested interest and (4) has the time to make a reasonable decision, then that person should be allowed to determine whether or not she or he receives a specific treatment. Liberty or autonomy requires both the right to and capacity to make a choice. In health care, such a choice is called informed consent.

Informed consent is a useful political and legal idea and one that Christians should support. In essence, informed consent is a parallel to the right to vote, as autonomy is a parallel to the political concept of liberty. Indeed, it is a manifestation of liberty. As with voting, an autonomous decision does not necessarily lead to a desired outcome. Persons must be free to make bad choices, not because this will make them better in the long run (a teleological argument), but simply because free choice is a central value of the U.S. social contract and that contract is worth protecting.

An example of informed consent and autonomy formalized as procedure is the advance directive. When persons lack capacity, since the society so values the right to autonomy, legal constructs have been developed in the name of this right. Together these procedures are known as advance directives. Again, though this "pretend autonomy" is not an accurate portrayal of the circumstances in which a sick person exists (for she or he does not have capacity to think or to communicate what is thought), the procedure does *tend* to protect the weak and vulnerable and should be maintained. Further, advance directives generally promote freedom.

Advance directives exist in three forms, though jurisdictions vary in the precise use of the terms. The three types are the durable power of attorney, the living will and the general directive. The first two have a stronger legal status; the latter is really more a statement of preference. Beyond these, and with the power to override them, is the judicial order. This is not actually an advance directive, but is a directive that comes into play when there is unresolved conflict over decisions or when no one takes responsibility. General directives are broad, usually unspecific, wishes expressed prior to incompetence about one's treatment. They may or may not have any legal significance. Certainly they are not considered with the same weight as a living will or durable power of attorney.

The *durable power of attorney for healthcare decisions* is a statement made prior to incapacity, which designates an attorney-in-fact to make choices on treatments. Sometimes in bioethics literature, this person is called a surrogate decision-maker. This person is permitted to make choices in the best interest of the patient or as a substituted judgment according to what the patient would have decided if able. Sometimes the decision is based on that which would be made by any rational person and sometimes that which would be made if the specific patient were his or her communicating rational self. The latter assumes a wider range of choices for "rational" persons. Should an attorney-in-fact not be designated, the usual order for surrogate decision making is spouse (or, in some cases, significant other), adult children, parents, siblings and other relatives. Conflict can arise rapidly and Christians should endorse the durable power of attorney procedure for avoiding problems during already difficult times. Having said this, Christian ethics among believers should be strongly communitarian and require that the preparation does not end with designation. In other words, it is imperative that persons discuss preferences prior to a crisis (be it with a spouse or other person who is so designated) and that they use the values of the body of believers.

The *living will* is usually understood to be a directive about specific treatments, primarily about the withdrawal of or limits to specific treatments when death is imminent. The document has to be witnessed by persons who are not related to the patient nor involved in the medical treatment of the patient. It comes into play when one is deemed legally incompetent. Generally, the living will can be revoked verbally. Also, it is important to understand that the term *living will* may mean different things in different states and that a form signed in one state may not be binding in another.

The more or less common agreement about the civil validity of the ethical concept of autonomy, and procedures to protect it (like informed consent and advance directives), can mask the fact that persons are not merely political creatures. Since there is general agreement about autonomy, and there is not about other significant values, autonomy, in the form of documents like advance directives, tends to trump other considerations. The "autonomy" argument is not only insufficient on its own but also can be misused. Decisions that are described as autonomous may, in fact, be compelled by those with power to control the decision-maker. Free choice may give way to utility. This is all the more likely as shared notions of prudence and virtue are generally lacking. Thus the utilitarian calculus weighing the total pain (including emotional, economic, the experiences of family members and staff, etc.) against the total benefit of continued life (especially lower so-called quality of life) gets translated inappropriately into the language of futility which is, in turn, used to abrogate free choice and/or the protection of the right to life for the member of the social contract.

In addition, though individuals do (or should) exist as equals before the law, they also exist as members of families, as persons suffering from diseases, as individuals with different degrees of medical knowledge, as people with differing mental capacities. This is why, though Christians can and should endorse the use of the concept of autonomy, they should do so cautiously and while asserting that autonomy is an insufficient basis for decision making.

In practical terms, even if not legally, there is a continuum of autonomy, from completely incompetent to having the normal, reasonable ability to make a rational decision to making a radically autonomous choice. At one end of the scale is the person who either completely lacks the mental ability to make a decision or cannot communicate that decision to others. This would include a young child or a person in a so-called vegetative state or a person with aphasia. Such a person would be readily acknowledged by any court as legally incompetent. Such an individual has eclipsed autonomy—eclipsed because the capacity may be hidden rather than missing.

Another category is those who would likely be deemed legally incompetent, but who have some ability to contribute to the decision-making process. These persons have diminished autonomy. Some of these are teenage children who have partial understanding but not a legal right for decision making.

Some persons may have diminished intellectual abilities due to developmental disability, traumatic brain injury and so on. In addition, others may have diminished capacity because of emotional fragility. They may defer to someone else out of fear or weakness or submissiveness or a sense of being overwhelmed by circumstances. Such persons should be consulted about the decision to be made, but should not have the final say unless a genuine capacity for understanding and for making a decision based on a reasonable evaluation of future outcome and consistency with current character is evident. Because this category of "diminished but capable of contributing to the decision" is not legally recognized, laws and judicial rulings in the United States have created a functional mess, for instance, with young teenage girls being able to choose abortion, but not make decisions about other major and minor treatments or even over-the-counter medications.

The third and fourth categories on the scale are made up of those who would be deemed legally competent. The competent can be differentiated by the recognition, or lack thereof, of community obligation.

The third category is made up of those in strong relationships that generate covenantal communities, who have morally mature understandings of their lives and will consider the implications of their decisions for others when making choices. Though this sounds like a high threshold, there is no reason to believe that teenagers, the uneducated and others who might be demeaned by cultured elites could well have this capacity and should have their right to decision making respected. Such persons recognize that the political concept of liberty really cannot function without some genuine care for others. This can be referred to with the seemingly oxymoronic moniker "interactive autonomy." This is the preferred approach for Christians. It is autonomy limited by obligation.

Finally, those in the fourth category make their decisions supposing no obligation to others—family, hospital staff, other persons with disabling conditions and so on. In a society that has accepted popularized versions of Freudianism and various other developmental theories, it should come as no surprise that freedom is not infrequently defined as "being oneself" with this individuation in turn meaning to separate from parents, siblings and other communities of obligation. This isolated autonomy is manifest in the replacement of marriage as a religious covenant with the marriage as role contract. It is seen in hospital rooms when someone looks at the injury survivor and declares, following an event like traumatic brain injury or spinal cord injury, "I cannot use up my life in a relationship like this." In its most severe form, this kind of segmented thinking becomes the true isolation of the individual. Such persons might want to discuss a moral decision with others, but will not recognize that even about oneself others should have some say. It might be argued that such persons are legally competent, but ethically incompetent. Under the United States social contract, the state should not compel such persons when decisions do not do any direct and significant harm to others. Christians could not endorse such an attitude among believers.

Legal categories:

1. Incompetence
2. Competence

Pragmatic ethical categories:

1. Eclipsed competence (total incompetence)
2. Diminished competence (limited competence/limited incompetence)
3. Interactive competence (competence but within community)
4. Isolated competence (competence without community)

Decisions about using alternative medicines, allowing an abortion, participating in experimental protocols and numerous other health care choices require consideration of autonomy. Arguably, the most important example of patient decision making in health care, and the one central to debates about autonomy, is the ending of life-sustaining treatment. Though decisions about euthanasia are always complicated, it is morally helpful to distinguish choices by ethically significant categories. For euthanasia these can be outlined with questions:

- Is the act voluntary? (Autonomy as right)
- Does the "agent" have capacity? (Autonomy as capacity)
- What means would be used?
- What is the severity of the agent's condition?
- What is the site of the moral standards?

An agent can accept a moral action (voluntary), can reject it (involuntary), or not state an opinion (nonvoluntary). If the act is autonomous in the isolated or interactive sense, that is, permission has been obtained without coercion (including not only physical, but psychological, religious and economic), then the individual has the right to refuse treatment. This is autonomy as a right to choice or liberty. The right to refuse treatment does not make it morally correct; it does mean that that the moral demand for freedom is stronger than the demand to restrain the individual for compelled treatment. Such an act of euthanasia would be called *voluntary*. Nonvoluntary refusal of treatment is not possible. To state the obvious, if permission cannot be obtained, then permission is not given.

Sometimes for those who cannot communicate, consideration of what she or he would have wanted or what any reasonable person would choose may be appropriate to consider, but the potential vested interests of the surrogates should always be questioned. Under the Patient Self-Determination Act, which allows the refusal of life-sustaining treatment, no one who is an involved professional caregiver should participate in the final decision. When permission cannot be obtained, in order to protect the social contract by protecting the contract-makers, the choice should default toward life. There is a bias toward living that is not the same as vitalism (the reduction of human life to physiology), but that recognizes that biology is an inextricable part of life on this earth and a clear indicator of personhood (to use the vernacular). Finally, involuntary withdrawal of actual life-sustaining treatment should be strictly prohibited.

Physician-assisted suicide, now legal in Oregon and Washington in the United States, is primarily a means of demonstrating that the act of euthanasia was conducted for and by the patient as an autonomous moral agent. It therefore supposedly buffers the practitioner from violating professional moral constraints on facilitating self-killing and from legal action. The right to die—an absurd concept as no one needs such a right nor can it be denied as death comes to all—is equated with liberty by those who mistakenly promote the Western notion of hyperindividualism. The error is analytical as much as moral; they think they can master every moment with choice by making decisions without consideration of the impact on the broader society, by determining rightness and goodness purely subjectively. Still, this error should not become a reason to deny the right to reasonably refuse treatments.

The choice to refuse treatment is not the same as the choice to demand it. Specific treatments might cause greater problems than no treatment at all. More likely, a given procedure or drug would not be efficacious and so there is no reason to spend the money and time on such. Resources are wasted and there is a lost opportunity cost for providers obligated to care for other people besides the one demanding the services. Such treatments would be futile, and can morally be ended or not initiated even if contrary to patient or family wishes. Let it be emphasized that futility must be medically defined, not using the quality of the individual's life.

The second aspect of a euthanasia choice is capacity. As noted above, capacity is both a legal and pragmatic status. The protection of the legal concept of autonomy, even when in actuality the patient is not clearly autonomous, such as when she or he is eclipsed or diminished, occurs with advance directives or the designation of a surrogate decision-maker. Capacity is defined by rationality with the ability to communicate. Both isolated and interactive individuals, as defined above, have capacity. Christians are morally opposed to persons making treatment withdrawal decisions in isolation, but immorality does not constitute lost capacity.

The third aspect of the euthanasia choice is the means to be used. While some might assert there is no outcome difference between removing a treatment that results in death and an active intervention that results in death, there is a difference for the society. The abbreviation of the time to die by killing is not worth the cost to society in permitting the active termination of the legally innocent. Evangelicals are generally strongly opposed to active euthanasia. This is consistent with opposition to abortion. Arguably, it is inconsistent with support for capital punishment, as Roman Catholics with the whole-life ethic argue. The only counter argument is that capital punishment, when exacted of someone who is absolutely and clearly guilty, is rendered because the individual has opted out of the social contract. This claim would seemingly open the door for the rational person who wanted euthanasia claiming that she or he was "opting" out of the social contract. While these may or may not be inconsistencies, the correction should not come at the cost of society tolerating the killing of legally innocent persons and, thereby, making others vulnerable. If someone wants to commit suicide, that individual should not ask for state assistance nor expect encouragement, but rather moral condemnation even if not legal sanction. The state should endorse the protection of the contract-maker, even from himself or herself on matters of life and death.

Between active and passive means of euthanasia are those that are partial. Though generally considered illegal, they are not uncommon. Sometimes called a *slow code* or a *gray code*, the partial means of euthanasia occurs when a person, usually older and without a "do not resuscitate" order, "codes" or goes into cardiac or respiratory arrest and efforts to revive are not rigorous. Appropriate conversations prior to the crisis and proper documentation would make most partial means of euthanasia unnecessary.

A fourth variable is the severity of the patient's condition. Commonly, a distinction is made between near-term terminal and nonterminal illnesses. Usually, it is assumed that among those with nonterminal diseases and disabling conditions only persons with the most serious chronic disorders would want suicide. Not surprisingly, persons with disabling conditions generally do not view their existence as a complete burden. Further, existential crises are not limited, nor do they selectively target, those with physical disabling conditions. Christians ought not to ever despise this life. Being disabled is not dying and suicide should not be considered a moral or legally sanctioned option. When the severity is such that death is imminent, though, there is no reason to compel additional treatment.

Another distinction about condition is between acute and chronic. Sometimes temporary severity leads to the momentary loss of competence. Uncontrolled fear or despondency on the part of the moral agent have traditionally been deemed reasons to question the validity of a moral choice. Contracts signed under duress or in the midst of crises are challengeable on the grounds that one party is forced to act out of desperation. Persons in acute conditions or even significant others caring for them may be disoriented to the point of temporarily losing perspective or even rationality and, when such is the case, should not be allowed to make critical decisions. A reasonable waiting period is appropriate prior to any withdrawal of treatment. This period will vary depending on the condition—from hours in an ICU following a genuinely significant traumatic brain injury requiring full life support and with little higher brain function to months following a spinal cord injury that leads to paralysis.

The fifth variable is the community within which the decision is made. Again, Christians should have higher expectations for Christians. It may be that those of the world will more readily choose to stop treatments or life-support or may, conversely, cling ferociously to life when all treatments are futile. Such a decision, if not a threat to others, should be tolerated for the greater good of liberty. This does not mean that toleration of physician-assisted suicide, any other form of active euthanasia or passive euthanasia against the chronic but not terminally ill should be accepted. To the contrary, these should be fought as violations of the social contract obligation to protect contract members.

CONCLUSION

The concept of autonomy as a right in the modern West is based on the assumptions of social contract theory. Certainly, Christians can be comfortable with the legal concept of the autonomous individual. Arguably, the idea of political autonomy has its roots reaching into Christian Protestantism's idea of the person who stands alone before God. A strong case for the source of the concept can also be made for ancient Greek notions of the ideal human, the late medieval economic urban man and English common law. Regardless of which or to what degree (the fact is, they probably had an interactive effect on one another through time), the evangelical can accept the idea as functional for the political arena. Though an over-simplification, autonomy can be understood as the individualized form of the broader political concept of liberty. Without sounding pejorative, autonomy is a useful political fiction. No one can actually be a law unto the self (or order unto the self); no one actually exists independently of all others, but it is good for the state to pretend such is the case.[10]

Evangelicals can function in societies without legal autonomy, but freedom for the religious community and autonomy for individuals is clearly preferable. Certainly, the concept fits well with the post-Reformation revivalist evangelicals who place significant emphasis on the need to make a decision for Christ. Indeed, the evangelical can understand every moral decision—be it an effort to resolve a dilemma or a decision to develop a habit of holiness—as a little decision for Christ, a reiteration of the initial decision to count the cost, to accept him, and accept entry into his moral community.

Still, having endorsed the idea of autonomy as a political concept does not mean that it is the best way to frame decision making outside of the political and legal spheres. While health care certainly is overlapped with politics and law, it is also an arena for the family, economic considerations, academic training and formal religious organizations. Given that, Christians should recognize that any individual decision-maker in a health-care setting is not, in reality, completely independent of all others, or "auto-nomous."

A limit to autonomy arises in that suicide should not be a right. Simply put, the physical body of each individual belongs to God and must be treated accordingly. Saul was, therefore, wrong to seek assistance and wrong to initiate his own death. But, this argument is not compelling for the secular world and should not even be brought into the public square except to ex-

[10]Jon Gunnemann, private conversation, 1985.

plain how the community of faith treats its own. The reason within the Christian community differs from the reasoning of the social contract society, but the moral conclusion should be the same. Those in the image of God or those who are makers of the social contract should be protected, valued for their intrinsic worth.

For addressing choices with other believers, the Christian might make an appeal to the images the Lord uses. He says that he is the vine and we are the branches; this clearly takes the believer beyond a sort of hyperindividualism. Or, the believer might consider images of the body, particularly useful in bioethics, recognizing that those in the community of faith genuinely need one another. The person who comes to Christ chooses, as an individual, to withdraw from the way of the world and to enter into a different community. Moral decisions, then, are confirmations of that decision to re-identify with the body of Christ. Within the faith community these decisions or confirmations of relationship with Christ must be expressed in all aspects of living and dying.

The argument for the world is different. The reasonable citizen, including the reasonable Christian, opposes medical suicide because of the nature of the social contract. While the Christian may be a libertarian on many issues, she or he cannot endorse the termination of the contract makers, as membership of rights-holders is the foundational concept for the functioning of the state. Human life precedes the state and justifies its existence. In other words, the social contract requires that the state protect the physical well-being of the individual, even in a diminished condition. Vigilance is called for as the risk for the abuse rises with vulnerability. The Christian, therefore, must advocate for the real distinction between intentional killing and death as a secondary effect to palliative treatment (principle of double effect) and not allow intentional obfuscation of the difference. The line is difficult to draw—but so is the line between dependence and autonomy and still it is a useful fiction that protects the individual and the community.

Christians can express their support for protecting life while recognizing that physical death is not the ultimate evil by encouraging the use of Advance Directives, or at least the Durable Power of Attorney. Within the Christian community, this can be understood as simply part of the general recognition of one's finitude and obligations to prepare one's heirs. An advance directive is an act of kindness that minimizes, though by no means eliminates, the flood of decisions that need to be made by next-of-kin as someone is dying.

For believers, such preparations should not be understood as rights to be exercised, but expressions of love for God and for others within the community of faith and for those others who may be in significant relationship with the dying person. It is, to return to the words of Christ, a way to assist others who have to count the cost of difficult decisions.

14

Assisted Reproduction and Sexuality

HUMANS AS MALE AND FEMALE

Jesus endorsed heterosexual, monogamous marriage as a pattern of creation, goodness as God intended. Yet, he also commended celibate singleness, going so far as to say that some are eunuchs for the kingdom of God. Evangelicals have tended to emphasize the legitimacy of marriage over celibate singleness. Presumably this is because the couple becomes a "church within the church" *(ecclesiolae in ecclesia),* but what of other aspects of marriage, specifically child-bearing? Should the order of creation, that husband and wife are fruitful, govern bioethical decisions for couples who otherwise appear unable to have genetic offspring?

> Now while he was in Jerusalem at the Passover Feast, many people saw the miraculous signs he was doing and believed in his name. But Jesus would not entrust himself to them, for he knew all men. He did not need man's testimony about man, for he knew what was in a man.
>
> Now there was a man of the Pharisees named Nicodemus, a member of the Jewish ruling council. He came to Jesus at night and said, "Rabbi, we know you are a teacher who has come from God. For no one could perform the miraculous signs you are doing if God were not with him."
>
> In reply Jesus declared, "I tell you the truth, no one can see the kingdom of God unless he is born again."
>
> "How can a man be born when he is old?" Nicodemus asked. "Surely he cannot enter a second time into his mother's womb to be born!"
>
> Jesus answered, "I tell you the truth, no one can enter the kingdom of God unless he is born of water and the Spirit. Flesh gives birth to flesh, but the Spirit gives birth to spirit. You should not be surprised at my saying, 'You must be born again.' The wind blows wherever it pleases. You hear its sound, but you cannot tell where it comes from or where it is going. So it is with everyone born of the Spirit."
>
> "How can this be?" Nicodemus asked.

"You are Israel's teacher," said Jesus, "and do you not understand these things? I tell you the truth, we speak of what we know, and we testify to what we have seen, but still you people do not accept our testimony. I have spoken to you of earthly things and you do not believe; how then will you believe if I speak of heavenly things? No one has ever gone into heaven except the one who came from heaven—the Son of Man. Just as Moses lifted up the snake in the desert, so the Son of Man must be lifted up, that everyone who believes in him may have eternal life.

"For God so loved the world that he gave his one and only Son, that whoever believes in him shall not perish but have eternal life. For God did not send his Son into the world to condemn the world, but to save the world through him. Whoever believes in him is not condemned, but whoever does not believe stands condemned already because he has not believed in the name of God's one and only Son. This is the verdict: Light has come into the world, but men loved darkness instead of light because their deeds were evil. Everyone who does evil hates the light, and will not come into the light for fear that his deeds will be exposed. But whoever lives by the truth comes into the light, so that it may be seen plainly that what he has done has been done through God." (Jn 2:23–3:21)

PART ONE: THE TEXT

You *must* be born again. The phrase is central to the self-understanding of evangelical Christians.[1] In this passage Jesus asserts that one must be radically transformed, to the point of having a genuinely changed identity. The person is not only recognized as having different characteristics but is morally identified as different than others, according to evangelical theological claims; she or he is a genuinely transformed being. If any human is going to be Christ's follower, then the individual must simultaneously remain the same being and yet become a genuinely new person at the same time.

The often used metaphor for conversion is butterfly metamorphosis, and it is appropriate. As with the lepidopteran's change, conversion radically alters the character, even while maintaining continuity with the past. Christians,

[1]"Born again" describes a posttransition condition. For believers, it is also a declaration of an ongoing relationship between the individual and God. Besides describing evangelical self-understanding (or because of it), the phrase also serves as the means of significant caricature. Even theologians and church leaders, who should know better, such as William Temple, seemingly disregard the centrality of the idea to Christianity because they dislike some of the cultural specifics of what was North American blue-collar evangelicalism. Needless to say, those arguing for the "twice-born" theology have succeeded while the so-called mainline/old-line denominations have gone into significant decline.

further, assert that though the transformation to the final heavenly form of the individual *(telos)* is incomplete, it is a transformation that has direction—it is movement toward the intended end *(telos)* of the Creator for that being.

Jesus, in the imperative "you must be born again," does not want to imply that this is reducible to a mere change of mind or affiliation with a new organization, though it does include such. Rather, the transformation is a complete redirecting through a submissive relationship to God. While the conversion is active in the sense that it is something to which the individual must agree and in that the results include changed behaviors and affiliations, it is passive in that the fundamental change is wrought by and sustained by the Deity.[2] Certainly it appears that Jesus is claiming (and evangelicals would strongly assert) that the "must" of the imperative indicates that it is only this relationship that will allow such a genuine transformation of the individual into what he or she is intended to be by his or her Creator.

Jesus goes on to use the image of travail to imply not only the significance of the change, but its difficulty. In a sense, the moment of transition is just that, a moment. It requires little but accepting what is offered. Yet, it has vast implications—the loss of the womblike comfort of self-delusion and denial. This may mean that some things, including some relationships with other people, have to be abandoned or radically modified. The transition, though frequently painful, is also full of hope. Rebirth represents entry into a realm of vastly expanded possibilities.

Jesus certainly wants to use an image that allows for spiritual rebirth as a beginning, that may involve some endings, but rebirth is not the end of the individual. Besides old relationships changing or being redefined, new relationships must be established. The convert, indeed, enters into a new primary community. This is not only rebirth of the individual, but also rebirth into a new family with siblings and parental (authority) figures. This latter point is reinforced when, in 1 Peter, another reference to being "born again" is linked to the longing of newborn babies for milk, a sign of the child's need and the motherly ability of the body of believers (1 Pet 1–2). Evangelicals assert that this change, one as dramatic as the transition of biological birth, actually occurs in this life. Indeed, to be defined as an evangelical, one must acknowledge that this initiation of new life occurs prior to biological death.

---

[2]A point of theological disagreement arises among evangelicals over how much agreement must be sustained on the part of the individual. This is one difference between Calvinists and Wesleyans, with the "mixed" Baptists agreeing with Calvinists on the point of "eternal security."

This experience, along with the doctrinal affirmation of the exclusive salvific power of Jesus Christ, the epistemological authority of the Scripture within the community of faith, and accountability to God directly and through other believers are defining characteristics of evangelicalism. New birth is what establishes the salvific and sanctifying relationship and is the principle legitimating experience for the individual holding the evangelical Christian worldview.

Numerous passages in the Text use the image of conception and childbirth to metaphorically convey spiritual and moral truths.

> Under the apple tree I roused you;
> there your mother conceived you,
> there she who was in labor gave you birth.
> Place me like a seal over your heart,
> like a seal on your arm;
> for love is as strong as death,
> its jealousy unyielding as the grave.
> It burns like blazing fire,
> like a mighty flame. (Song 8:5-6)

Drawn from the Song of Solomon, this passage is traditionally assumed to be either the voice of God speaking to Israel or God the Son speaking to the church (the New Israel). The conception of the Beloved, her birth, and the wooing of her by the Lover all occur in the same location, thus designating each as a moment of import and, presumably, increasing significance for each until the yet-to-occur consummation of the love between the Lover and the Beloved.

In a second notable section, reference is made to the sadness that will come upon Jesus' death for the disciples, yet it will be followed by a truer joy than had ever been experienced by anyone before. The physical resurrection of Jesus they are soon to witness will be the assurance of their hope for the final resurrection to come.

> I tell you the truth, you will weep and mourn while the world rejoices. You will grieve, but your grief will turn to joy. A woman giving birth to a child has pain because her time has come; but when her baby is born she forgets the anguish because of her joy that a child is born into the world. So with you: Now is your time of grief, but I will see you again and you will rejoice, and no one will take away your joy. (Jn 16:20-22)

A third passage is similar in its use of the image, but refers to the end of the world as the birth of the new heavens and the new earth, which are the child that is born. This is, in Christian tradition, the consummation foretold in the Song of Solomon and the completion of the promise made by the empty tomb.

> Many will come in my name, claiming, "I am he," and will deceive many. When you hear of wars and rumors of wars, do not be alarmed. Such things must happen, but the end is still to come. Nation will rise against nation, and kingdom against kingdom. There will be earthquakes in various places, and famines. These are the beginning of birth pains. "You must be on your guard. All men will hate you because of me, but he who stands firm to the end will be saved. (Mk 13:6-9, 13)

In all these cases, suffering and patience yield joy. All of these uses of the image of childbirth center on the change for both mother and infant initiated in the woman who grows "great with child" (Lk 2:5 KJV) and through her holding her baby until finally he or she, in the proper time, is free to live out his or her potential.[3]

The symbolism, as is often the case with Christian imagery, relies on points being made about penultimate goods that, in turn, point to the even greater ultimate Good. Relational structures are repeated. Labor as earthly work is good, but laboring for the Lord is even greater. Marriage is a blessing from God; the two become one even while maintaining their individual being, but marriage as part of the church to Christ is even better. Similarly, being born is good—it is never an evil—yet being born again is greater. Good examples of this good-to-best analogy are found in Isaiah (in a passage that has been deemed predictive of Jesus' sacrificial crucifixion) and in the Gospels.

> But Zion said, "The Lord has forsaken me,
> the Lord has forgotten me."
> "Can a mother forget the baby at her breast
> and have no compassion on the child she has borne?
> Though she may forget,
> I will not forget you!
> See, I have engraved you on the palms of my hands." (Is 49:14-16)

> As Jesus was saying these things, a woman in the crowd called out, "Blessed is the mother who gave you birth and nursed you." He replied, "Blessed rather are

---

[3]The notion of proper time for spiritual birth is implied in Romans 5:6-8 and the idea of the wrong time for birth found in Job 3:2-12.

those who hear the word of God and obey it." (Lk 11:27-28)

Three things are often forgotten—or disregarded—about the image of rebirth offered through Scripture. The first is theological, specifically about the spiritual process that includes rebirth. The second has to do with the relational character. The third with the status of the reborn. First, rebirth implies the capacity to grow toward maturity. Whatever the particulars may be, and evangelicals differ on those, justification initiates the process of sanctification. Rebirth is not just payment for sin; it is conversion or transformation. One is supposed to mature, not stay a baby—and the unrealized potential exists for that maturity in the newborn and, indeed, in the preborn.

To be born again is to appropriate the power of the atonement.[4] Though various subtraditions within evangelicalism emphasize one or the other interpretation of the doctrine of atonement, evangelical theology actually requires that three basic understandings be present

- *Penal substitution.* Christ is the Priest and Sacrifice who restores the just order intended in creation. God is angry at our sinfulness, but through the substitution of Christ sin is displaced by justice—though justice rendered in love so that its consequences, undeservedly, come mercifully to those who acted unjustly. Sometimes misunderstood by those who mistake Christianity for a tritheistic instead of a monotheistic religion, this is God choosing to offer up himself in order to restore his created intentions.

  > Such a high priest meets our need—one who is holy, blameless, pure, set apart from sinners, exalted above the heavens. Unlike the other high priests, he does not need to offer sacrifices day after day, first for his own sins, and then for the sins of the people. He sacrificed for their sins once for all when he offered himself. (Heb 7:26-27)

- *Christus Victor.* Christ is the victorious conqueror of death, which serves as an emissary of evil generally. According to any doctrinally orthodox Christian theology, evil is real and evil is powerful, not merely human mistakes or ignorance. Christ's crucifixion and inevitable resurrection (for, in Christian theology, these should be recognized as one event, with the rising of

[4]The three understandings of atonement are often "explained" to evangelicals through hymns. Three traditional examples are Robert Lowry's "Nothing but the Blood" for penal substitution, Eugene Bartlett's "Victory in Jesus" for Christus Victor, and the traditional African American spiritual "We Are Climbing Jacob's Ladder" for moral exemplar. Note that all three of these hymns actually include images for more than one understanding of the atonement and, subsequently, of the justification experience.

Jesus certain following his sacrificial death) "is" the victory of meaning over anomy and absurdity. Believers are at war with evil but can be victors with Christ.

> This is how we know that we love the children of God: by loving God and carrying out his commands. This is love for God: to obey his commands. And his commands are not burdensome, for everyone born of God overcomes the world. This is the victory that has overcome the world, even our faith. Who is it that overcomes the world? Only he who believes that Jesus is the Son of God. (1 Jn 5:2-5)

- *Jesus the True Exemplar.* Besides restoring the divinely intended order and providing personal victory to the individual believer, Jesus provides the capacity through the Holy Spirit to those who follow him to be more than they could have ever been while still broken by/captive to sin. Jesus was the One who was tempted but did not give in—the One who set the moral standard, a standard that can be increasingly lived out as one accepts his Lordship.

> At one time we too were foolish, disobedient, deceived and enslaved by all kinds of passions and pleasures. We lived in malice and envy, being hated and hating one another. But when the kindness and love of God our Savior appeared, he saved us, not because of righteous things we had done, but because of his mercy. He saved us through the washing of rebirth and renewal by the Holy Spirit, whom he poured out on us generously through Jesus Christ our Savior, so that, having been justified by his grace, we might become heirs having the hope of eternal life. This is a trustworthy saying. And I want you to stress these things, so that those who have trusted in God may be careful to devote themselves to doing what is good. These things are excellent and profitable for everyone. (Tit 3:3-8)

The believer should in humility accept the payment for sin. The believer should joyously join in triumph over the power and consequences of evil. And the believer should accept Jesus as the model for living. In the metaphor of being born again all three are operative. The idea is that one was something less than what one was intended to be, then one was brought forth by God, and now one is expected to mature toward the holy ideal.

The second forgotten aspect of the born-again metaphor is more immediately pertinent to bioethics. The community of mother/child arises out of the community of husband/wife, out of relationship. In addition, the child is in relationship with the mother from the moment of conception. Birth requires the direct participation of three individuals: the child, the mother and the father. The individual is part of a family. The family is not only a spiritual reality, it is a biological one. The parents bind themselves in sexual relations. The ultimate physical act of affection (sexual intercourse) belongs with the ultimate legal act (civilly validated marriage, when possible under the laws of the state), the ultimate social act (public marriage commitments) and the ultimate spiritual act for a man and woman (marriage before the body of believers).

The relationship of child and mother is also a legal, social and spiritual relationship. Women differ from men, perhaps most significantly in the biological norm of carrying and giving birth to a child. The mother carries the child within her, composed of the genetic material of both parents and various physiological inputs from her during gestation. Though the Scripture entitles God "Father," it also uses female metaphors and similes to describe the characteristics of God. God is like the mother who gives birth to the newly reborn individual, having developed the new babe in the womb of wooing or prevenient grace. Jesus implies such when he states, "O Jerusalem, Jerusalem, you who kill the prophets and stone those sent to you, how often I have longed to gather your children together, as a hen gathers her chicks under her wings, but you were not willing!" (Lk 13:34). This echoes passages from Isaiah, including

> As a mother comforts her child,
> so will I comfort you;
> and you will be comforted over Jerusalem. (Is 66:13)

Nicodemus asks, "Can a man enter again into his mother's womb?" The picture offered by the Jewish leader is of his mother, of a real person, who had physically suffered following months of bringing him, Nicodemus, to term. The relationship of mother and child in the womb is unique among all human relationships. It is unique in its closeness and in its costliness to the woman, not unlike the costliness to God of becoming incarnate and dying for his children.

Pregnancy and birth are an offering by a woman to her child. She becomes, as the parent, a servant to the child. The child after birth, at least as proscribed by virtually every cultural order throughout history, is to also become the servant of the parent, even as the parents continue to support and guide the child. The Christian ideal is mutuality, which allows for the distinct fulfillment of roles of the family community even while valuing each individual as himself and herself.

The problem for those at the end of modernity with these two concepts as applied to parent-child relations is twofold. First, they do not recognize the nature of servanthood. The important liberty of the social contract has become a hyperautonomy that does not allow for the virtuosity of servanthood (hence the language of pro-abortion advocates that excludes responsibility for a living entity in the name of self-power). And, second, they do not recognize that mutuality of relationship must be mutuality of servanthood. Relationships cannot move from the mere contractual to true covenant and love unless all serve all—husband and wife, parent and child. The mother who groans through childbirth can be filled with joy because she recognizes both the tremendous good that she already has given and will be able to offer the newborn and the good that the child will offer her. When properly expressed (though in a fallen world this is not always the case), both parent and child are more than they might otherwise have been by virtue of their serving one another. As with the other major component of the family, marriage in which the whole is supposed to be more than the sum of the parts, so it is or should be with parent-child.

It is the desire for the covenantal relationship, the living bond that values the individual even while making the whole more than the sum of the parts, that all properly directed humans seek. The desire is innate. Not surprisingly, then, when "natural" childbearing is not possible, people seek artificial alternative means—even while others fear the implications of this natural, covenantal bond and terminate a pregnancy (but abortion never yields joy, even if it gives temporary relief).

The third aspect of the rebirth analogy is the different spiritual status for the person who has been born again. All the uses of the metaphor or analogue require that one is better off and, indeed, ontologically or relationally different following birth or rebirth. To recognize that the status of the born is different from the preborn is stating the obvious. For, regardless of the ability to survive, there is at least a difference of relationship for the child with the gestational mother and the outside world before birth than after. This difference does not make the preborn valueless or, to use contemporary language, not a person. The Lord desires that each and everyone would be born again. God seeks the one who is spiritually preborn. The believer should see in every nonbeliever a preborn Christian, one who might accept and become a full brother or sister, and likewise should see in every preborn human a child who might continue to live to the glory of God. Whenever possible, then, Christians should assist those who are pre-reborn or preborn come to the fullness of life.

PART TWO: CHRISTIAN BIOETHICS

For Christians, biological birth, given the use of the analogue for Jesus' words on being born again, should be understood as (1) a stage in a process that had begun earlier, (2) a dramatic change, (3) an experience occurring in community, certainly including the father but most significantly the mother and child (and most costly for them physically and perhaps emotionally), (4) usually desirable for the parents and always for the child, and (5) a transition that substantially changes the child and the parents. Alternatives to birth, such as miscarriage, sterility and abortion are marked by sorrow, not hope.

Jesus chose to draw a parallel between the status of the believer and a child who has been biologically born. A superficial reading might lead to the conclusion that the neonate has a higher worth than the prenatal child and, therefore, that the believers are higher in status than the nonbelievers. Certainly the status is different, but it is not higher. Or, of greater practical important, the differences do not constitute a devaluing of the prenate but an elevation of the newborn.

God does not want those who are not saved to be damned. He does not want them to suffer. He does not want them to drift through life in anomie (1 Pet 3:8-10). God values those who are not in the church. Further, the church is supposed to value those who are not yet born again. Even the human enemies of Christians are, theoretically, to be viewed as potential brothers and sisters, not mere objects to be discarded. To use a significant example, God called Saul of Tarsus while he was persecuting the church—indeed, even while he was participating in the killing of the first recorded Christian martyr. It would be demonstrably erroneous to claim that God did not value Saul/Paul prior to the Damascus Road experience. Rather, he was so wanted that Jesus pleadingly asks from the mysterious bright light, "Saul, Saul, why do you persecute me?" (Acts 9:4). Paul later generalizes this divine seeking with the phrase, "While we were yet sinners, Christ died for the ungodly" (Rom 5:8). Simply put, the presaved person matters to God and should matter to the Christian.

Applying the analogy, though there is a difference between being in or out of the mother's womb, that difference is not so extreme or fundamental in nature as to morally permit the termination of the life of the preborn except in conflict of life with life. The killing of the preborn is no more justifiable for Christians than the extermination of non-Christians, the spiritually preborn. Any so-called Christian endorsing abortion is more like a Crusader against the infidel, declaring "God can sort them out," rather than a New-Testament follower of Jesus. Christians should never again participate in nor silently tolerate such barbarism. Likewise, Christians cannot be silent about the harming of the preborn or marginalized human being. Indeed, if necessary, followers of Christ must give voice in the form of protest and political activism to those silenced in the name of convenience, economic expediency or (supposed) emotional well-being.[5]

The only New Testament passage that might deny the worth of a preborn human being—and even that must be said with the greatest hesitancy—is the report of the words of Jesus in reference to Judas. "The Son of Man will go just as it is written about him. But woe to that man who betrays the Son of Man! It would be better for him if he had not been born" (Mt 26:24). This is a statement more about the person's actions than about the ontological status of the individual himself. Certainly evangelicals assume that even Judas, had he only sought forgiveness, could have entered the kingdom by God's grace. The judgment of Christ at this point is from the eternal perspective when all potentials are either realized or failed.

This does not mean there are not situations in which someone might be so overwhelmed by his or her own predicament that she or he wishes to have never been born. These are most dramatically presented in Jeremiah and Job. This passage of Jeremiah was written in reference to the torment directed toward the prophet precisely because he was doing what God wants him to do. The Job passage represents the words of a man who has been deprived of everything, yet clearly was not morally worse than (and probably was better than) his peers.

> O Lord, you deceived me, and I was deceived;
> you overpowered me and prevailed.
> I am ridiculed all day long;
> everyone mocks me. . . .
> Cursed be the day I was born!

---

[5]It should be noted that some evangelicals do not believe it is ever correct to participate in the world's politics. The argument for participation on the issue of abortion is contingent upon the believer's acceptance of any political activity, including voting. If such is accepted, then abortion certainly is a matter warranting a political response.

> May the day my mother bore me not be blessed!
> Cursed be the man who brought my father the news,
> who made him very glad, saying,
> "A child is born to you—a son!"
> May that man be like the towns
> the LORD overthrew without pity.
> May he hear wailing in the morning,
> a battle cry at noon.
> For he did not kill me in the womb,
> with my mother as my grave,
> her womb enlarged forever.
> Why did I ever come out of the womb
> to see trouble and sorrow
> and to end my days in shame? (Jer 20:7, 14-18)

> Why then did you bring me out of the womb?
> I wish I had died before any eye saw me.
> If only I had never come into being,
> or had been carried straight from the womb to the grave! (Job 10:18-19)

But again, from the Christian perspective, there is no such thing as a wrongful birth because there must be someone to be wronged and there would not be if that one had never been born. There is intrinsic good to human life. Even egregious circumstances for the baby do not warrant killing. And so Isaiah declares:

> Woe to him who quarrels with his Maker,
> to him who is but a potsherd among the potsherds on the ground.
> Does the clay say to the potter,
> "What are you making?'
> Does your work say,
> "He has no hands"?
> Woe to him who says to his father,
> "What have you begotten?"
> or to his mother,
> "What have you brought to birth?" (Is 45:9-10)

To put this another way, there may be rights that an unborn child does not have or at least that would not be available until birth makes them readily accessible. The right to life, however, ought not to be one of those "different" rights. It may be that the right to life is not as expansive for the preborn as the already born in that the life of the mother may take precedence in those extremely rare cases when lives come into conflict. However, this is a diminishment based on the most basic right for the woman, not other rights—even otherwise important, significant rights.

Generally, evangelical arguments against abortion are not based on specific exegetical work on biblical passages about abortion because there really are not any that provide a specific command one way or the other. This does not mean there is no guidance, and the early church found that guidance in arguments on caring for the lost, the orphan, and the rejected. A few key Scriptures, though, do need to be noted.

- *Exodus 21:22-25:* In this passage, most translations conclude that the punishment is for the miscarriage. Since the punishment is less than "life for life," the preborn must not have been considered human or fully human, it is argued. This is the only passage that might legitimate abortion under desperate circumstances, and then not for birth control. Having said that, there is no reason one passage should "overrule" the general tenor of the Text. Further, translation of this passage is problematic grammatically.
- *Psalm 51:* This passage, a statement of David's repentance, includes a reference to being conceived in sin, thereby implying individual identity as a preborn.
- *Job 3:1-19:* Job, while bemoaning his numerous tragedies, wonders whether he would not have been better off having perished at birth; the argument is made that for some, abortion may be preferable to a difficult life (the "every child wanted" argument).
- *Jeremiah 1:5:* The passage indicates intention from God and identity before birth.
- *Isaiah 49:1-5:* Similarly, the Lord calls Isaiah "from the womb," indicating identity.
- *Luke 1:41:* John the Baptist leapt in Elizabeth's womb on hearing the voice of Mary, the mother of Jesus, which implies some state of spiritual "awareness"—though perhaps not consciousness in the actual sense of the word.
- *Luke 1:30:* By far, the single, most-important passage, this refers to the status of Jesus as a preborn; Mary, after all, would have been a perfect candidate (not married, pregnant, financially burdened, hearing voices about

the pregnancy, obviously intelligent and talented, facing social marginalization, claiming pregnancy caused by someone other than her betrothed, the pregnancy relationship with the preborn was not intentionally sought) for an elective abortion. For Christians, Jesus was Jesus in the womb.

Further biblical/theological reasons that evangelical Christians oppose abortion include some of the following (these are not mutually exclusive):

- Doctrine of creation (all humans are created in the image of God)
- Doctrine of the incarnation (the Lord assumed human condition, first prenatally)
- Obligations of neighborly love (the preborn child is in need of hospitality)
- Obligations of enemy love (the obligation to care for those who are placed in our path, even the difficult, including the inconvenient or burdensome preborn)
- Virtuosity of peacemaking (nonviolence is usually the best course in face of difficulties; abortion is an extraordinarily violent response to what may be a difficult situation for the mother)

Unlike almost any other issue in bioethics, though little direct reference is made in the Text, the church has addressed abortion since its inception, and that history warrants some consideration. The pre-Constantinian church prohibited abortion among believers and condemned it among those of the world. Here are a few samples from the first four centuries of the faith:[6]

- Didache: "You shall not murder a child by abortion, nor kill the newborn."
- Epistle of Barnabas: "You shall not murder a child by abortion, nor kill the newborn."
- Athenagoras *Plea* 35: "We say that women who induce abortions are murderers, and will have to give account of it to God."
- Tertullian *Apology 9.6*: "In our case, murder being once for all forbidden, we may not destroy even the fetus in the womb. To hinder a birth is merely a speedier homicide."
- Minucius Felix *Octavius* 30.2: "There are women who . . . [are] committing infanticide before they give birth to the infant."

[6]The most accessible work on the subject is Michael Gorman, *Abortion and the Early Church: Christian, Jewish and Pagan Attitudes in the Greco-Roman World* (Eugene, Ore.: Wipf and Stock, 1998). This list is drawn from his work.

- John Chrysostom "Homily 24 on Romans": "[Abortion is] murder before the birth . . . or rather . . . something even worse than murder."
- Basil "Letter 188.2": "Those too who give drugs causing abortion are murderers themselves, as well as those receiving the poison which kills the fetus" (though he does encourage leniency for the recipient woman).

The pre-Constantinian arguments usually relied on assigning the act of abortion to one or both of two categories: abortion as injustice and abortion as vicious (as "of vice"), corrupting lethal violence.[7] For the former, the Christian should reject the act as the inappropriate rendering of the preborn as less deserving of moral concern than others created in the image of God. For the latter, the unborn child is seen as an object of immoral violence and Christians may not participate in the killing of an innocent without corrupting themselves. Obviously the two approaches are similar, but the second actually depends on a stronger assertion about the virtuosity of Christians, that they generally should be nonviolent toward human beings except under extraordinary circumstances that involve proportional loss.

When the church yoked itself to the state (or vice versa), abortion remained prohibited, but the reasoning behind the prohibition changed. Rather than being primarily a virtuous expression of the community for any who were marginalized (in this case, literally the voiceless), modifications of Roman law were used. The argument to protect the weakest became an academic argument based on philosophical speculation on the status of the preborn. Though historical processes are never simple, generally these changes were founded in a shift in emphasis from protecting the marginal to preventing the concealment of illicit sexual behavior.

After the toleration of Christianity, the trends begun by the apologists (philosophers who defended Christianity before unbelievers on the basis of arguments drawn from previous Greek and Roman philosophical works) became dominant in the moral reasoning of the church. Rather than the story of the gospel as a way of life, the gospel became a text from which ecclesial authorities could draw philosophical propositions. Over time, this left room for non-Text-based, scientifically immature philosophical speculation on the status of the preborn.[8]

---

[7]Gorman, *Abortion and the Early Church,* see especially chapters 4-5. See also *The Church and Abortion: In Search of New Ground for Response*, ed. Paul T. Stallsworth (Nashville: Abingdon, 1993), including his use of other material from Gorman (for instance, p. 42 n. 32).

[8]Importantly, these "prescientific" arguments that use "science" to prove their philosophical case

By the time of the Scholastics (thirteenth century), the claim sometimes was being made that the male ensouled the physical body at forty days after conception, while the female ensouled at the eightieth or ninetieth.[9] This left room for abortion prior to those times or at least lessened the moral significance of the act. In practice, abortion remained strongly prohibited within most Christian communities, though tacitly accepted by some in Christendom. Officially, it was deemed a form of immoral contraception (which, it was claimed, either hid illicit sexual behavior or interfered with God's command to be fruitful and multiply). Unfortunately, the differentiation in the social status of females and males in the womb was also reflected in a lack of concern for the pregnant woman. That which allowed abortion philosophically actually helped diminish the status of women in the church.

Even into the early modern era, women—under pressure from husbands or from other impregnators who wanted to maintain their own social position—would make the choice to abort. When women made the choice, shame and fear were the driving emotions. Nineteenth-century feminist Elizabeth Cady Stanton declared that "when we consider that women are treated as property, it is degrading that we should treat our children as property to be disposed of as we see fit." The remedy she thought would be "the complete enfranchise-

---

remain central for the prochoice (proabortion) and prolife camps in the United States. A far more important issue on abortion in the post-Christian West is the status of the preborn as a voiceless member of the social contract. Finally, at the political level, this is a legal argument about who counts.

[9]Supposedly derived from Aristotle, through Thomas Aquinas (the days are usually 40 for males, with more variance for females—80, 90 or otherwise). The time was needed, apparently, to assemble the components in which the soul would function. John Haldane and Patrick Lee provide a very good description of Aquinas on ensoulment: "[Aquinas] also held that, unlike the souls of brute animals, the human soul is directly created by God. In various places he argues that the rational soul has intellectual powers of conceptual thought that are independent of matter, and hence the operations of these powers are not performed with a bodily organ. Therefore, the rational soul must have its existence independently of matter. But what has existence independent of matter cannot come to be through the coming into existence of a matter-form (or body-soul) composite. Thus, Aquinas held that God immediately creates the human soul and (at the same time) infuses it into the body. That said, the human rational soul is created and infused into the body only when the human parents have, by their generative act, produced a material substance that is disposed to receive and to be informed by a human soul. In one place Aquinas follows Aristotle in saying that the rational soul is infused at 40 days for males, and at 90 days for females (*Commentary on the Book of Sentences*, Bk. III, dist. 3, q. 5, a. 2, *Responsio*)." (in John Haldane and Patrick Lee, "Aquinas on Human Ensoulment, Abortion and the Value of Life," *Philosophy* 78 [2003]: 255-78 <http://www2.franciscan.edu/plee/aquinas_on_human_ensoulment.htm#_edn18>). Haldane and Lee also note that one should be hesitant in appealing to Aquinas as an authority on abortion morality.

ment and elevation of women."[10] Unfortunately, she was wrong, not about the need to enfranchise women, but in thinking that women would be less prone to be self-centered than men.

Today in the West, shame and fear are occasionally still factors, but usually the justification is the right to self-governance and the pursuit of happiness.[11] The argument of contemporary "feminists for life" is compelling at this point.[12] Such actions, while justified with self-empowerment language, are more likely either a manifestation of false consciousness (the oppressed accepting their position of oppression) or an effort to hide what is considered a personal failure. Certainly, the vast majority of abortions are not matters of physical health and only if the term is so expansively defined as to become meaningless can they be defined as matters of mental health. Most abortions, the overwhelming majority, are moral choices—bad moral choices.

How, then, should those who follow Christ respond? Unlike some social issues, this is not one that can be simply dismissed as a moral mistakes by isolated individuals. In other words, the politicians who for the sake of holding office say that they are personally opposed to abortion but would not restrict it are either lying or ethically incompetent.

While social engagement to end the civil endorsement of abortion is fully appropriate, the use of violence is not. Some will claim that, like slavery before it, the response of believers should be defense—even if violent—of the victims. The arguments of Paul Hill, who killed an abortionist, are not appreciably different from those of John Brown, the abolitionist who stormed the Harper's Ferry Arsenal and helped precipitate the American Civil War. The application of just coercion criteria, though, denies any appropriateness for violence against abortionists. Likewise, they eliminate any justification used by proabortionists to kill the unborn, except in the case of protecting the life of the mother. Deadly violence is wrong in both cases, because they prematurely claim killing is a necessary last resort.

---

[10]Feminists for Life collection of comments on abortion by Elizabeth Cady Stanton, Letter to Julia Ward Howe, October 16, 1873, recorded in Howe's diary at Harvard University Library <http://www.feministsforlife.org/history/foremoth.htm#ecstanton>. Stanton also stated, "There must be a remedy even for such a crying evil as this. But where shall it be found, at least where begin, if not in the complete enfranchisement and elevation of women?" (*The Revolution* 1 [March 12, 1868]: 146-47).

[11]United States women who are not married are more likely to have an abortion than a live birth (Centers for Disease Control, "U.S. Pregnancy Rate Down from Peak; Births and Abortions on the Decline" October 31, 2003 <http://www.cdc.gov/od/oc/media/pressrel/fs031031.htm>.

[12]Feminists for Life <www.feministsforlife.org>.

However, other means of nonviolent coercion may be acceptable, much as they were when used during the civil rights movement against institutionalized racism. Economic pressure such as boycotting physician groups that employ abortionists, the removal of abortion as a covered service in insurance programs and so on would be acceptable. Speaking out against abortion should not be marked by the condescension. Even if bitterness and animosity are tolerated on the public square, they are not acceptable for believers.

While shame language, though said in sorrow and not in self-righteousness, is appropriate when directed at those who actively encourage the act of aborting, it should not be used with the women seeking abortions. They should be lifted up whenever possible, given care as needed. Similarly, those who have had abortions and are coming to believers with their sorrow and guilt should not be shamed, but rendered genuine concern. Opposition to abortion must be yoked to acknowledgment and response to the lopsidedness of the moral burden for the woman. Abortion cannot be understood as an ethical problem unless both the status of the preborn and the status of the woman are considered. Focusing only on the former is both a reasoning and a moral error, as is the opposite for those who are proabortion.

Evangelicals should turn to their own heritage. A substantial portion of the evangelical church participated in the first wave of feminism in which the nuclear family was validated at the same time that women were treated with greater respect. Nineteenth-century feminism was often evangelical, prohibitionist and prolife. Women are also, as much as the preborn, *imago Dei.* While the distinction between male and female is one of reproductive capacity, it is not the only characteristic of that distinction. The difference of male and female is one aspect of the whole image of the Divine, presented in the complementary nature of male and female individuals. In other words, males need females and need to respect them and attempt to understand how they might be marginalized by a difficult pregnancy.

The believer should advocate for the preborn, not because they have identical status with the already born, but because the individual with status as a preborn human is worthy of concern in and of himself or herself. Evangelicals must acknowledge that at least early in a pregnancy the preborn are not the same in ability, relationship and so forth as the neonate. To not acknowledge such diminishes the strength of the moral position against abortion, since the difference is factually demonstrable. Such does not, however, diminish Christian opposition to abortion on demand. Even if the status of the preborn (or, more precisely, the so-called nonviable preborn) is different, it is not such that the unborn person does not deserve concern and care. Further, development in the womb is on a continuum, not something biologically divisible into trimesters. To use the language of the world, why should a lesser capacity (for the early stage preborn) or an awkward and inconvenient relationship (with the mother) mean that this clearly unique and distinct Homo sapien being is not a member of the social contract? To exclude the preborn becomes a threat to all who are on the margins of society. For this reason alone, evangelicals should oppose all abortions except those that are necessary to save the life of the mother.

At its simplest, the preborn children are sojourners; when abortion is actively proposed they are alone (even while in the womb, sadly). In many cases they are emotional orphans, abandoned by their fathers and, now, even their mothers. As such, they (as all the broken) require care and concern. Of course, evangelicals have been susceptible to charges of selective moral outrage and the charges have the ring of truth. To offer a fuller witness to the life-changing impact of rebirth, evangelicals should actively include other sojourners—the poor, the mentally ill and the woman considering abortion—without excluding concern for the preborn.

The woman who seeks an abortion is or may feel like a sojourner—though in her case it is more a matter of cultural, psychological or spiritual aloneness. Ironically, women may feel alone when they are experiencing the opposite problem as well. Sometimes women want to conceive and cannot. This becomes all the more morally complicated when considering what conditions would lead to toleration or even encouragement of the use of birth technologies. Does the reason for failing to conceive and bring to birth—due to sterility, celibacy, lesbian or male homosexuality, etc.—make a moral difference in supporting or tolerating biotechnical intervention?

In Scripture, there is at least one clear example of a faithful follower of Yahweh using alternative means to have children. Abram is given, by his wife Sarai, the handmaiden Hagar that the latter might bear a child in the name of the former. This model of surrogacy is neither clearly condemned nor condoned in the Text, though the consequences of their inadequate faith are dramatic. The offspring is despised by Sarai, as is his genetic and gestational mother. The story does not indicate anything clearly about surrogacy except that (1) there will often be emotional ties that cannot be minimized by the presence of contracts and that (2) the powerful will take advantage of the weak.

> Now Sarai, Abram's wife, had borne him no children. But she had an Egyptian maidservant named Hagar; so she said to Abram, "The LORD has kept me from having children. Go, sleep with my maidservant; perhaps I can build a family through her."
>
> Abram agreed to what Sarai said. So after Abram had been living in Canaan ten years, Sarai his wife took her Egyptian maidservant Hagar and gave her to her husband to be his wife. He slept with Hagar, and she conceived.
>
> When she knew she was pregnant, she began to despise her mistress. Then Sarai said to Abram, "You are responsible for the wrong I am suffering. I put my servant in your arms, and now that she knows she is pregnant, she despises me. May the LORD judge between you and me."
>
> "Your servant is in your hands," Abram said. "Do with her whatever you think best." Then Sarai mistreated Hagar; so she fled from her.
>
> The angel of the LORD found Hagar near a spring in the desert; it was the spring that is beside the road to Shur. And he said, "Hagar, servant of Sarai, where have you come from, and where are you going?"
>
> "I'm running away from my mistress Sarai," she answered.
>
> Then the angel of the LORD told her, "Go back to your mistress and submit to her." The angel added, "I will so increase your descendants that they will be too numerous to count." . . .
>
> So Hagar bore Abram a son, and Abram gave the name Ishmael to the son she had borne. Abram was eighty-six years old when Hagar bore him Ishmael. (Gen 16:1-10, 15-16)

The desire to have children is powerful. It is generally intrinsic to human adulthood, though social, psychological and population factors can diminish the desire. It should come as no surprise that persons want their own children, and so seek biotechnological solutions to infertility.

The same human desire drives people today that led Sarai to seek a surrogate and pushed Tamar to bear a child by her kin. Er, Tamar's husband, died and his brother Onan was sent to impregnate her, as she wanted and as the society expected a child in Er's name. Apparently God expected it as well, for when Onan "spilled his seed"—that is, practiced birth control by withdrawal—he was killed.[13] Later, Tamar deceived her father-in law into believing that she was a prostitute so that the familial obligation to her of making her a mother would be fulfilled.

[13]This passage is sometimes erroneously used as an example of the prohibition of masturbation. The passage is not about that behavior which must be evaluated by other references, in particular those about lust.

> Judah got a wife for Er, his firstborn, and her name was Tamar. But Er, Judah's firstborn, was wicked in the LORD's sight; so the LORD put him to death.
>
> Then Judah said to Onan, "Lie with your brother's wife and fulfill your duty to her as a brother-in-law to produce offspring for your brother." But Onan knew that the offspring would not be his; so whenever he lay with his brother's wife, he spilled his semen on the ground to keep from producing offspring for his brother. What he did was wicked in the LORD's sight; so he put him to death also. . . .
>
> About three months later Judah was told, "Your daughter-in-law Tamar is guilty of prostitution, and as a result she is now pregnant."
>
> Judah said, "Bring her out and have her burned to death!"
>
> As she was being brought out, she sent a message to her father-in-law. "I am pregnant by the man who owns these," she said. And she added, "See if you recognize whose seal and cord and staff these are." Judah recognized them and said, "She is more righteous than I, since I wouldn't give her to my son Shelah." And he did not sleep with her again. (Gen 38:6-10, 24-26)

Lot's impregnating his daughters is another example of sexual relations not approved, but seem to be partially excused due to the difficulties faced in continuing the family. The fact that the offspring are progenitors of tribes often in conflict with Israel may indicate divine disapproval or be understood by the author as a natural consequence of an immoral act. The tribes of Moab and Ammon, as with the Ishmaelites, were simultaneously cousins who were in a special relationship with Israel and also frequent enemies. Their existence being traceable to dubious sexual behavior permitted Israel to hold a certain degree of disdain toward these related tribes.

> Lot and his two daughters left Zoar and settled in the mountains, for he was afraid to stay in Zoar. He and his two daughters lived in a cave. One day the older daughter said to the younger, "Our father is old, and there is no man around here to lie with us, as is the custom all over the earth. Let's get our father to drink wine and then lie with him and preserve our family line through our father."
>
> That night they got their father to drink wine, and the older daughter went in and lay with him. He was not aware of it when she lay down or when she got up.
>
> The next day the older daughter said to the younger, "Last night I lay with my father. Let's get him to drink wine again tonight, and you go in and lie with him so we can preserve our family line through our father." So they got their father to drink wine that night also, and the younger daughter went and lay with him. Again he was not aware of it when she lay down or when she got up.

> So both of Lot's daughters became pregnant by their father. The older daughter had a son, and she named him Moab; he is the father of the Moabites of today. The younger daughter also had a son, and she named him Ben-Ammi; he is the father of the Ammonites of today. (Gen 19:30-38)

It would seem that birth technologies under some circumstances are acceptable but often problematic. From an evangelical perspective, if occurring as an expression of heterosexual monogamous marriage, and if there is no intentional (or highly probable) wasting of embryos, then the application of Assisted Reproduction Technologies (ART) may be morally appropriate. Some justification exists for accepting the percentage of fetal loss that might occur in natural fertilization in an ART process, but Christians should seek to minimize such as with ART there is control that does not exist in the natural process, and with control comes responsibility. If no human preborns are intentionally or carelessly killed, then ART may be acceptable for society. Moral acceptability for Christians would additionally depend on the impact on the family. The negative experience of Abram, Sarai and Hagar was not due exclusively, or even primarily, to the sexual liaison with the surrogate, but the shift in family structure. Of course, this was surrogacy through sexual relations, which is not acceptable to Christians.

Except for extraordinary circumstances having to do with the continuation of a family line, the Old Testament does not endorse sexual relationships outside of heterosexual marriage. The New Testament is far more rigid. Only within monogamous heterosexual marriage is sexual intercourse deemed moral, though in the New Testament unmarried celibacy is equally legitimate and sometimes considered practically preferable. The spiritual significance of perpetuating one's biological line diminishes almost to the point of disappearing in the New Testament.

Other forms of sexual expression are defined as wrong for three reasons: (1) They violate the command of God (deontological). (2) They violate the covenant between man and woman intended at the day of Creation (virtue as an expression of the created order). (3) They tend to undermine social institutions that mediate the power of society, specifically the nuclear family, and that are needed to maximize social good (utilitarianism).

Generally speaking, many in U.S. society would disagree. Abortion, sex outside of marriage and the use of birth technologies under almost any circumstances are all matters of taste in the United States. With the strong language of rights, some argue that sex outside of marriage is needed for fulfillment, or at least should not be impeded as a matter of liberty, and that producing or not producing children is self-expression and any means of doing so is legitimate. Abortion is a method of protecting personal liberty and the opportunity to pursue happiness. Birth technology use by anyone is part of that pursuit.

This kind of argumentation is inevitable. With birth control, especially the pill, sexual behavior was separated from childbearing. With artificial reproductive technologies, childbearing is separated from sexual intercourse. Some of this separation may be acceptable to Christians and some may not. Evangelicals generally are not opposed to birth control because, unlike the traditional Catholic argument, evangelicals tend to claim that the primary reason for sexual relations is the binding of wife and husband—as with the binding of Christ and the church—rather than a reproductive command (Gen 1:22). And some scientific discoveries, especially about various forms of sterility, require less simplistic reasoning about sexual relations being all but exclusively about having children.

Nonetheless, abortion and birth technologies that result in the death of the unborn are neither supported for Christians nor should they be casually tolerated in the broader society. Legitimate arguments can be made that Christians should tolerate sexual immorality among those of the world, at least as long as it is not a direct threat to their own families (especially children) and communities. Abortion and the killing of "leftover" human preborns would not qualify as something to quietly tolerate.

Jesus uses the image of rebirth to declare the newness of life into which one enters by accepting him as Lord. One gains a new relationship to God as Father, "Abba" (Mk 14:36; Rom 8:15; Gal 4:6), and Christ as elder brother. The analogue tells the evangelical that human life matters, that birth is a significant transition into new relationships, but that prior to birth one still matters enough that God would have all be delivered in new relationships with him. Christians must absolutely oppose abortion on all grounds except the life of the mother. They may accept ART that is not intentionally or highly probably destructive of preborns.

PART THREE: CHRISTIAN BIOETHICS AND THE WORLD

Abortion and the casual killing of preborns leftover from ART is a denial of hope and trivialization of human life. Most often in the West, though not always, this killing occurs in the name of personal fulfillment, and the life of the preborn is lost by a family or a preborn is discarded in a laboratory. The justification for both actions is quite similar, though since the consequences are not necessarily the same they must be differentiated. ART is problematic, but can be acceptable. Abortion, except to save the mother's life, is immoral and should be illegal for the sake of the social contract.

Though principally an immorality directed against the vulnerable individual, abortions (and uses of ART that include the casual discarding of "leftovers") negate some hope for all lives, not just the ones who are killed. Abortion does this primarily by being an action built on the assumptions of a careless utilitarian (at best) or crass hedonistic (at worst) moral reasoning, namely that human beings can be trivialized to the point of being mere objects to be manipulated. This is precisely what a mother does not do when she experiences the joy of serving her child by bearing the infant to birth. For Christians, then, birth is an intrinsic good because God creates humans as a good and that goodness is ideally manifest in the love and care of parent for child and child for parent. For U.S. society, the morality of abortion should not be decided by what is good but by what is right. Under the U.S. social contract, individuals have the right to exist and killing them is wrong.

The hiding of sexual immorality with abortion is no longer a significant moral concern of the broader society. Sexual immorality is now accepted and must be tolerated in a social contract society that emphasizes freedom. The prevention of such immorality remains (or should remain) a moral concern for those in the community of faith, but is not paramount when addressing outsiders. Of course, from a Christian perspective, the ultimate physical act of affection (sexual intercourse) belongs with the ultimate legal act (civilly validated marriage, when possible, under the laws of the state), the ultimate social act (public marriage commitments), and the ultimate spiritual act for a man and woman (marriage before the body of believers). Yet preventing sexual immorality cannot be the basis of the Christian opposition to abortion in the civil arena. Indeed, consistent opposition to abortion requires that condemnation of promiscuity be limited simply for the practical reason of wanting to work with the pregnant woman. Shaming is pointless and may encourage a second moral failure (abortion) to cover the initial sexual impropriety. In the public arena, evangelicals may want to vehemently disagree with immoral sexuality, and their congregations must set standards for leadership and members. On the other hand, for the sake of liberty under the social contract, believers have to tolerate those of the world who disagree.

When addressing the world on abortion, the primary moral language must be that of the right to life and the right to liberty. The right to liberty cannot be had at the expense of an innocent life, for life takes priority over liberty. Some assert that the ambiguity of the preborn's humanity means that the right to life for the preborn should not overrule the clear humanity and associated rights of the mother. Certainly, at the earliest stage between the period of conception and the natural limit of twinning, it is debatable as to whether the preborn is a distinct human being (since she or he could still twin). There is no doubt she or he is uniquely human—not of another species. But ontological status uncertainty does not create moral uncertainty. One of the most incompetent pieces of ethical analysis ever offered in a public forum was that presented in *Roe v. Wade* in the United States in which uncertainty about status of the preborn led to moral certainty about killing the preborn. The exact opposite is most logical. If definitely human and likely a unique human individual, then default toward life.[14] Similarly poor ethical reasoning is evident in comments from politicians along the lines of "I am personally opposed to abortion but do not think I can ask others to share my views." This is akin to antebellum political leaders saying, "I don't have any slaves, but those plantation owners should be entitled to do what they want."

Of course, one reason why such poor reasoning is used to cover up the immorality of abortion, and in a related way the casual discarding of extra embryos from ART, is that abortion is a marker for broader cultural claims.[15] While the language of "culture wars" may not be appropriate, especially as the simplistic uses of the concept imply that all the issues line up a certain way and that there are only two sides, there are nonetheless cultural "locations." This is evident in the choice of symbols the two sides of the abortion debate use.

Proabortion/prochoice advocates:

- Opposition called: "antichoice"
- Lapel symbol: a coat hanger

---

[14]From two different ends of the American political spectrum, one can follow formulations of this argument in Ronald Reagan, *Abortion and the Conscience of the Nation* (Nashville: Thomas Nelson, 1984) and the writings of Nat Hentoff of the *Village Voice*. For the latter, see "The Indivisible Fight for Life," originally presented at the Americans United for Life Forum in Chicago, October 19, 1996 <http://groups.csail.mit.edu/mac/users/rauch/nvp/consistent/indivisible.html>.

[15]See Kristin Luker, *Abortion and the Politics of Motherhood* (Berkeley: University of California Press, 1984).

- Discarded fetus: "Products of Conception"
- Process: "Termination"
- Cultural argument: Need for "individual empowerment," either as a matter of individual rights or as a corrective to oppression or abuse
- Economic argument: Pregnancy is used to control women; pregnancy and single-motherhood impoverishes women

Antichoice/Prolife advocates:

- Opposition called: "proabortion" (some refer to as "murderers")
- Lapel symbol: rose and little feet
- Discarded fetus: "Preborn"
- Process: "Killing"
- Cultural argument: Denies value of women as women, that is, humans with capacity to be mothers; denies value of nuclear family
- Economic argument: Abortion is a money-making endeavor for some chief advocates

Without question, at least the starting assumption of the prolife movement is correct—the entity is living. The biological criteria for animal life are satisfied: growth/development, movement, response to stimuli, respiration, animal cell structure and member of a reproducing species. The last point might be debated, in that some would argue that the entity is not really human. While an "ontogeny recapitulating phylogeny" argument might be made to prove the entity is not a real human, it finally is unsatisfying because the entity is never anything but a developing human being (let alone that such an argument is not good evolutionary science).[16] That is like claiming that a tadpole is not a frog because it lacks legs and has a tail.

The entity goes through developmental stages—that is, change within continuity. After all, even insect metamorphosis is one individual being transformed through a continuous process. Proabortionists attempt to assign a single point for the beginning of humanness. Some favor the experience of others (e.g., quickening), available tests (e.g., brainwaves) or passing out of the birth canal—completely out—or, for those holding the most extreme posi-

[16]A poignant comment on this is found in Robert P. George, "Where Babies Come From," *First Things* (October 1990).

tion, even up to four weeks after birth ("postnatal abortion").

Typically, the denial of rights for preborns has been resolved by proabortionists in one of two manners: either the preborn/fetus is defined as a nonhuman or the concept of societal member (and the possession of associated rights) is shifted from the "human" to the "person" and "person" is then defined to exclude the preborn.

Of course, it is not only the status of the preborn that matters but also that of the mother. Certainly, any social argument about abortion must also include respect for the rights of women—as a familial, cultural and political concern. Abortion, supposedly a mechanism for empowering women, actually denies the legitimacy of what is distinctively female—childbearing—trivializing it relative to Western models of success. Women are not just persons; they are female persons.

The implications seem to go well beyond the solitary decision a woman makes about her body after consulting with her physician or what a lab does with the unimplanted embryos. This is not, in other words, just a medical choice. It has huge implications for the definition of *human* and, hence, social contract membership and rights in the West at the end of modernity. It speaks volumes about how persons with disabilities will be treated. It has powerful implications for the euthanizing of those not strong enough to put up a significant fight. Also, it seems to have power to shape the culture.

Few moral issues in American history have served as such an enduring cultural and moral declaration about the marginalization of the vulnerable as abortion—others have been slavery and related civil rights concerns and genocide against Native Americans. Though not involving wholesale slaughter or ethnospecific slavery, women's suffrage and rights also was an important declaration about social membership. The challenge for Christians is to assert a moral standard against an attack at core, social-contract values without fundamentally threatening these same values by their own behavior.

Christians must recognize that in the West the dominant understanding of humanness among those of the world is that of an autonomous decision-maker—and it is and should be acceptable to evangelicals when in the sphere of politics. The believers should only expect the world to treat individuals—all individuals—as equal before the state. This is best achieved by disinterested procedural justice operating on the assumption that all biologically distinct and unique human beings count for basic rights of life and liberty. In the political expressions that affect bioethics, social contract theory protects the rights of individuals to make decisions about how they are treated. It restricts the paternalism/maternalism of the state and of others who have inordinate power. It has a lot of advantages over other constructs that might be used to justify the power of the state or the elite.

Still, the social contract does limit liberty. Persons cannot hurt other persons and may not act in a manner that would reasonably put others at significant risk. The state may protect the borders from invaders and may police within the boundaries. In other words, one of primary functions of the state in the social contract is the protection of the lives of the individual contract makers. For this reason, the state may protect incompetents. By protecting the most marginalized "individual contract makers" the state declares its intention to protect all.

Some find abortion more acceptable if there are extenuating circumstances. Proabortionists use the exceptional cases in the media, while downplaying, though not denying, the primary function of abortion as a means of birth control. Some of these extraordinary reasons, though not adequate to justify abortion, raise significant questions about how women are treated at a particularly vulnerable point in life. The reality of these difficulties for the pregnant woman should be acknowledged. Of course, these reasons may not be mutually exclusive (e.g., a disabled child might be defined as an economic burden). Still, abortion is at best like killing a careless trespasser and at worst like killing an innocent bystander (even in the case of incest and rape). Prohibitions of abortion may arguably disadvantage the class of persons who might get pregnant. Though this is a lesser concern than the deprivation of life for the unborn, it should be taken into account in political responses to abortion.

The law is currently shaped by two major Supreme Court cases. *Roe v. Wade* allows for abortion through an interpretation of a right to privacy in the Fourteenth Amendment, asserts the trimester model of pregnancy, while claiming state interest after viability can interfere with maternal freedom, though not with protection of the health of the mother. The other case is *Planned Parenthood v. Casey,* which maintains *Roe v. Wade* but eliminates the trimester model in favor of an "undue burden" standard and leaves open the moving of permissibility of abortion on the basis of shifts in viability. Further, from this and other cases, the state can impose restrictions (e.g., informed consent). The ruling in favor of the Partial Birth Abortion Ban Act of 2003 by the Supreme Court in 2007 *(Gonzales v. Carhart)* will have an increasing impact as viability moves earlier through technological improvement. The current administration, though, is pushing to minimize protections.

Further political action is required. That may mean those opposed to abortion will have to politically dirty their hands, though must be cautious to not allow their hands to become stained by the desire for self-aggrandizing political power. Three points of concession may be temporarily made, conceded as a pragmatic step in protecting all contract makers. The three points for possible temporary concession are allowing abortions for: (1) rape or incest, (2) disability that will probably result in near-term death for the preborn and (3) abortion prior to twinning.

Abortion of preborns created through incest and rape is immoral, as the child is not guilty of the crime committed by the father. Certainly, even those of the world would agree that "the soul who sins is the one who will die. The son will not share the guilt of the father, nor will the father share the guilt of the son" (Ezek 18:20). Still, pragmatically conceding such in the law would be a good first step, if other abortions were outlawed. Most abortions would end; it would be worth the temporary concession, not in moral reasoning but as a political effort to save lives. To use a comparison, if one could save a train of Roma and Jews from being taken to extermination camps, but not everyone on the final car of the train could be saved, that would not mean that those who could be saved should not be. The absolutely perfect should not be made the enemy of the relatively good.

Allowing abortion when the preborn child would die in the near-term is a form of passive euthanasia that would, with strict examination, be temporarily acceptable to believers. Ultimately, this might remain acceptable. What would not be acceptable in the long run is abortion of the disabled simply because they are disabled. This will call for significant political activity and will call for significant support of women with unwanted pregnancies as well as strong advocacy for disability rights.

Prior to the point of possible twinning, the human entity may be more than one developing human being. In other words, the entity is distinctly human, but not necessarily uniquely a given human. Contrary to the other two possible concessions, this one should not be made even for pragmatic political benefit. Abortion technologies have "improved" and now the so-called morning-after pill is available. It is likely that this will not be curtailed anytime soon. Nonetheless, unlike the other two situations in which the woman is a victim or the child is injured/sick, this method (assuming there is not rape or incest) is a means to eliminate possible consequences of a bad decision. That would not be a position someone advocating for the rights of individuals should take.

The political conflict over ART is related to that over abortion but is far less precise, if for no other reason because the motive of the parents who may discard a preborn is not to prevent birth, but to have a child—though not the child they reject. They see themselves as having a problem that can be medically defined and medically treated. Illness or sickness is usually physiologically or anatomically defined, but one always marked by social and cultural categorizations. Baldness may or may not be a sickness, but some men want to cure it pharmaceutically. Certainly, sales of erectile dysfunction drugs indicate that a not unusual consequence of aging is considered a disease. Is infertility a sickness? If affecting a couple, is it a family sickness, or is it to be defined individually? Certainly a "normal" (for the species, gender and age) biological function is diminished or lost if the infertility occurs prior to age thirty-five. In addition, an almost universally desired relationship (by God's creative plan or by evolutionary process or both—depending on one's theology of creation) with one's offspring is absent. The problem is not just medical. Many persons want to pass on their genetic material through offspring. Other social options exist (e.g., adoption), but these require a genuine commitment to family as something beyond blood.

A family is a group of genetically related persons (or persons who act as if they are genetically related), defined by ancestors or descendants, who work for common productive and reproductive ends. To state this in an oxymoronic way, individuals do not exist individually. All societies depend on families as mediating institutions or for primary governance. It could be argued that the state should support families. Perhaps. At least, it can be asserted that the state should defer to families or not work against them. ART is extremely profamily in that sense, but opens the door for significant conflicts over the structure of family.[17]

Some of the ART techniques are:

- IVF: In vitro fertilization (fertilization in glass and implantation in uterus)
- ICSI: Intracytoplasmic sperm injection (form of IVF with sperm injected into egg)
- ZIFT: Zygote intrafallopian transfer (fertilized egg guided into fallopian tube)

[17]Some key cases: *Stern v. Whitehead* (1988), *Davis v. Davis* (1992) and Ricardo Asch, at University of California, Irvine, who "stole" eggs or embryos from at least 75 couples (1997).

- GIFT: Gamete intrafallopian transfer (guiding unfertilized transferred egg and sperm)
- AI: Artificial insemination (can be done with "primitive" techniques)
- Cloning: Asexual (in the technical sense) reproduction: taking genetic material and inserting it into other living cells, followed by replication[18]

The reasons to use ART are basically to obtain a child with a known genotype *and* (likely) phenotype and to maintain a biological link with the offspring. As with Abram and Sarai, secular arguments for alternative birth technologies should address possibilities of significant problems. These may not be insurmountable, but they should not be denied. A simple list includes:

- High degree of embryo waste
- Disproportionate numbers of abnormalities
- Premature deaths
- Sex bias following preimplantation genetic diagnosis
- Possible ethnic bias, given the ethnicity distribution of children up for adoption
- Technology is only available to specific socioeconomic classes
- Altering family structure, especially concept of parenthood (genetic, gestational, rearing, sociolegal parenting are separated)
- Eugenic selection
- Use of preborn as research medium or pharmaceutical resource[19]

CONCLUSION

Evangelicals believe in the eternal significance not only of the persons who are born physically and reborn spiritually but also of those who are preborn biologically and those not in a child-Father relationship with God. As such, believers should not participate as practitioners in abortion and should fight

[18]See Robert Orr, "The Temptation of Human Cloning," *Today's Christian Doctor* 28, no. 3 (fall 1997), pp. 4-7.

[19]One grave danger to unfettered development of ART techniques would be research or therapeutic cloning or other abuses of preborn humans. Somatic Cell Nuclear Transfer is cloning developed, supposedly, for therapeutic reasons. The technique involves killing embryos. Recently alternatives have been suggested. Often ignored is the fact that the best, current therapies have been from adult stem cells, not from embryonic clones. Further, to suggest that developed technologies would not be used for eugenic purposes is either disingenuous or naive.

any effort to force those in training for nursing or medical specialties to be trained in elective abortion. Believers should develop alternatives for pregnant women that go beyond platitudes and casual words of encouragement to genuine Christian hospitality. This may be through refuge crisis centers, but should also include opening their homes and providing financial support during and immediately after the pregnancy, as well as adopting unwanted children. Those who engage in political activities should participate in or support protests, election efforts, and so forth. Economically, they should boycott those who make support for abortion or the abuse of reproductive technologies as a central moral claim. As appropriate, they should challenge those using ART and those who practice the technologies to be consistent in their claim about wanting to create and protect life. Still, believers should do these things as people who are reborn, avoiding hatred and violence in the effort to overcome hatred and violence toward the most vulnerable.

15

Biotechnology and Eugenics

HUMANS AS CREATORS

Humans are creators but are not the Creator. From a Christian perspective, they are not even cocreators, but subcreators, stewards for the Master. As such, they have great responsibility. Humans are both part of nature and above nature, which in turn should lead to the cautious use of new biotechnologies—recognizing both the human creative task and the tendency for humans to think far more of their capacities and judgments than they ought to do. Biotechnologies for agricultural purposes are legitimate, if proper precautions are taken, especially about unintended release into ecosystems. Human biotechnology requires greater caution, at least at the individual level. Human biotechnology for the curing of diseases in individuals, even by correcting a genetic line, is acceptable stewardship, while altering for "improved" normality (what is usually called "positive eugenics") is not.

> I am the true vine, and my Father is the gardener. He cuts off every branch in me that bears no fruit, while every branch that does bear fruit he prunes so that it will be even more fruitful. You are already clean because of the word I have spoken to you. Remain in me, and I will remain in you. No branch can bear fruit by itself; it must remain in the vine. Neither can you bear fruit unless you remain in me.
>
> I am the vine; you are the branches. If a man remains in me and I in him, he will bear much fruit; apart from me you can do nothing. If anyone does not remain in me, he is like a branch that is thrown away and withers; such branches are picked up, thrown into the fire and burned. If you remain in me and my words remain in you, ask whatever you wish, and it will be given you. This is to my Father's glory, that you bear much fruit, showing yourselves to be my disciples. (Jn 15:1-8)

When Jesus spoke these words, the listeners, even most of those who resided in Jerusalem, had some practical idea of what he was speaking.[1] At the very least, they knew what a grapevine looked like—how the roots passed through the dry soil to the water deep beneath, how the vines twisted up posts, and then the grapes in their season weighted down the branches that held them tightly. Their knowledge did not penetrate as far as the biochemistry of photosynthesis or the genetics of breeding, but they did have some idea about what kind of grape would produce what kind of taste.

The specificity and, paradoxically, greater generality of late modern language and knowledge lacks the localism of the past, even the recent past. The understanding of agriculture assumed 2000 years ago would have been of a different kind than that of most persons at the end of modernity. The people who heard the parable would have known the grape as part of the vine, not as something selected from the fruit case of a supermarket—as something connected, not an individual entity detached. Jesus wanted (and wants) his believers to recognize they are parts of a whole at the same time that they are individuals.

The early Christians understood this horticultural image. Further, they recognized the significance of grapevine and wine as religious images. Elsewhere in John, Jesus claims to be the living water, the bread of life, the light, and the door/gate for the sheep. These images were meant to be not only convenient sermon illustrations, but also analogues about the desperate physical need for water, the strength that was based on daily nutrition, the mind's need for light to see and to survive, and the community's need for safety. Likewise, the image of the grapevine was meant to convey more than connection; the vine was understood to produce through the branches, to yield its fruit, and so should his followers through him.

Production defines the significance of the fruiting branch and, similarly, Jesus wants his followers to understand they are to produce fruit. Paul says as much in Galatians:

> [T]he fruit of the Spirit is love, joy, peace, patience, kindness, goodness, faithfulness, gentleness and self-control. Against such things there is no law. Those who belong to Christ Jesus have crucified the sinful nature with its passions and desires. Since we live by the Spirit, let us keep in step with the Spirit. (Gal 5:22-25)

---

[1]Special thanks for ongoing sabbatical conversations while I was Visiting Ethics Scholar in Molecular Biology, University of Missouri; see preface.

Being born again is not so much an end as a beginning. One is supposed to mature, come to fruition in the faith. The *telos* that God has for each person is not achieved with redemption, but in rebirth initiated as a cooperative venture in the use of the divine grace as one moves toward true holiness. Simultaneously one is transformed and yet is the same. This willingness to encourage change, even while recognizing necessary limits, has ancient roots in the faith. For instance, Tertullian, an ante-Nicene father, notes:

> Now nobody denies what nobody is ignorant of—for Nature herself is teacher of it—that God is the Maker of the universe, and that it is good, and that it is man's by free gift of its Maker. But having no intimate acquaintance with the Highest, knowing Him only by natural revelation, and not as His "friends"—afar off, and not as those who have been brought nigh to Him—men cannot but be in ignorance alike of what He enjoins and what He forbids in regard to the administration of His world.[2]

As Tertullian points out, this "is the one ground of condemnation, that the creature misuses the creation."[3] This misuse arises from ignorance, but willful ignorance, ignorance that is subsequent to the broken relationship with God. Tertullian is referring primarily to those of the world, but to a lesser degree it also applies to believers. For even knowing the will of God for our final existence with him does not provide absolute knowledge of the particulars of every situation. To believe otherwise is to fall into the same arrogance as some reductionist followers of scientism today and the Pharisees of Jesus' time. What can be said about the goal or *telos* of human existence is that persons are not to merely revert to the prelapsarian condition of Adam and Eve, but to become like Christ (the new Adam of 1 Cor 15). The goal of life is to satisfy not only the creative intention of God, but also the redemptive. And, somehow, the redemptive order includes proper consideration of the natural world.

The grapevine was a good that served the people of ancient Israel. The natural world was not something that served the people of Israel, and had intrinsic worth as the creation of God. This does not mean adoring some false, static image. Rather, Israel then and evangelicals today have a duty to both use and preserve the creation, to transcend Nature and to be part of it.

[2]Tertullian "On the Shows or De Spectaculis (the Theatre)," chapter 2, trans. the Rev. S. Thelwall, Twenty One TNT <http://www.21tnt.com/archives_sermons/antenicene.htm#onbaptism>.

[3]Ibid.

Humans are stewards fulfilling the intended divine *telos*.

Obviously, then, Christians are not opposed to changing something so that it might become more fruitful, including themselves. Likewise, they are not opposed to altering naturally occurring plants or animals in order to obtain fruit. The domestication of corn and of dairy cows would not seem problematic in the least to evangelicals. Nor should such be a problem for anyone, at least not logically, as no culture that has survived into the twenty-first century is not so structured as to encourage, under some circumstances, changing human environments. Yet there are limits to such transformation, for while evangelicals support the idea that humans can be creators, it is always as subservient to the Creator. The management or intentional changing of human order or the natural order ought to serve the divine plan. Paul explained this in his use of the graft on the tree (Rom 11:17-24).

This willingness to alter nature—both human nature and the natural world—until recently seemed more pronounced in the Western world than elsewhere. The causes of this are numerous—everything from resources to the development of guns to survival of certain Greeks texts. The factor that has been most commonly cited is religious. The monotheistic religions of the West allowed for altering the natural order because God is considered distinct from and rules over that order. The Protestants accentuate this, according to the traditional Weberian claim, which explains to no little extent why industrialization and expansive agriculture took off in the English-speaking world.

By the end of the eighteenth century, the acceptance of the possibility of improving oneself and transforming one's surroundings combined with Anglo-American pragmatism into a generally shared affirmation of the possibility for progress. Personal and social improvement became the motif of the evangelical tapestry in the nineteenth century, as for most Americans. From the leaders of the Second Great Awakening through the social reforming evangelist Charles Finney to populists like William Jennings Bryan, evangelicals believed in mastering nature and mastering themselves in the name of progress—progress that would raise the poor and the oppressed and win souls to Christ. The improved individual improved the society, and the improved society would improve the individual.

From the end of the nineteenth century and up through the New Deal the cultural emphasis was on progress, even with the difficulties immigrant populations faced, cynicism following World War I and the 1929 crash. Evangelicals may have helped spur the cultural assumption on in a small way prior to World War I, but they were by no means alone in making the claim that progress was a social good and that progress included the mastery of nature—both human nature and the natural world. Lest one think this was only the position of commercial interests or naive revivalists, consider the music of Woody Guthrie, who sang of the Dust Bowl but still commended the damming of the rivers of the American West and Tennessee Valley. The entire New Deal was undergirded by the belief that the educated elite could direct the whole society toward an earthly promised land with "patures of plenty."

World War II brought caution. Evangelicals had already become suspicious of those who held power over technology and, with the shift from postmillennial to premillenial thought, began to question the idea of progress altogether. This was especially true about biotechnologies. Evangelicals had opposed sterilization and other efforts by American eugenicists to improve the race, which was one reason why they tended to oppose atheistic evolutionary models (as Bryan had pointed out, the theories as presented tended to leave no room for the intrinsic dignity of the human). World War II solidified this doubt. Technology had its place, evangelicals claimed, but only when viewed cautiously and with recognition of the vested interests of decisionmakers. So today evangelicals are not opposed to the alteration of humans through technologies, specifically biotechnologies, but only if such, is done with extraordinary caution. The desire to make improvements calls for caution, for without such, hubris surely follows (and the attitudes of some involved in biotechnologies manifest that very form of pride).

Change is not intrinsically good, only change toward the divine end or *telos*. One clear implication of Jesus' words is that there may be many branches, but there is only one vine that sustains life and only one standard for altering humans or altering nature: whether or not such change is in the divine will. Humans, properly, are not the Creator or even cocreators, but always subcreators under the authority of God—at best, stewards with important responsibilities, but never owners who can arbitrarily set the standards.

Evangelicals have viewed nature as something that praises God on the one hand, and as something that can be used to achieve human purposes compatible with the divine purpose on the other. Humans are allowed to "garden," but responsibly. That means that changing nature and even changing humans genetically is acceptable, but only with the greatest caution. This may mean the creation of new chimeras or even new reproducing species, as long as they serve a good purpose and do not create any genuine threats to humanity or nature. It means, too, that humans can be genetically altered to control disease, but never for positive eugenic purposes that would alter the species and deny the reflection of the *imago Dei* in each individual.

PART TWO: CHRISTIAN BIOETHICS

Intentionally or not, philosophers and bioethicists tend to strongly differentiate human and nonhuman biotechnologies. To some extent, this makes sense. After all, in virtually all societies, especially those shaped by Western culture, humans are clearly distinguished from other animals and the rest of creation. This is formally noted for the U.S. social contract in the founding documents, including the Constitution.

Believers should agree with neither those who claim that only humans matter nor those who make claims for rights for animals that equate species. Christians should recognize that humans bear the image of the Deity, and that makes each and every person different from nonhumans. Believers should also recognize that they are of the dust, formed from the earth as the nonhuman animals.

> I also thought, "As for men, God tests them so that they may see that they are like the animals. Man's fate is like that of the animals; the same fate awaits them both: As one dies, so dies the other. All have the same breath; man has no advantage over the animal. Everything is meaningless. All go to the same place; all come from dust, and to dust all return. Who knows if the spirit of man rises upward and if the spirit of the animal goes down into the earth?" (Eccles 3:18-21)

How humans fit or do not fit into nature determines to no little degree what is thought about the application of biotechnologies—both in the humans species and in non-humans. Recognizing that people are both in nature and above it implies dignity for human beings and allows respect for the natural order and its component parts. As far as biotechnology goes, this both/and approach allows for some alteration of humans and nonhumans on the condition that fundamental character is not destroyed for the species and, in the case of humans, for the individual.

The problem with considering humans completely above nature is that the natural world is then viewed solely instrumentally. Whoever has power or authority can "claim" the natural world, as did conquerors of the past. Colonists who indiscriminately took land, miners who carelessly polluted streams and loggers who clear-cut wide swaths across mountains should not be condemned with historical revisionism, but the flaws in the reasoning should be clearly recognized. Nature does not, according to the Scripture, belong to any human, though it may be used respectfully by humans for legitimate purposes. The respect required includes consideration of the goodness the Creator declared when he made the natural world.

The problem with considering humans only a part of nature is that they cannot be held accountable any more than any other natural thing for living out biological impulses. If the reductionist claim is correct that a human is no more than one additional, random evolutionary expression, not fundamentally different from anything that has gone before or will come after, then everything is natural and accidental. The only compelling moral claim is to not destroy other natural components if the absence or alteration of those components would consequentially destroy oneself. Yes, there may be aesthetic experiences, but these are either mere chance and immaterial or related to survival, which returns to survival and reproduction as the only justification of morality—which means morality itself is not real but instrumental only. Good and bad, right and wrong do not exist as actual values, or do so only as subsidiaries of survival and reproduction. The primary moral duty—if humans are part of nature and nothing else—is to evolve, as individuals or as kinship groups or in whatever way is most efficient in perpetuating genetic material—to be, as is popularly declared, the carriers of selfish genes.[4] And they do so while realizing that their race will inevitably end as the cosmos drifts toward nothingness.

Of course, nature can be defined in grander terms, as if nature transcends the natural. For a pantheist, there is no fundamental distinction between humans and any other beings. This might lead to broad respect for life, but there is no reason to provide respect on the basis of human dignity. This might, for some, mean the elevation of nonhuman animals, but just as likely will lead to disregard for other *Homo sapiens*.

If, instead, humans are simultaneously encapsulated and not encapsulated within nature, then they can value themselves, their kin, the rest of humanity, individual nonhuman creatures, ecosystems and nature itself. Of course, if nonbelievers wish to assert that humans are parasites or toxic invaders of nature, like purple loosestrife along an inland pool or emerald ash borers de-

---

[4]Richard Dawkins's language. He asserts there are other moral implications in Richard Dawkins, *The Selfish Gene* (Oxford: Oxford University Press, 1999).

stroying the trees of forest canopies, then any possibility for significant discourse is limited. Or if nonbelievers assert that nature is only for instrumental use, then commonality is unlikely to be found on issues of biotechnology or any environmental concern. Evangelicals do not (or should not) think that human life, or any life, or the whole of creation is morally neutral, nor should they claim nature is divine. They should value the lesser good of nature and assume responsibility.

Evangelicals can and should, then, be strong advocates for ecosystem protection in that nature joins with humans in praising the Creator. Further, nature mismanaged will mean the resources humans need, which have been provided by God, are unavailable. Beyond this, an obligation to future generations necessitates appropriate care of the environment. Besides the wellness of the system of which humans are, indeed, a component, evangelicals should support the protection of individual animals when possible. Evangelicals can and should support the animal welfare movement. On the other hand, they should challenge the logic of animal rights as an ultimately self-defeating assignment of status and responsibility to creatures against the latter's own nature. In doing so, evangelicals give priority to the environmental system over the individual animal.

This does not mean that humans or components of nature should never be changed. In fact, it is a gross ecological error to assume that nature is static. Whether one wants to use the language of evolution or not, it is clear that individuals and species change. When humans participate in the change, they should ask, what will the change be—what will be gained and what lost? In other words, from a Christian point of view, creatures and creation have *teloi*, purposes for existence. For instance, there is nothing wrong with domesticating certain animals and plants, such as cattle and corn, but destroying complete megaecosystems while establishing a monoculture is clearly reprehensible whether done by intention or carelessness.

Similarly, humans may make reasonable changes in their own biology, but not to the point of actually destroying the species or substituting for it something someone in power considers preferable. The problem is not only that it is intrinsically wrong (which could be debated) but also the lack of knowledge creates far more risks than probable benefits. Further, it is a logical necessity that those who are not altered will do the altering—the ungenetically changed will do the changing. This is fraught with danger arising from the hubris of the elite. If nothing else, the last one hundred years demonstrates quite clearly that political leaders, commercial giants, and prominent scientists do not always make the best—and often make the seemingly worse—decisions for the commonweal. The idea that, like corn and cattle, humans would be domesticated, and soon utterly dependent (like corn and cattle) on the good wishes of the overlords should be strikingly unappealing. Supposed positive eugenics would inevitably be used by decision-makers for their own purposes—be they evil purposes, to use Christian language, or for the genetic benefit of their own offspring, to use neo-Darwinian language. Change, then, if directed by humans, is not necessarily evil or good, but rapid change controlled by a limited few can be astoundingly dangerous.

Likewise, keeping everything as unchanged as possible is neither right nor wrong intrinsically. It does mean that some will suffer who might not otherwise if new technological solutions were discovered. To think that the way things are is the way they should be is referred to as the *naturalistic fallacy*.[5] Or, it may reflect another reasoning fallacy, what can be called the *temporalistic fallacy*, that what is is what was and/or what will be. Change will occur and there is a place for humans to participate in change. Still, the human manipulation of that change—whether altering nonhumans or humans—must be for defensibly good reasons, not just change for the sake of change.

How the decision making about new biotechnologies takes place depends not only on the specifics of the technology but also on the operative functional religion underpinning the decision. Functional religions are worldviews that structure moral decision making for a community, large or small, through authority and claims of epistemological validity. A substantive religion is a functional religion in which there is a notion of deity or deities. All squares are rectangles but all rectangles are not squares; all substantive religions are functional religions but all functional religions are not substantive religions. A comparison can be drawn between evangelical Christianity as a substantive religion, scientism as a nonsubstantive functional religion and syncretistic New Age "green" spirituality as a substantive religion.

- Worldview: A comprehensive, single, general explanatory arrangement by which events of "reality" can be explained; indeed, worldview defines what is "reality."
  - Christianity—God loves and engages his creation.

---

[5]G. E. Moore, *Principia Ethica* (London: Cambridge University Press, 1922).

> Scientism—The universe is random and accidental, though its patterns are not accidental given that they exists.

> Syncretistic "green" spirituality—Reality is pantheistic or panentheistic.

- Meaning: A means by which one gains purpose in "reality."

> Christianity—God loves individuals and has desires for each specific life which, as one follows, provides individual purpose.

> Scientism—There is no real meaning, though the claim is made that "truth" is meaning and that the reductionist epistemological method provides truth. (This is the principle flaw in scientism, as meaning is completely arbitrary; the critique of so-called postmodern critics of science as a life philosophy, rather than the scientific method *per se,* seems accurate.)

> Syncretistic "green" spirituality—A version of natural law, which purports all find meaning if individuals correspond their lives with the elimination of pain for all creatures and seek to "fit."

- Legitimation: The social structures that endorse reality and one's place in it.

> Christianity—This is the community of faith, primarily; to a lesser extent for U.S. Christians also, Western political theory—specifically Lockean-Jeffersonian-Madisonian social contract theory—allows, even if it does not endorse, the Christian worldview.

> Scientism—Science in the academy with life purpose judged (supposedly) by the epistemological method of science (though actually by the personal taste of academic peers).

> Syncretistic "green" spirituality—Most legitimation is sensory, especially the sensation of pain; if an act avoids causing pain to sentient beings (presumably except humans who may, at least on occasion "deserve it") then an act is verifiably legitimate.

- Theodicy: the explanation of failures and suffering.

> Christianity—Cause is primarily sin—individual or corporate (including an assumption of "falleness" in the creation, in all organizations, and in all individuals.

> Scientism—There is no final explanation of suffering, only that it "is." Sickness, disease, etc. are triggered by attempting to violate physical laws or simply because the "time has come." (This is a major problem for

scientism, as the suffering of the poor and otherwise marginal is finally just something that happens and, certainly, has no eternal significance; when advocates of the philosophy of scientism cry out about injustice they are living off the moral capital of the past, usually the Christian past, of their own lives or cultures.)

> Syncretistic "green" spirituality—Suffering is generally defined in anthropomorphic terms which are applied to the nonhuman world so that all suffering across species is equated; most suffering is attributable to humans; thus humans become, essentially, the original sinners.[6]

- Socialization:
  > Christianity—This is primarily through the church, family and friends.
  > Scientism—This is primarily through academia, in which they are disproportionately represented, and to a lesser extent in the media (though, the popular media could hardly be described as "scientific").
  > Syncretistic "green" spirituality—Socialization tends to occur through shared protest and "education" events and through web-based communication.
- Ritual:
  > Christianity—Worship with words and acts declaring that God loves and engages his creation.
  > Scientism—Primarily publication and engagement in "righteous fights"—often with straw men of Christianity they can easily kick over, rather than significant Christian leaders who have the same level of education.
  > Syncretistic "green" spirituality—Often includes modification of "ancient" worship activities sometimes called *neo-pagan* (supposedly appropriated from Native American and pre-Christian European worship) as well as ritualized protest activities.
- Authoritative leaders:
  > Christianity—Usually clergy; with evangelicals there is significant power in the laity to determine the "correctness" of the clergy, so author-

[6]For example, "A rat is a pig is a dog is a boy" said Ingrid Newkirk, president, People for the Ethical Treatment of Animals; she also equated 6,000,000 animals raised in confinement barns and eaten to the Jews who died in the Nazi Holocaust.

ity, except in rigid sectarian groups, is limited; some would argue that Christian media figures are highly influential—and they are, but not authoritatively.

> Scientism—The authority comes primarily from location in universities and, to a lesser degree, endorsement by the public media; especially important are charismatic leaders, for unlike in substantive religion where there are local clergy and local communities in which regular conversation about morality occurs and in which standards are accepted or endorsed, those favoring "scientism" flock to national or international populizers who then gain significant intellectual and even moral authority among their devotees (e.g., Dawkins, Singer, Sagan).[7]

> Syncretistic "green" spirituality—Authoritative figures tend to come at two levels: those active in the public square who are slightly less extreme, and those participating in illegal activities, and sometimes terrorism (the distinction between PETA and ALF/ELF serves as an example).

Most grand disagreements over nature are arguments that are finally religious. Atheists and believers must—if they are honest—acknowledge that they make a leap of faith. The atheist leaps to a commitment—again, if honest—to reductionism that finally means life is absurd. The syncretist green leaps to the demonstrably false conclusion that all (or most) life forms experience ultimate reality in similar ways. The Christian believer leaps to a Deity who provides purpose—not only for them but also for nature. Once making that jump—a leap that is neither rational nor irrational, but beyond rationality—the follower of Christ has a basis for morality in the eternal purpose of the Deity. Standing with one foot in finitude and one in infinity, Christians can value and appropriately use the other components of nature and evaluate the value and the risk of the genetic alteration of their own biological nature. Atheists finally have no honest basis for evaluating the right or wrong, the good or bad of genetic alteration and syncretistic pantheists tend to disregard scientific understanding of the natural order.

The religiosity or spirituality of genetic change can be described with a five-category moral typology.[8]

---

[7]The most interesting argument for a foundation for morality is "emergent" evolutionary values. One of the best presentations is by Ursula Goodenough, *The Sacred Depths of Nature* (New York: Oxford University Press, 1998).

[8]A similar typology was developed by Paul B. Thompson (*Spirit of the Soil: Agriculture and Environmental Ethics* [Routledge: London 1995]) with "productionism, economics, stewardship

- *Prohibitive.* The first category, including those most vehemently opposed to agricultural, pharmaceutical, and human biotechnology, are often pantheists. The tendency is to elevate the value of either nature or individual nonhuman animals, resulting in the practical diminishing of status for humans (e.g., supporters of the religious Gaia theory). Such persons tend to be strongly deontological, on the basis of values developed out of westernized Hinduism, though finally shaped as mystical (privatized and syncretistic). They will oppose biotechnologies, since any alteration is a violation of the intrinsic value of the individual nonhuman or human. In addition, humans are often deemed incompetent as decision makers about nature. Also, they tend to use strong cyclical notions of time, which is an opposition to the idea of progress.
- *Hesitant.* The next category includes persons who have an image of the earth and/or the organisms within it as cocreatures with humans. The moral language of such tends toward that of familial obligations, mutual respect and the virtuosity of working with nature. These people may or may not favor some pharmaceutical uses, but tend to be strongly opposed to agricultural transgenic organisms, partially because of the potential environmental problems, but also because of the danger to small farmers in the United States and developing world (they generally favor the decentralization of agricultural production). They will tend to use a strong version of the precautionary principle and often include individual nonhumans in the evaluation (e.g., Franciscan Christian interpretations, the poet-farmer Wendell Berry, some old-line Protestant groups).
- *Hesitatingly Accepting.* The middle position of the typology is based on a theological understanding of the superiority of humans that generates an obligation of stewardship. These tend to strongly support pharmaceutical uses and may accept (hesitatingly) uses of biotechnology that assist endangered species, clearly reduce damage to ecosystems, or help small farmers in developing nations. They are likely to support genetic corrections to treat genetic diseases or disease risk factors. Genetically modified organ-

---

and holism" as worldviews. The one included in this work was developed independently, using the H. Richard Niebuhr "Christ and Culture" typology as a model.

Arguments about the "spirituality" of genetic modification in the Western context tend to be drawn from the work of Aldo Leopold, Rachel Carson, Louis Bromfield, Wendell Berry, Holmes Rolston, Baird Callicott, Lynn White, Gary Comstock, Calvin DeWitt and, increasingly from outside the United States, Peter Singer and Vandana Shiva. This list is abbreviated and other names, perhaps more influential on the various parties, might be added.

isms (GMOs), then, would be acceptable, but only if judged using a milder version of the precautionary principle (e.g., most evangelical Christian groups, Hindu and Buddhist biotechnology supporters).

- *Openly Accepting.* The fourth group is utilitarian in reasoning, but recognizes the need to include nonhumans and ecosystems into the calculation for the sake of humans. These will allow for any genetic alteration that "pays off," though are willing to include serious risk evaluations for consideration (e.g., some U.S.-based scientific organizations, many mainstream agricultural organizations).
- *Unfettered.* The final group completely demystifies nature and sees its components as objects to be manipulated to any end by those with the power to do so. These often assert the compete legitimacy of both human and nonhuman genetic alteration. Paradoxically, those in this last group will sometimes assert that they are the most "natural" in allowing individual humans or social groups to "fight" for their survival. Further, they tend to assert that there is a technological imperative; an inevitability to development and use of new technologies that help humans fit the new niches that are constantly generated.[9] They might frame their argument by asking, "why leave it up to luck?" The most extreme may be strong libertarians or social Darwinists (e.g., the reported behavior of the government of the People's Republic of China and, perhaps, Singapore).

Again, these are ideal types (to use sociological language). Persons may have mixed allegiances and will use a variety of moral arguments, especially given that such arguments may not be mutually exclusive. Certainly, too, there are examples of those who do not fit into any category cleanly. Still, the typology provides a pattern for analysis that can assist in moral conversations between persons with different claims about the legitimacy of nonhuman and human biotechnology.

Christians must be located in one of the three central moral types. Recognizing sins, especially those that take shape as hubris, greed, and bigotry, means that believers should be strongly cautious. Caution does not mean that technologies should not be adopted; rather, they should be accepted as morally legitimate after reasonable evaluation of the risk and benefit (probabilities of occurrence and severity of occurrence) of specific applications of the technol-

[9]Hans Jonas uses the term *technological imperative*, though not in the sense of inevitably positive change.

ogy as well as general approaches to the research. Though each specific biotechnology would differ to some extent—for instance, accepting an in utero treatment that would cure or improve a preborn's health would be vastly different from one used to determine the "need" for an abortion. Amniocentesis might be used for both, so it would depend on the intention of those conducting and receiving the test as to whether it should or should not be conducted. Similarly, stem cell technologies with adult somatic cells are not problematic, while embryonic stem cell research is definitely a moral problem as it encourages the diminishing of value for human life generally, and preborn life specifically, as well as kills the given individual unborn child. In other words, some technology could be adopted but applied in limited ways.[10]

Generally speaking, evangelicals are open to technologies (their mastery of organizational and communication technologies are indicative). Some among those who are innovators of biotechnologies are believers (notably Human Genome Project leader Francis Collins) and their moral evaluation of the technologies has generally been balanced. The testing of a balanced approach is one that (1) is a benefit to individuals, but (2) not harming other humans (including the unborn and future generations) nor (3) significantly harming the natural order. What is unacceptable to believers is the alteration of the human genome for positive eugenic purposes or the intentional destruction of unique ecosystems. No human being is smart enough to decide what should constitute superhumans, and no human being is smart enough to widely control nature. Still, those genetic alterations that are not ethically prohibited should be cautiously accepted or tolerated by believers. When uncertain, Christians can publicly call those doing research and regulating the technology to protect social contract makers and the broader natural order.

One approach to providing protection to humans and nature is the biblical model of sabbath. Some want to prohibit any and all biotechnologies—for humans or nonhumans. At the other end, some want any possibility open to execution in labs and applied in medicine or agriculture as the market demands or the various labs doing the development determine. A preferable choice when uncertain is the sabbatical which is like a moratorium in that it calls for cessations of activities, but is like continual review in that it calls for

[10]Most commonly, five levels of willingness to adopt a new technology are described: (1) innovators, (2) early adopters, (3) early majority, (4) late majority and (5) laggards. This is drawn from the most important book in the field, Everett Rogers, *Diffusion of Innovation*, 4th ed. (New York: Free Press, 1995). Rogers is criticized in a variety of ways, but the trends or tendencies in adoption do seem to generally hold.

continuing development of technologies. Periodically, perhaps every six years, a pause for genuine reexamination of the application of technologies and impact on nature and cultures would be honestly considered—though it would also be acceptable for evangelicals to support cautious continual review or, for some technologies, moratoriums. Good can be done with biotechnologies, but it is essential to determine how the supposed good is defined—what kind of grapes will grow and whether they will be used for good wine or turned into bitter poison.

PART THREE: CHRISTIAN BIOETHICS AND THE WORLD

Roughly speaking, one can divide intentional genetic alteration into four major eras. First, through selection from nature and subsequent cultivation, humans chose plants that were more suitable to their needs than others that existed in nature. This occurred, according to anthropologists, at least ten thousand years ago (some Christians might challenge the timeframe, but at least it occurred millennia ago). Animal domestication followed. People selected, favoring the offspring of certain animals, but did not generally crossbreed for traits. Second, about 250 years ago the selective breeding of cattle for milk and meat production was refined into a "rational" process. This change, not accidentally, coincides with the beginnings of the Industrial Revolution in the West. Third, at the beginning of the twentieth century, the explanations of Mendel became generally known and were intentionally applied in breeding and hybridization. This effort has paid off in that broiler size (for cooking chickens), milk production, etc., have risen dramatically. The development of penicillin through specialized mold growth and polio vaccines are two of the most dramatic, but by no means only, biotechnological developments of this era. The last years of this third stage have included artificial birth technologies, specifically artificial insemination from high quality stock. The last years of the twentieth century mark the beginning of the fourth era, that of the direct alteration of the genome in humans and nonhumans.[11]

[11]Based on personal conversation with Michael Roberts, Ph.D. This does not mean that Roberts agrees with this characterization of stages. See also Michael Roberts, "U.S. Animal Agriculture: Making the Case for Productivity," *AgBioForum* 3, no. 2/3 (spring/summer 2000): 120-26. Roberts notes that "[c]attle originated around ten to twelve thousand years ago by domestication of the now extinct species *Auroch*. There were several separate domestications of cattle." Roberts cites J. Diamond, *Guns, Germs, and Steel: The Fates of Human Societies* (New York: W. W. Norton, 1997).

All breeding, in the second and third stages, was an effort to alter the genetic structure of the plant or animal in order to obtain a more desirable phenotypic expression. Now, however, the desired traits are being achieved by microscopically manipulating the genetic structure. At one level, this is no different from any other effort at selective breeding. Yet especially the speed at which the change occurs as well as the possibility to implant characteristics from other species, and even other phyla and domains, does have different implications. The quantity of change has become so dramatic that it makes a qualitative difference.

Biotechnologies are different from other technological changes that have appeared over the past 300 years. This is not the equivalent of the invention of the printing press (that might be compared to the availability of computers and the worldwide web). Rather, biotechnologies should be compared to the discovery of fire. It is that dramatic of a shift in knowledge and technology. What makes it different?

- Speed of change.
- An overemphasis on immediate market benefit that will not allow the "invisible hand" to operate (to use capitalistic language of Adam Smith).
  - Nonhuman agriculture is pushed by approximately five large organizations apparently seeking vertical integration or vertical monopolization.
  - Human biotech is pushed by social elite seeking "children" suitable to their standards.
- Absence of or inadequate environmental checks.
- Possible cataclysmic consequences, far beyond the understanding of much of the public.

Genetic modification is proceeding on two related fronts in the United States: the alteration of human genetics for their well-being and the development of nonhuman organisms to serve human ends (and, to a lesser extent, for environmental purposes). Sometimes these overlap, such as when animals are altered in order to create pharmaceuticals or tissues for transplants. The technologies have vast potential for improving human health through nutritional improvement, with medical applications, as well as many other ways. They also create stunning potential for dangers, not only direct biological hazards but also the cultural and moral danger of eliminating boundaries between humans and other species, thus creating a possible threat to the U.S. social contract. "[S]cientists and technologists not only attempt to manipulate beliefs about the *natural* world but also operate on the *social* world and, in particular, manipulate the interests of others."[12] This is what the various sides are doing in the GMO and human biotechnology debates. They are operating in the market and political forums with advertising and, sometimes, coercion. They are using protests and political pressure. They are using religiouslike justifications to win popular support.

The current status of GMO use in the United States and the world is confused, to say the least. In the United States, the vast majority of processed foods contain genetically engineered plant substances. Persons opposing GMOs have concerns about safety, environmental release and farm reorganization, but this opposition is not winning in the market in the United States. They might argue it is because people have been deprived of information. In most of Western Europe, Japan and some places in Africa consumers or governments have limited the adoption of GM foods and/or crops for production. Much of the opposition focuses on food production, with a mixture of anti-American, antitechnology, and antiglobalization rhetoric. Those who assert that traditional methods of agriculture production fit the human ecology and natural ecology and that GMOs simply make small producers more dependent on multinational corporations make a stronger case. Others in the developing world have not responded negatively with some asserting that GMOs represent a second Green Revolution that will feed the masses, empower local communities and prevent environmental destruction caused by pesticides and farm expansion into wilderness.

In the United States the most significant GM crops are various species that are Bt, *Bacillus thuringiensis*, modified and those that are resistant to pesticides (most often called "Round-Up-Ready" after a brand of glyphosate). Bt is a naturally occurring bacterium that produces a toxin that kills various plant pests, including the European corn borer, an invasive species introduced into North America. The Round-Up-Ready products of Monsanto, for instance modified cotton or corn, survive spraying for weeds, thus eliminating plant competitors. Additional GMOs are designed for frost and drought resistance, or to grow in consistent sizes to ease harvest and packaging. Besides these,

[12]John Law, "The Case of the Portuguese Maritime Expansion," *Technology and the West: A Historical Anthology from Technology and Culture*, ed. Terry S. Reynolds and Stephen H. Cutcliffe (Chicago: University of Chicago Press, 1997), p. 122.

researchers are trying to produce "farmaceuticals" through genetic alteration (hogs to produce human insulin being a good example), as well as improving the taste and nutrition of foods (golden rice being the most famous effort). Another goal is making better fibers for clothing.

The response of the public and governments to manufacturers' and researchers' excitement about the possibilities has, not surprisingly, been uncertainty. It has even assumed formal status with the *precautionary principle*, which states that in the absence of clear scientific evidence to the contrary, the status quo should not be changed when the alternative may have dire consequences. Taken to an extreme, this principle is absurd as change cannot be avoided; even the effort to keep the status quo requires change to respond to everything else around continuing to develop or decay. Still, when properly "cautious about caution" the precautionary principle is useful. Some of the consequences that are feared and benefits that might accrue with GMOs include, but are not limited to, the following:

- Environmental hazards:
  - Escaping GMOs becoming invasive species with no predators or controls (kudzu effect)
  - Increased pesticide use with pesticide resistant GMOs
  - "Gene jumping" to related species, which eliminates or severely alters the native species (hybridization/introgression)
  - Increased resistance among pests to an inserted gene, thus encouraging the spread of the unwanted plants (weeds) or animal pests
  - Creation of chimeras as animal cruelty (e.g., creating "obese" chickens and hogs)
- Environmental Benefits:
  - Decreased pesticide use because the GMO can "out-survive" the pests
  - Potential for cleanup of oil spills, toxic waste and so forth thorough GM microorganisms
  - Alternative fuel (less polluting in obtaining and using) through production of high energy GMOs
  - Protection of endangered species genomes
  - Protection from erosion (lower water consumption and so on)

- Human Health Risks:
  - > Farmer
    - Increased pesticide use because of "Ready" GM crops
    - Health risks of GMO with much higher exposure for farmer
  - > Consumer
    - Allergens
    - Creation of new infectious disease
    - Creation of new carcinogenic agent or other long-term risk
    - Technologies developed that can be immorally applied to humans (e.g., bioweapons, eugenics)
- Human Health Benefits:
  - > Farmer
    - Less exposure to pesticides
  - > Consumer
    - Healthier foods
    - Increased availability of food (e.g., in drought areas)
    - Distribution of basic nutrients (e.g., vitamins)
    - Pharmaceuticals from GM plants, animals, bacteria or fungi
    - Tissues for xenografts
    - Technologies developed that can be morally applied against humans (to cure diseases)
- Economic/Social Risks:
  - > For farmer
    - Vertical integration (corporation control from production [e.g., seed and fertilizer] through production of processed products) as excessive centralization of power
    - Loss of family farm though control of planting and purchase
  - > For others
    - Market control over options in consumer market
    - Monopolistic control over costs for consumer
    - Danger of crop monoculture collapse
    - Corporate or state control over species through inappropriate application of patent law

Indigenous people groups

Lose control over production

Theft of indigenously developed genetic material (developed over centuries through village/tribal agricultural breeding programs)

Technologies developed that can be immorally applied against humans

- Economic/Social Benefits:
  - > For farmer:

    Ease of production

    Higher yield

    Higher quality/more consistent raw products
  - > For others

    Easier management of products

    More desirable products to buy

    Protection of human freedom (including freedom to invent and develop products for market)

    Scientific knowledge as a moral good (for society and for prestige of researchers)

    Technologies developed that can be morally applied to humans

Anti-GMO advocates have used three particular events as anecdotal evidence to discourage the spread of the technology. These were the appearance of Starlink corn in products intended for human consumption, the laboratory determination that Bt corn could kill or inhibit the development of monarch butterflies and the appearance of genes from GMOs in Mexican grains grown far from any sanctioned planting. This latter concern was exacerbated by the preliminary determination that the genetic behavior of the modified crops was atypical in that the genes were not located where the corresponding naturally occurring genes would have been. All three have been addressed and have been more or less resolved. It should be noted there was some similarity to the notorious "alar on apples" scare. Even so, that does not eliminate some of the more general concerns that are legitimately raised, especially with the spread of GMO beyond plant zones, etc.

There is no coherent secular argument for not altering, unless it has to do with risk. The intrinsic worth of nature is unverifiable, but the instrumental worth can be approximated on the basis of possible benefits and possible costs for all concerned. Costs can be economic, aesthetic, physical health and so on. The calculation of risk should include not only the probability of an event (positive or negative) occurring but also the severity of the consequences should it occur. This, in turn, must be compared to other alternative options, including doing nothing, even as a range of uncertainty remains. And, of course, someone must be responsible for the risk.

Accountability or culpability is the responsibility for consequences. The accountability is rarely entirely any single person's, but is usually spread, and the more it is spread the more likely no one will be held accountable. It can be described with an equation:

$$A = B + E + (I + P)$$

A = accountability (= culpability)
B = benefit accrued to agent (directly and/or indirectly)
E = level of expertise by agent (what is known or what should be known)
I = influence in act (usually a function of "earliness" in process)
P = power to act (e.g., formal, bureaucratic)

Ongoing risk assessments and periodic pauses in research or rigorous continuous discussion about the biological and cultural implications are necessary. Matters like identity preservation, ownership of intellectual property, indigenous peoples' ownership of traditionally bred varieties, as well as potential environmental and health risks, require consideration along with consideration of potential dangers and benefits. Perhaps, as suggested above, periodic sabbaths, when a pause is taken, would be warranted. Regardless, those in the scientific community, corporations that sell GMOs and the government should have the highest culpability and must be held economically and personally responsible.

Similarly, some human biotechnologies make sense while others do not, given the risks and/or given the fundamental values that are violated. For instance, specialized or personalized designer drugs that match an individual's genomic make-up would be quite useful, if finally cost effective. But actually changing the human being is different. Unlike nonhuman animal and plant alterations, changing the human genome is both more permissible and less permissible: more permissible if the benefit is to correct significant diseases; less permissible, even warranting prohibition, if used to improve normality. Add to the list of those especially culpable any who would use human technologies for their own offspring.

The responsibility seems highest in the special case of human genetic alteration. The mapping of the human genome has occurred not only for the sake of scientific knowledge, but also in the hope of developing technologies. The funding of expensive computerized laboratory equipment and extraordinary expertise means there is general social acceptance, even if not clear understanding. A historical parallel is King John II of Portugal calling for a scientific commission for the purpose of converting esoteric scientific knowledge into a set of widely applicable practices to develop maps for the purpose of navigation, trade and ultimately colonization.[13] Those maps are not entirely unlike the Human Genome Project that produced a map for human biotech.

The effort, now successful under the separate leadership of Francis Collins and Craig Venter, has been to obtain information. The map allows the determination of not only presence but location of various parts of the genome. The efforts have made the technology as simple as possible. Some participating labs hoped to maintain control over the information gathered so as to prevent abuse and/or make profit over medical applications developed on the basis of the information, primarily through the use of patent and copyright law. However, as if by the proverbial technological imperative, the momentum seems all but uncontrollable. Rules appear unlikely to stop the dissemination of the information and development of technologies. Indeed, while Collins has promoted continued cautious development, Venter has strongly asserted the need to proceed as fast as possible.

Social acceptance remains the main barrier to the next step, especially as the instrumentation grows simpler, and the technology spreads through the academic and entrepreneurial sectors. Indeed, the question is now less whether the instrumentation can be developed, but whether it should be used, just as the technical possibilities for the ships of Portugal became less of a concern than the colonialization by the Iberian nations and the rest of Europe of other areas of the globe.

The effort to legitimate human genetic alteration, for therapeutic and even for enhancement purposes, is in no way more evident than with the appointment of bioethicists to the boards of companies aggressively promoting genetic alteration. The society cannot trust organizations to monitor themselves with human or nonhuman biotechnology, and so they hire "experts" who gain their position not by their morality but by their philosophical expertise that can provide an imprimatur. There is no reason to think such sanctions will

---

[13]Ibid., p. 134.

protect society. Simple rules and elaborate rationalizations will not be sufficient against concentration of expertise and money. Criminal punishment as an option will be required if significant restrictions are to be maintained.

Legitimate concerns about human genetic technologies include

- careless genetic research techniques that
  - lose control over a dangerous genetic alteration (for instance, a created genetic disease)
  - use humans as mere objects, rather than subjects; possible examples include
    - embryos for embryonic stem cell research
    - humans as objects of research
      - voluntary (e.g., paid volunteers, those concerned with others' suffering)
      - avoluntary (e.g., the unconscious, those whose tissue is taken and used without their permission)
      - involuntary (e.g., coerced students, persons in dire financial circumstances)
- conflicts of interest in conducting research
- intellectual property status
  - patenting human genomic patterns that restrict reasonable development
  - patenting a person's genetic material without his or her permission or benefit (including that of persons from marginalized groups)
- alteration of human heritable, rather than somatic, genetics (in particular for "enhancement")

Several of these concerns intersected recently, most notoriously in the Gelsinger case at the University of Pennsylvania, though others have also occurred. But it is the last concern that is the most significant. The people who stand to gain the most economically or with prestige are not the best to determine whether or not humans should be altered to meet the researchers' or corporation owners' or government leaders' standards of what is good. The seeming financial entanglement in the Gelsinger case is an indicator of what will certainly arise as technologies for positive eugenics develop. Another indicator is the financial gain sought by some in vitro fertilization facilities that readily acknowledge the use of preimplantation genetic diagnosis (PGD) for sex selection. It is not that financial benefit should not accrue to those with high levels of skills and ownership of limited resources and not that society should not benefit in some way, but that such should not occur at excessive cost to either the ones seeking the therapy or those upon whom experiments are conducted or to society or the natural world rather than the ones who would profit.

It is obvious that therapeutic correction of genetic disorders is a legitimate alternation of nature. It should be equally obvious that alteration of human beings to conform to the ideals of academicians or rich entrepreneurs or government bureaucrats is morally repugnant. The former clearly benefits some and harms none. The latter clearly puts at risk all with clear benefits only for a few.

The boundary cases indicate how problematic human genetic alteration could be. Say that homosexuality does have a genetic precursor, not for the behavior but a risk factor for the behavior. Would parents have a right to alter their child's genetics? Or, conversely, would a homosexual couple who had adopted a child have the right to alter a child to be more likely to have homosexual interests? Homosexuality is, in all likelihood, partially genetic, perhaps congenital, and certainly a conditioning caused behavior. It is also a matter of choice. Christians assert the activity is immoral, even though the tendency itself is not. It is conceivable that in some states in the U.S. Christians would be allowed to alter their children and in others they would be deemed bigots and abusers. The political complexity of deciding who would get to decide what is apparent.

In the case of human alteration, a range of the moral legitimacy of genetic engineering can be drawn. At one end is that which should be encouraged; at the other, that which should be clearly prohibited. Positive eugenics, the alteration of geneline for enhancement should be prohibited. Efforts to alter the individual's genetics for appearance, sport skills, gender and so on should be strongly discouraged even if the altered trait will not be passed on. Some biotechnology to improve quality of life, like increasing longevity, should be allowed and perhaps encouraged. The eliminating of genetically based diseases should be actively sought.

Researchers, scientific organizations and profit-seeking corporations should have a say and should be respected for the significant knowledge they can provide for ethical analysis. However, the society must depend on its social contract and maintain that as the basis for legitimating biotechnology research, not turn to biotechnology as the basis for building society, as if such would not be laden with the errors of hubris, greed and bigotry.

CONCLUSION

Altering nature is a fundamental characteristic of the human animal. Arguably all animals, and, for that matter, all life forms change their environments as they work their way into niches and attempt to expand them. Humans certainly have a large ecological niche and are more able than other animals to alter their environment. There is no continent or region on a continent that humans have not occupied. So, two things can be definitively stated about humans: (1) they will change their environments and (2) they will do so without proper consideration of all the implications. The moral imperative, in this case, must constrain the technological and biological imperatives because GM technology is fundamentally different from most that have gone before, in the potential to alter the ecology and in the potential to change the human species for the worse.

The Lord allows husbandry of the vineyards. Analogically, this may be understood as permission to alter and control nature, but to do so only within limits—limits of what is genuinely good. Altering nature is acceptable to Christians, but only within the constraints of reasonable environmental evaluations. Altering human nature is not acceptable, but genetic change for disease control is.

While evangelicals historically have been willing to promote "progress" through social change and technological development, and today may have a deep desire to end suffering with genetically based cures and increased agricultural and pharmaceutical biotechnologies, they should promote reasonable caution. The potential dangers call for some restraint, especially of those seeking money, prestige, or some kind of personal glory without due consideration of possible consequences. The irresponsibility of a few could have devastating effects.

16

Gift-giving and Receiving

HUMANS AS DONORS

Human communities are shaped by gift-giving relationships. Organs, blood, tissues, gametes and participation in research, for instance, are often given for the well-being of others. Their use after being given, however, is often determined by the market on the basis of supply/demand. Christian giving should be governed by the standard established by Christ. The society, though, may abandon gift-giving for human biologicals in favor of either compelled donations of some kind or a more open market process.

> And he took bread, gave thanks and broke it, and gave it to them, saying, "This is my body given for you; do this in remembrance of me."
>
> In the same way, after the supper he took the cup, saying, "This cup is the new covenant in my blood, which is poured out for you. (Lk 22:19-20)

PART ONE: THE TEXT

Gifts are never given without expectation—expectation about how the gift is understood and how the recipient will respond. While the gift, at least if it is truly a gift, does not require a specific response of economic value (quid pro quo), the giver usually at least hopes for appreciation. The relationships that helped define the giver and the recipient before the gift are shifted, reordered. So it was with Jesus' life. He gave with expectations, hoping for a particular type of response. This gift of his life upon the cross is central to the Text. Indeed, the gift on the cross is the narrative peak of the gospel story. Even a first time reader, unguided by the community and unaware of the narrative's conclusion, would understand the crucifixion event as the crisis that defines the story—would recognize a self-offering, freely chosen giving for the well-being of others. The believer understands this as the point toward which Jesus' life was directed. The Christian account relies on the idea of the incarnate God (God in physical form, coincidentally and fully human and divine) dying as a gift. All other parts of the story—from the nativity through the teachings and healings through the resurrection to apocalyptic return—depend on this self-offering.

The idea of the divine gift is so essential that it is summarized in doctrinal creeds that are actually synopses of the story, and it is central to the ritual of the church. Weekly, at many fellowships of believers, the sacrament of communion is offered. In congregations that do not participate weekly in the rite, there is almost inevitably a verbal affirmation of the gift given by Jesus.

When a gift is given, the recipient can respond in several ways, each of which can communicate different messages:

- Accept the gift and respond with a gift of greater worth
  > indicates a desire for an escalation, wanting greater largesse in the future, almost functions as a bribe

  > demonstrates that the return giver is wealthier or has more prestige

  > indicates that the initial gift is part of a greater intangible gift that the recipient has received from the first giver (e.g., status associated with being the initial recipient, other kindnesses)
- Accept the gift and respond with a "balanced" gift (equal or equivalent)
  > establishes or verifies peership and trust
- Take the initial gift callously with no regard for the giver or appreciation
  > sees it not as a gift but as if a rightful possession, done by one who does not value the relationship, either because it is not needed or wanted

  > creates power imbalance with recipient claiming higher status

  > creates resentment in giver

  > arises out of misunderstanding of the significance of the giving/gift (especially common in crosscultural gift exchanges)
- Accept the gift with a gratitude offering of something of lesser worth returned
  > done out of civility [shallow or genuine] ; a thank you, for instance

  > done in recognition that the initial gift cannot be properly reciprocated,
- Reject the gift
  > done almost always to reject the relationship, at least the form of relationship implied by the offering

Obviously, these are not absolute distinctions. If, say, a graduation present of money is received and the recipient casually, almost flippantly, says thanks, then that may be a mixture of accepting the gift with feeble gratitude because the graduate does not know better and a character failure marked by callously taking.

The gift of Christ calls for a response and only one of these types is appropriate—accepting with a gift of lesser value in return. The first type of response is impossible as, obviously, no one can give a gift of greater worth to the Christ. No one has anything of infinite worth to give. The gift of Christ is such that an equivalent corresponding gift is utterly beyond possibility. An attempt to match the gift would only indicate a misunderstanding of what has been offered or would be presumptuous. The potential recipient would indicate, in trying to equate a finite response to the infinite gift of God's sacrifice, both a lack of recognition of what has been given *and* a lack of recognition of who is in what role in the relationship. Likewise, accepting the gift of Christ as if it is owed to the recipient, as with most versions of universalism, is a trivialization of the gift.

There are only two possible coherent responses to Christ's offering: to humbly accept it with gratitude or reject it and despise it. Rejecting God or disregarding God are not insults delivered to a petty tyrant, but rejection of kindness from a Rescuer extending a hand to a drowning woman or reaching into a burning building to pull out a man with lungs full of smoke or, more precisely, a kind adult offering parental love to an orphan made belligerent by the mistreatment of others and foolish mistakes of his or her own.

The giving of Jesus was not of a contractual nature, but covenantal. It asked and continues to ask for more than an economically or functionally defined equivalent in return. The only proper expressions of gratitude, given the line of the Christian narrative, are thanksgiving to God and gift-giving to others, continuing on in a life-long pattern. Both are necessary. The former is a responding gift of gratitude. The latter is an acknowledgment of the change wrought by the divine gift. Jesus chose to assume the posture of weakness and shame. He was not compelled to do so by his own sin but elected to for ours and calls us to help others in the midst of their weaknesses with the giving of our resources, our skills and ourselves. Recipients of the gift owe him gratitude and that gratitude to his unparalleled gift-giving shapes all other responses of gift giving. This thankful gift-giving in response to Christ's gift is what transforms a mere good-enough work into something truly good (for, in reality, no truly *good* work precedes the relationship of redemption). The giving of Christ binds the willing recipient of his gift, obligates him or her to Christ first, but then to other recipients of the gift, and finally to all those who might receive that gift—that is, all of humanity and even the nonhuman natural world (Rom 8:15-25). The extent of this obligation is as wide and deep as a person's life. It encompasses all relationships.

Though to the world the Christian gift-giving response may look like charity in the crass, popular sense, from the believer's perspective this is a matter of sharing, true charity.[1] The strengths that the Holy Spirit has provided, often using the weaknesses of the recipient, are the means by which one gives. The world's charity is far preferable to hoarding, but it is not divine love expressed. It too often demands excessive grandiosity tinged with degradation of the recipient, where for the mature believer *agape* is the response of gratitude, a necessary Christian virtue. So, for instance, the one who was a thief before his or her coming to Christ—and who might even still be illicitly using those previously developed skills—is told to work, to do "something useful with his own hands, that he may have something to share with those in need" (Eph 4:28). Not only, then, is there an obligation not to *do* the bad, but to *be* good, not only to not steal (nonmaleficence), but to be a giver (beneficent).[2] For the sake of the believer's soul as well as those served, there is a need to grow in sharing. For that reason, Paul commands the wealthy to not be arrogant or to put hope in any possession, but "to do good, to be rich in good deeds, and to be generous and willing to share. In this way they will lay up treasure for themselves as a firm foundation for the coming age, so that they may take hold of the life that is truly life" (1 Tim 6:18-19). Giving as Christ gave helps the recipient and the giver; it is a means of grace for both.

It is important to note that, like offerings to the baals, some giving can be illegitimate. The goodness or rightness of an act is not defined only by the personal cost. Gift-giving and sacrifice are not intrinsically good; rather, their goodness depends on the object of the giving both in the literal sense of who receives the gift and in the sense of the attitude or intention of the giver.

---

[1]Love is not a zero-sum calculation. More love is created in the individual who loves God first. Thanks to Mt. Zion (Mercer County, Kentucky) Bible Study for the conversation on this.

[2]These terms are used to allow comparison with bioethical principlism—but there is a significant difference for believers in that nonmaleficence is primarily deontological (something to do or not to do), but beneficence is primarily virtuosity (a way to be).

When sacrificial gift-giving is appropriate, it simply must be done—it is not spiritual heroism (an act of supererogation). The believer, quite simply, is to give whenever she or he can and whenever such giving will be truly beneficial. Sometimes such giving may be sacrificial, but it is not thereby heroic. For Christians it is not a question of whether or not sharing is expected, but whether or not there is any limit at all on that sharing. Jesus, the God come to Earth, after all gave up divine attributes in order to become our Servant and expects believers to assume his attitude of giving.[3]

Five assertions can be made about Christian love and giving.

First, the indiscriminant giving of oneself is not loving, for love is always particularized. Love that will not be shown can hardly be considered love, unless the concept is limited to shallow affection, only recognized internally and, then, only as a feeling. Rather (and this can serve as a working definition), *Christian love* is the affections properly directed and the will practically expressed.[4] As John noted of Christ, and then extended to the believers:

> This is love: not that we loved God, but that he loved us and sent his Son as an atoning sacrifice for our sins. Dear friends, since God so loved us, we also ought to love one another. (1 Jn 4:10-11)
>
> This is love for God: to obey his commands. And his commands are not burdensome, for everyone born of God overcomes the world. (1 Jn 5:3-4)
>
> And this is love: that we walk in obedience to his commands. As you have heard from the beginning, his command is that you walk in love. (2 Jn 1:6)

Second, the discrimination of love means that giving differs according to the nature of the relationship between giver and recipient. For instance, the role of parent calls for a higher level of giving to his or her child than does the role of casual acquaintance to that same child. Perhaps more revealing, the obligation of the parent for giving to the child is higher than for the child giving to the parent, though time may change the extent and content of giving as the capacity of the child as a giver expands.

Third, love is not a blind passion but a practical expression of true affection. Love is properly guided by prudence or wisdom. The obligations of love,

---

[3]See Philippians 2, especially the section called the Carmen Christi (Phil 2:5-11), the hymn to the incarnate Christ. The claim of Paul in taking up and quoting (or in writing) this early hymn is that Jesus is God but takes up the nature or "form" (in a philosophical sense) of a servant. An argument could be made that the giving of Christ was supererogatory or that it could be claimed such was the fulfillment of his nature.

[4]Based on Augustine and John Wesley.

the giving of the giver, vary according to love's object. The cost and expression of love may not be the same for every act; in other words, love calls for proportion and pertinence. To use a ridiculous example, it would not be proportionate to give one's life in order to prevent a friend from getting a parking ticket, but it might be to save him or her from being hit by a car. Considerations of pertinence come into play in that love includes not only the impact on the individual to whom the gift is given, but the broader communities to which giver and recipient belong.

The wisdom of love means the risk of gift-giving must be minimized relative to the relationship's value and the worth of the giving. This is a sort of utilitarian or, more properly, prudential reasoning. It is a balancing of risk and benefit, of pain and pleasure. While utilitarianism is not acceptable as the dominant form of moral reasoning for a Christian, it can function at a secondary level. Christians are not compelled to give when the gift itself would be counter-productive or not of benefit to the recipient. As the sacrament can be taken inappropriately and become a judgment on the recipient, so other gifts can harm if the receiver is unable or unwilling to properly receive (1 Cor 11; Mt 7:6). Also, the believer is not to give, except under the most extraordinary of circumstances, to the point of his or her own destruction. What is not acceptable is a calculation of the risk that includes a self-evaluation that others are intrinsically more valuable to God or that one is of more value to God than others. The virtue of gift-giving is marked by what the world would consider extravagance, but prudent extravagance.

Fourth, Christian love transforms the individual who genuinely gives gifts. So, for example, the recipient of an act of true charity (as *caritas/agape*) like food or rent money is helped, but the giver is helped even more. Such giving is a means of grace—that is, a way the Holy Spirit acts in the individual; as she or he loves others the love of God opens the capacity of that person to love more greatly, finding more room in the expanding heart. This is why charity, in the common sense in late modernity, is sometimes not *caritas*. The individual who gives self-righteously or condescendingly in order to secure his or her social status actually is hurting his or her soul. Having said this, it is still preferable to ignoring the suffering altogether.

Fifth, love may be initiated, but always incompletely expressed, in justice. Justice should be indiscriminant—hence, the procedural justice of the U.S. social contract is supposed to be blind. Also, those who are not loving can express justice, but those who are loving should never be unjust. The Christian who seeks justice in the state is only partially and insufficiently expressing his or her love. Justice is never the sum or total of love. For the believer, the impartiality of justice must always be founded and followed by the partiality of love.

Giving is central to the story of salvation and to the lives of those who accept their place in that story. Jesus asks his followers to go beyond rules of justice, even good rules, to the virtuosity of love—*agape* (Greek) or *caritas* (Latin)—not love or charity in the modern, almost trivial senses, but giving of the self as an expression of the self.

PART TWO: CHRISTIAN BIOETHICS

Jesus Christ literally gave his body and blood. Further, he said in reference to his offering:

> My command is this: Love each other as I have loved you. Greater love has no one than this, that he lay down his life for his friends. You are my friends if you do what I command. I no longer call you servants, because a servant does not know his master's business. Instead, I have called you friends, for everything that I learned from my Father I have made known to you. (Jn 15:12-15).

The analogue is a powerful one for believers. His gift was a gift of life to the believer, given at the cost of his dying. Are Christians, then, compelled to give in a similar manner? Yes, but the analogy is faulty if interpreted to mean Christians give their physical bodies rather than giving themselves fully in love to God and, then subsequently, to others. Jesus' gift of physical life is astounding, but even more so that the Eternal sacrificed while incarnate. Similarly, the sought response is that each individual give himself or herself as a potentially eternal offering to the Christ. Such is always inadequate, except that Christ himself deems it a sufficient expression of gratitude.

The exchange of Jesus' life was not a direct one-to-one correspondence with the saving of a specific individual, though it was for specific individuals. Evangelicals debate the form of this specificity. Some argue that atonement was limited to those who accept Christ. Those favoring universal atonement assert the particular offer was for each person, that Jesus comes to all so that each individual, in particularity, can see him and accept or reject him. Either way, the gift is efficacious only for those who receive it. To use language currently popular with some, it makes the cross all the more scandalous that the universal God would have particular concern. Paul puts it this way:

> For Christ's love compels us, because we are convinced that one died for all, and therefore all died. And he died for all, that those who live should no longer live for themselves but for him who died for them and was raised again. (2 Cor 5:14-15)

The oft-stated evangelical claim—"if you were the only sinful person who had ever lived, Christ would still have died for you"—is accurate. He would have, but he did not. Such words are meant to encourage one to recognize the worth God puts upon each person's well-being. According to evangelicals, Christ did not die for only one person.

His was a particular offer of universal love. The person who accepts the gift of Christ's offering of himself does so in his or her particularity. This, then, leads that saved individual as the particular person she or he is, to offer Christ's eternal love to others in particular ways. The Lord's is discriminating, but it is not a limited resource—it discriminates in that it is given to individuals, but is not limited by time or space as is human giving with such things as money, assistance, hospitality—or organs, blood and tissue.

Organ and blood and tissue donation and research participation are near sacramental. For Christians they are, when honestly given, eternal declarations in a temporal form, eternal truth in temporal actions. As the communion bread is a bounded, temporal object yet alters one's life here and now and for the life to come, so body parts for transplant or research participation can radically alter the recipient's and the giver's lives for years and decades into the future.

Because the gift of the believer is always less than the gift of the Savior, it is never actually a sacrament. Still, it approaches the same significance as the believer lives more and more in accordance with the very image of Jesus. The giving act, as with the sacraments as gifts from God, becomes a means of grace for the persons who truly seek to follow Christ. Paul puts it this way:

> Who has ever given to God,
> that God should repay him?
> For from him and through him and to him are all things.
> To him be the glory forever! Amen.

> Therefore, I urge you, brothers, in view of God's mercy, to offer your bodies as living sacrifices, holy and pleasing to God—this is your spiritual act of worship. Do not conform any longer to the pattern of this world, but be transformed by the renewing of your mind. Then you will be able to test and approve what God's will is—his good, pleasing and perfect will. (Rom 11:35–12:2)

Yet if the standard of giving is the Sacrament, is not complete sacrifice required? After all, Jesus said, "Greater love has no one than this, that he lay down his life for his friends" (Jn 15:13). The answer is, sometimes. Sometimes Jesus hid and sometimes he was willing to face abuse and scorn, even unto the point of death. Likewise, sometimes Christians are called to martyrdom, and sometimes they should live a mundane, but holy life. The giving of bodily substances does not rise to the level of required martyrdom. Christians should risk their lives for the faith or for another person who is facing great danger only if there is a reasonable chance of success and only if it is the last resort (before death or desecration). Live donation that results in the inevitable or highly probable death of the donor does not satisfy the criteria, but some significant risk may well be acceptable—especially if there are other reasons for the gift (like friendship or family relationship).

While the Eucharist should be frequent, it should not be taken so often as to allow the ritual to impede one's continued functioning in the world of the worldly.[5] In a similar sense, the giving of tissues and blood must be limited by the extent the giving would impede other moral obligations. The sacrifice demanded is not of one's biological life, but of something greater—of one's entire being. That may or may not require the giving of the physical body. That may or may not mean the giving of organs or tissues or marrow or blood. Other obligations and relationships may take priority as sacrificial demands are placed upon the believer. In the Romans passage, in fact, the sacrifice of the believer is a sacrifice of living.

Paul grappled with this matter in asking for financial support for the poor Christians in Jerusalem. One is to give, but not to the point of self-destruction. Gift-giving is necessary, but imitating Christ in giving does not require killing oneself for research or for the donation of organs. It is too likely that such could occur out of false guilt or a desire to glorify oneself. If a deadly offering of the self, then the act of donation may well be immoral. Accepting martyrdom glorifies God through the offering of oneself as a gift; seeking out martyrdom is a presumptuous messianic claim. Paul wrote, in 2 Corinthians:

> And now, brothers, we want you to know about the grace that God has given

[5]Evangelicals do not accept the doctrine of transubstantiation. Some evangelical groups do erroneously assert that baptism is salvific, but this would be a similar error. It is an important but not fundamental mistake. The sacraments themselves are means of grace, not the grace itself—for that is the expression of the Holy Spirit.

> the Macedonian churches. Out of the most severe trial, their overflowing joy and their extreme poverty welled up in rich generosity. For I testify that they gave as much as they were able, and even beyond their ability. . . .
>
> For if the willingness is there, the gift is acceptable according to what one has, not according to what he does not have.
>
> Our desire is not that others might be relieved while you are hard pressed, but that there might be equality. At the present time your plenty will supply what they need, so that in turn their plenty will supply what you need. Then there will be equality, as it is written: "He who gathered much did not have too much, and he who gathered little did not have too little." (2 Cor 8:1-3, 12-15)

Christians considering live donation of organs must look at the nature of the gift-giving as it impacts the recipient, the giver and broader communities. Required are prudential decisions about survival and efficacy, as well as about the roles that bind the individuals together. A Christian is not compelled to give his or her liver or heart when such a gift would inevitably or almost certainly kill the giver. The believer's life is a good gift from God that should not be alienated or lost intentionally, though it may be put at risk for another. The demand of gift-giving to others does not require the cost of intentionally defying the gift of biological life from God.

Arguments about the prudence of dangerous live donation or research bear similarity to just coercion theory. Organ donation, research participation, blood donation and even gamete donation can be examined using these criteria.

- The cause is just (saving the life of the potential recipient would qualify, as would gaining significant biomedical knowledge or providing essential training; having genetically related offspring would not).
- The intention is right (the reason must be to save another for the other's own sake and not to achieve some other immoral end such as prestige or money; Christians may have to accept that those of the world could have different intentions, so that donating blood or even solid organs for money might be acceptable if the distribution of the blood and especially the organs remains tied to the ability to pay for surgeries).
- The persons deciding have legitimate authority (if the donor is the one deciding to donate, then the authority is proper; Christians cannot accept the compelling of donation, a self-contradictory concept).
- There is a reasonable chance of success (it is necessary to be cautious with parents who have one healthy child and another needing a transplant and

may be willing to "try anything"; the probability of succeeding must be high given the grave risk being assumed in live donation [some assert that no organ and tissue live donation should occur, except perhaps for kidneys, since the efficacy of the procedures is debatable, especially in light of the costs; but "reasonable" does not mean 50 percent +1]; the same demand for a reasonable chance of success is true for research but in this case, success would be gaining genuinely useful information);

- The last resort (all reasonable interventions have been attempted or carefully considered, including xenographs and artificial or genetically modified materials when appropriate; in the case of resarch, this would mean proper prior computer and animal testing).
- The action is proportional (the saved life and the donor's life will not be of such a diminished condition that the donation is excessive for the benefit gained; the likely length and quality of the recipient's life can be taken into account, though secondarily; in the case of research, life-threatening studies should not be, for instance, for baldness or ED correction).
- There is discrimination (in just coercion theory, this refers to the required effort to avoid hurting noncombatants; it could well be argued that the "war" with disease should not be extended into another battlefield—that is, the body of the potential donor or research participant—except when great benefit is likely and significant cost to the donor or participant is unlikely).

The use of these criteria helps the believer recognize some of the strict limits that should be placed on the donation of human substances. In particular, Christians should be extremely wary of the harvesting of organs or the soliciting of research participation from the rejected and vulnerable of society. Selecting the socially vulnerable is so instrumental as to be, to use Kantian language, treating the person as a means only. Though some dangerous donations may be morally permissible, extra protections are necessary.

At least eight categories warranting special protection are (1) prisoners, (2) the mentally ill, (3) the developmentally disabled, (4) children, (5) the preborn (arguably a subset of "children"), (6) the desperately poor, (7) victims of crime and (8) those sick with unrelated disorders but desperate for additional care.

1. Prisoners as donors present several specific moral problems for evangelicals. Obviously, most of the difficulty arises because of the all but inevitable coercion. This is the primary concern, legitimate or not, with prisoner

donation in the People's Republic of China.[6] But, even in the United States there are significant moral risks with condemned prisoner organ donation or participation in clinical or basic research. First, if a hospital is considered a "total institution" in which vulnerable people can be controlled, there is no doubt that a prison is even more so.[7] Liberty in choosing or choosing not to donate is less likely. Second, the harvesting of solid organs from the cadavers of prisoners who have been executed or allowed to die seems to endorse the legitimacy of capital punishment. While there is significant disagreement about capital punishment among believers, the reckless application of the penalty is certainly morally reprehensible. Third, if the yield of cadaver organs is intended or at least planned, then there may be a tendency to actually seek or prioritize executions in order to obtain specifically needed organs. Fourth, if organ donation provides either a financial payment to surviving relatives or reduction of sentence for a live donation as incentive, then persons with suitable genetics or general health status would be treated more favorably than others and the punishment would no longer be determined by procedural justice. Fifth, believers are directly commanded to minister to prisoners; allowing them to be used as sources for organs or research would seem to raise questions about the real attitude of officials toward those believers are supposed to serve.

2 and 3. The mentally ill and developmentally disabled are categories of persons who are vulnerable because of their unrelated health condition. As such they deserve special protection. The primary "gift" that may actually be stolen from such is the gift of being a research subject—a gift they might not want or should not be asked to give. In the famous Willowbrook incident, now decades past, when severely disabled children were purposely infected with hepatitis, it was justified by the fact that they would receive better care than others in the institution and that infection in the general population was highly likely anyway. This was a situation in which the real needs of the children were used against them. The gross failure of the state

---

[6]See Michael E. Parmly, "Sale of Human Organs in China," Hearing Before the Subcommittee on International Operations and Human Rights, House International Relations," Washington, D.C., June 27, 2001 <http://www.state.gov/g/drl/rls/rm/2001/3792.htm>; Joshua Pantesco, "China Court Official Insists Organ Donation By Executed Prisoners Strictly Regulated," *Jurist,* Wednesday, March 14, 2007 <http://jurist.law.pitt.edu/paperchase/2007/03/china-court-official-insists-organ.php>; Human Rights Watch, "China: Organ Procurement and Judicial Execution In China," *Human Rights Watch Report* 6, no. 9 (1994) <http://www.hrw.org/reports/1994/china1/china_948.htm>.

[7]The term is borrowed from Erving Goffman.

health-care system was supposedly mitigated by a slightly less egregious failure of the state health-care system in providing research subjects with better care. Perhaps the state of medical knowledge about hepatitis was simply inadequate there and across the nation. Perhaps, too, the providers failed to protect the children (and asking parents in this situation was not sufficient), or they were so desperate because of administrative and state government failures that they chose an extreme solution. Even more extreme circumstances arise when such individuals are deemed unworthy of life or living a life of such low quality to have ceased to be persons and, therefore, can be used to obtain biological products or for research. It could quite clearly be argued that Christians should act as advocates for those with serious mental illness and developmental disabilities. The first place to begin would be to support those whose families are already affected so that all but truly necessary institutionalizations can be avoided. Perhaps believers could also, when possible, bring people into their homes. Or, when persons can live independently, they could help so that the individual might remain in a least-restrictive environment.

4. Parents are supposed to be guardians of their children's well-being. It is appropriate to leave questions of cadaver donation from children entirely up to the parents. Live donations and participation in research are different. This situation gets complicated when parents ask one sibling to donate to another, or make the decision for a child since she or he is a legal incompetent. This may be acceptable but should be reviewed by others who are disinterested in the specific parties. The state has a duty to protect all contract members. When the persons who are supposed to be acting to maximize the opportunity for the child to fulfill his or her *telos* under subsidiarity rules fail to do so, then the state should. This is also true if children are used in research. The difficulty in excluding all children from, say, pharmaceutical research is that children react differently to drugs than adults. Some research with children is necessary for the sake of all children, but the selection process should not be biased toward those vulnerable for reasons unrelated to the actual drug or procedure being considered. Generally, though parents are quite trustworthy and should maintain control over their children's well-being, their lowered ability to properly decide in complicated research and donation situations should elicit greater protections.

5. The preborn are especially susceptible to being taken advantage of for organ and tissue donation, use in dangerous research and use in the actual

production of pharmaceuticals. Usually those so used are morally dismissed as mistakes of nature, errors in judgment or leftovers (of ART). It should be repugnant to Christians that the weakest are defined as usable for research or even donation because they are first defined as refuse. Even worse, some advocate the creating of human entities for purely instrumental reasons and with no possibility of that human entity ever growing; such is completely contrary to the gospel understanding of human creation in the image of God.

Fetal tissue obtained following stillbirth is certainly acceptable for donation or research. Donation for research or therapeutics from abortions or "leftovers" from assisted reproduction efforts are, however, quite problematic. The use tends to diminish the moral significance of the preborn. It also is contrary to the American notion of the social contract. Certainly the murder of an adult for an organ is utterly repugnant, but the killing of large numbers of adults in the West for such a purpose does not seem probable. The killing of preborns for research and for biomedical products does, and is already being done. This is (1) a violation of deontological standards against the killing of innocents and (2) a slippery slope toward the mass devaluation of humans as individuals. Perhaps if specific donation decisions are completely distinct from the decision to participate in the antecedent event (the abortion or making of extra embryos), then the donation may be acceptable as a "tragic" gift. This was basically the argument with the initial Bush stem cell action. The potential good of the donation or research cannot justify the act that precedes the donation, though may make the donation hesitatingly acceptable after the fact. On the other hand, believers could equally argue that such should not occur given the risk that it would initiate (or endorse) the taking of tissue and proto-organs on a purely utilitarian basis.

6. The desperately poor should be protected from being forced to donate organs and tissues or themselves for research. Blood donations, including for money, by the poor are casually accepted, and since there is a minimal risk, may be tolerated. Organs are different; though it does not seem to be a problem in the United States, no one is free to enter a market out of desperation or to the extent that one's own body is alienated or taken away. This is similar to what Wesley, Wilberforce and Finney all argued about slavery—no one could legitimately sell oneself into oppression. Believers must oppose, and the state must prevent, such and should work to correct the social problems that seem to compel live donation sales. What may be hesitatingly acceptable, given the

current imbalance in who profits from organ transplants, would be reasonable compensation for cadaver donation. (This, however, would require significant protection of the vulnerable.)

7. Use of organs from murder victims is problematic, though to a lesser degree than using prisoners or the preborn in that there is no direct connection, presumably, between those harvesting the organs and those who did the killing. Should there be any tie to the recipient, the clear implication would be that the killing may have been performed in anticipation of the donation. That is unlikely or genuinely uncommon. Murder victims who have been cleared by the coroner and who have no connection to the harvester or recipient could be legitimate donors. While there is something sorrowful about such use, it can be redemptive.

8. Those sick with unrelated disorders but desperate for additional care may want access to special treatments or approval from providers and will, out of their vulnerability, offer up their bodies for research. The problems faced by such people may warrant their doing what they need to obtain those services. The lack of access is the fundamental problem and those who take advantage of desperate persons are acting in an immoral way. When the society allows such, it comes close to the same reasoning that would allow the sale of live organs by the poor.

Cadaver donations generally present no direct problem for evangelicals. The physical body devoid of life should be treated respectfully, but not any longer as a sacred temple—rather, more as a decommissioned church building. To not use it would be imprudent. Some other Christian communities and those in some other religions oppose organ donation. In defense of, though not in agreement with, those groups, evangelicals should oppose mandatory donations or any deprivation of familial control. Likewise, the remaining portions of the physical body should be returned following donation harvesting or dissection. The next-of-kin should retain quasi-ownership of the body, relinquishing control of the deceased's remains to the organ procurement agency only temporarily and conditionally. Also, the recipients or the organ procurement organizations should assume responsibility for any additional hospitalization costs while awaiting harvesting, including the time between brain death declarations (or the decision to *not* terminate life-support in order to maintain the organs) and official designation as a viable donor. Evangelical Christians should strongly endorse cadaver donation, albeit with conditions, among themselves; but they should not demand it of others in the society who may consider it as an unwarranted intrusion.

Cadaveric donations may become morally problematic if the line that defines death is shifted inappropriately or the legal defining of *person* is altered to facilitate organ procurement. A major concern with cadaver donation is the recent assertion that the standard for determining death should be shifted back to heart function. Brain-death definitions were substituted for cardiac function to no small extent to facilitate organ donation. The potential donor could be kept infused even after legal and biological death, and the procurement team did not have to rush to the point of risking mistakes and thereby the quality of the organs. The definition also was used to end treatment for persons who lived exclusively because they were mechanically supported. Now, the demand for the limited resource—solid organs—seems to be encouraging a return to the cardiac definition (usually called Donation after Cardiac Death [DCD] or Non-Heart Beating Donation [NHBD]) because it is believed more solid organs will become available. In doing so, persons who are not dead by any historical definition, albeit close, might be harvested. When life is likely present, one must default toward protecting the individual. When life is truly not present, donation is perfectly acceptable and desirable. The wide, definitional gray area does not eliminate the clear, moral black and white.

While live organ donation calls for great care, and cadaver donation sometimes has associated with it additional costs, blood donation creates so little cost and emotional difficulty that there should be no moral ambiguity at all for evangelicals. It is a giving of oneself, though only distantly analogous to the sacrament in that the costs are so minimal. It makes one temporarily vulnerable in minor ways. The weakness which one willingly assumes is the loss of time, slight inconvenience and minimal pain. Further, the biological loss, the missing unit of blood, is only temporary as the plasma is replenished in about a day, with the red blood cells being replenished in around four weeks and the iron for hemoglobin in about seven. In addition, the benefit for the needy user of the gift is significant in comparison to the costs to the giver. The community benefits of such an offering—potentially helping the donor and his or her family, encouraging others to be givers—make it worth it. This gift is clearly within the range of responses appropriate for the believer, and should be facilitated by church leaders. In fact, when possible, it should be expected. Though requiring greater caution, marrow donation is similar.

Human research is a legitimate service, a gift offering to help improve the condition of all. It is similar to blood donation in community impact, but can have higher costs for the donor. The good is usually not the survival of a given individual, but is for a class of persons—present and in the future—who might benefit from the gained knowledge. This is true for basic research, specific clinical research and for education. The uncertainty of succeeding and the uncertainty about future need means research participants should be subjected to far less risk for basic research and education than for something that might immediately benefit specific persons. In addition, strong protections are required, specifically because research is conducted disproportionately on the socially weaker (e.g., students, the poor).[8] As is often noted, lower social position and fewer advocates makes one more likely to be a subject in experimentation.[9] Christians should simultaneously encourage research while expecting the leaders of the state to protect citizens as an expression of the social contract.

Another type of donation that raises different questions about gift-giving is gametes donation and sale. Eggs are plentiful and semen is replaceable as with blood, but these differ in that they establish a different kind of relationship between the giver and recipient, one that endures through offspring. It is genetic rather than somatic. They establish a relationship that, by its nature, is incomplete. While Christians should tolerate this donation, it should not be strongly endorsed for the society and even discouraged among believers. The purpose of such donations is to get at least "some" of the genetics of the rearing parents, but preferable options would seem to be adoption or embryo adoption from ART leftovers. The consequences of gamete donation are not significantly different from those of a divorce with children—the spousal relationship is severed, but children remain connected to all the parents.

Prudence requires a calculation of risk and benefit, but also an accounting of the character of the recipients. Christians should support organ recipient standards and principle investigator qualifications that take into account the likelihood of the success with the limited resource (the solid organ,

---

[8]James Childress uses a version of the just coercion theory in justifying research participation. James F. Childress, "The Gift of Life: Ethical Issues in Organ Transplantation," *Bulletin of the American College of Surgeons* 81, no. 3 (1996) <http://www.facs.org/about/committees/ethics/childresslect.html>.

[9]Paul M. McNeill, *Ethics and Politics of Human Experimentation* (New York: Cambridge University Press, 1993).

the person participating in research, etc.). For organs, this would include considering social and psychological factors. A substance abuser who has no intention of abandoning, say significant alcohol consumption, cannot receive the gift of the liver in an appropriate manner. Paul notes that some take the sacrament unworthily and bring destruction upon themselves (1 Cor 11). The same can be morally true for persons using body donations or using others for research or using gametes. The limited nature of the resource generates increasingly strict criteria since some scarce goods cannot be equally divided (as Solomon once demonstrated with a sword in one hand and an infant in the other) and so should be dispersed by an equitable selection method that takes into account the likelihood of success (the nonwasting of the resource).

The state should recognize the responsibility to protect contract makers; evangelicals should recognize that all, even the weakest, bear the image of the eternal God who gave himself. That image of God must be protected by maintaining strong legal boundaries and this seems to be most effectively done by guarding a clear definition of death. The precise biological boundary between life and death has always been a difficult one to discern. The Christian's concern for the vulnerable should lead to general opposition to harvesting protocols that push through the vagueness of that boundary in order to increase organs (even with that being a noble cause). In the final analysis, giving can be virtuous, and as such should be manifest in even the most immature Christian. It should appear in the attitude of believers toward blood donation, organ and tissue donation, and participation in research, and then demonstrated in their behavior.

The Christian belief in resurrection has historically included the resurrection of the body. Yet, the body that is raised is a spiritual body, not the seed (the physical body) from which it springs (1 Cor 15). According to traditional understandings of heaven, the raised believer is a recognizable being, but that is not dependent on having particular drops of blood, kidney cells or the atoms of a decayed solid organ. As Paul implies in the famous chapter on *agape/caritas*, 1 Corinthians 13, even if the body is given over to be burned in martyrdom, the person can still rise from the dead by the strength of genuine love. While evangelical Christians do not place ultimate value on the physical body, the organic body is part of the whole while animated and is still worthy of respect following death as that which was the temple of God, bearer of the imago Dei. Still, there is no spiritual concern that organ donation from a cadaver, live donation when not life-threatening or use of oneself for reasonable research will impede entrance into eternal life.

For Christians, all true donation can be best understood as gift-giving.[10] Research volunteering has risks that run from virtually no more than living a normal life to far too risky for human participation, but it should always be voluntary and informed in order to be a gift. Similarly, organ transplants from live donors require great care; they should be, on the rare occasions when performed, voluntary and informed. Cadaveric less so, if the boundary of life is protected and quasi-ownership of the body by family is maintained. Blood donation requires little moral precaution and should be strongly endorsed; it is an easy gift to give since it is readily replaceable and performed at low risk. The connection between giver and recipient is almost always strong, even if the specific individuals who give and receive are not known by each other.

PART THREE: CHRISTIAN BIOETHICS AND THE WORLD

Much of the secular discussion of donation has been consciously shaped around the ideas of community, usefulness, memorial giving and the gift of life. Usually appeals are made to heroism (though occasionally shame avoidance), with some quasi-religious notions of charity building the social fabric, and utility arguments about parts being thrown away in the grave. Sometimes an appeal is made to the donor family that "a small part of *fill-in a name* will live on," thus providing a sort of (to use an oxymoron) abbreviated eternal life.

Most of these arguments do not encourage altruism in the true sense. Still, the giving is such that it serves either those one loves or strangers who would not otherwise be considered part of the primary circles of concern of the donor and, in so doing, strengthens the community in which they commonly hold membership. In fact, the community is strengthened by the minor hero status afforded to donors. Evangelicals may think of such giving as obligatory (at least blood and cadaver organ donations), but the broader society benefits from proclaiming the behavior of donors heroic. The positive behavior is accentuated and since the nondonors are usually not sanctioned or condemned, the society seems to be naming such gifts as supererogatory acts.

Research participation and the donations of blood, tissue or organs, be

[10]This term and material on gift-giving of blood are from Richard Titmuss, *The Gift Relationship: From Human Blood to Social Policy* (New York: Vintage Books, 1971).

they live gifts or from someone who recently died, tend to come easiest when a connection is made between the potential user and the potential donor. The willingness to sacrifice certainly rises in accordance with the degree of relationship. Even for Christians, generally, there is a higher obligation to share with those of the community of faith and with those of one's own family than with others. To expand on a model suggested by Adam Smith in *A Theory of Moral Sentiments*, sympathy is most strongly felt and requires the deepest response on the basis of both relational and geographical proximity, with additional consideration based on the suffering that elicits the sympathy. Yet most organ and tissue and virtually all blood donation is to people who are strangers, and the same is true with research participation. It is necessary, therefore, to commend the giving as herioc, thus creating status and generating a sense of community.

Richard Titmuss wrote the best discussion of the donation of human substances almost four decades ago.[11] In this landmark work, Titmuss examines the donation of blood in post-World War II Britain. He looks at the many forms of appeal and many personal reasons people have for donating. While it may be necessary to finally differentiate between blood, tissue, solid organs, reproductive substances and participation in research, the overview is generally applicable. Some of the important commonalties are these:

- The recipient, usually, is not known (at least prior to the gift).
- The giving is sometimes painful (physically and/or emotionally).
- The giving is relatively less severe for the donor than the consequences of not receiving for the recipient.
- All persons meeting certain medical criteria and within certain political boundaries are eligible as recipients (truer of blood than organs; not applicable to research in which knowledge is generalized over a population group).
- The gift is perishable (physically as tissue, blood, or organs; in research as time).
- Certain groups are excluded from donating by more or less rational criteria.[12]

Some might not want to donate because they do not want to allow the mediating organizations (e.g., the Red Cross, the hospitals, the physicians) the power to use a precious resource. Certainly, arguments have been made

---

[11]Ibid.

[12]Modified from Titmuss, *Gift of Relationship*, p. 74

that organ and blood use, in the past, were directed toward the powerful or those less likely to be disenfranchised by the health-care system. The most infamous case (though amidst the claims of special treatment there were also protestations to the contrary) was the use of a human liver on Mickey Mantle. Of course, in a concession to utilitarianism, the organ procurement advocates point out that donations went up after the incident and that meant that more people were served.[13] A more important example is the variation in donation and organ transplant surgery by economic class and ethnicity.

Not only can getting organs be financially costly, so can giving them, and that may discourage giving. Once permission has been obtained, the hastening of death declarations promotes the viability of the organs. Prior to that the donor is not less likely to receive intensive care, but more likely. The costs after designation as an actual donor are assumed by the organ procurement organization; the costs while waiting for a second declaration of brain death sometimes are not. The agreement of health-care providers to such extensions of life sustaining treatments is sometimes associated with their desire to maintain the body of the suitable donor. There is nothing wrong with this, if it does not interfere with the family's ministering to the dying and his or her ministering to them. Also, it requires proper compensation if the health-care providers would otherwise deem the treatments futile. Those who profit from the process should address this additional cost for giving. This burden should not be placed on the recipient, the donor or donor family, but on those who receive substantial payments for high technology medicine (institutions and practitioners) and those who receive the prestige associated with being experts—a significant benefit. Some organizations are attempting to address this hidden cost to giving.

Nonetheless, people do give, and society encourages the offerings. Titmuss describes eight different types of donors (here modified and expanded to nine).[14] The categories blur to some extent, but this may be because often mo-

[13]Mickey Mantle was added to the liver waiting list on June 6, 1995. He underwent surgery two days later; the mean average on the waiting list is sixty-seven days. Protestations aside, it is difficult to see how Mantle was sicker than others who died or in a better position to use the liver given his subsequent death. The one powerful argument that can be made by those favoring payment is that it would raise the total number of organs. Similar claims of favoritism have been leveled over the liver transplant for Steve Jobs in June 2009; the method appears to have been legal multiple listing based on the willingness and financial ability to travel anywhere in the United States at a moment's notice.

[14]The list is modified from Titmuss, *Gift Relationship*, pp. 74-79.

tives function simultaneously. The categories reveal as much about how the medical system works as what one wants to do or be when giving. While it appears that there is a strong distinction between those who give for some form of reimbursement and those who anticipate a social benefit or benefit for another individual, this may or may not be always true. Indeed even donors expecting some form of payback are often commended.

- Independent paid (impersonal market transaction)
- Professional (regular donation, often for pheresis or research)
- Paid induced volunteer (receives payment through third-party supported community effort; e.g., labor union, employer)
- Responsibility fee/replacement obligation (a reimbursement for blood used or experimental treatments received, e.g., family members giving blood following a procedure for a loved one)
- Family credit (given with the understanding that persons in the immediate family are commonly entitled to the accrued donation credits; a form of blood insurance with the premium paid with blood rather than money)
- Community/organization credit (given with the understanding that persons in the group are commonly entitled to the accrued donation credits; a form of blood insurance with the premium paid with blood rather than money)
- Captive voluntary (especially prisoners and members of the military who are "[d]onors in positions of restraint and subordinate authority who are called upon, required, or expected to donate."[15] The infamous hallucinogen experiments on soldiers is another example)
- Fringe benefit (persons gain nonmonetary, but personal benefits that could be translated into economic terms; e.g., a day off).
- Voluntary community (the closest to *caritas/*charity; give because it is what is expected of the virtuous community member)

Today some want to eliminate the demand/supply imbalance, especially with solid organs, by changing the procurement process from one of gift-giving to one of social requirement. This would seem to present problems for the social contract. Those at the edge of life would, then, have to intentionally opt into protection of their well-being and individual interests rather than have

[15]Ibid., p.84.

that be the default position of the state. The following list, garnered from numerous sources, indicates the various positions that have been suggested (terms are used in slightly different ways by some authors; see explanation below for use in this text).

- Voluntary expressed donation
- Routine inquiry
- Required request
- Routine referral
- Required referral
- Presumed donation
    - presumed unless previously rejected by patient
    - presumed unless rejected by family
    - presumed if family cannot be found
- Compulsory donation (expropriation/conscription)
- Sale of organs
    - cadaver organs
        - full market value
        - partial funeral or health cost reimbursement
    - anticipatory sale of organs
    - sale of "alive" organs
- Cloned organs
- Xenografts

Pure voluntary donation, in which the donor or donor family initiates conversation, is no longer the norm for solid organs, though it is for blood. The current requirement is that potential donors be formally asked either upon admission or sometimes during a hospital stay, if they would like to donate organs or tissue; this is usually called "routine inquiry." Often county clerks start this process at the time of driver's license renewal, long before hospital admission. A required request is a legally mandated request made by hospital staff when death is imminent. When a referral is made to the procurement agency and its staff makes the request (if mandated, the latter is called "required referral" and is advocated by those who believe the procurement agency staff members are more efficient at talking to families and obtaining organs). All of these approaches are acceptable for evangelicals, though they may not be raising the number of donors significantly.

Some have argued that the nation should move toward a model of presumed donation or presumed consent in which donation occurs unless someone opts out. This would provide protection of those with specific religious reservations or simply a personal aversion when such persons were intentional in expressing their opposition. The burden of proof, so to speak, would shift from the institution to the individual. This is not theoretically problematic to Christians, but does create a situation in which abuse is more likely and, therefore, would call for significant protections. It might be, then, when the sufficient protections were in place (for instance, a requirement to genuinely seek to contact family) that the system would not be practically different from required request, or it might help a bit.

Though finer distinctions are possible, there are three basic understandings of who should control the disposal of a dead body. First, the claim can be made that the body is the property of the person whose body it was. He or she should be allowed to have it burned or thrown in a hole in the backyard as long as it does not harm anyone else. If absolute, this leaves open the possibility of sales, either selling organs live or prospectively so the person whose body it is can enjoy the profit while alive. Second, the claim can be made that relatives have quasi-ownership. Currently the quasi-owners can decide some things, but there are limits, the most notable being that the body cannot be sold. If this became a stronger ownership right, then they could sell cadaver organs. Third, the claim can be made that the body, at least once the person has died, is now part of the commons and any usable parts should be made accessible for the common good. This would allow mandatory donation, which would not be donating at all but more like imminent domain. It would be an intrusion of the state into family functioning that would, no doubt, encourage similar intrusions in other areas as it legitimated the violation of subsidiarity. If the state can compel donation, can it also force participation in research, compel care or (far more dangerously) deny care for those it deems unworthy (especially those with disabilities, particularly mental "deficiencies")? Compulsory donation is immoral.

In the same way, compulsory participation in research is wrong. And, certainly, questions about research participation as a gift arise because abuse can and does occur. Sometimes students participate in research to garner favor or avoid wrath (real or imagined) of professors. Certainly it is rarely the rich who enter into research for pay, except if there is a possible heath benefit, so there is a danger that advantage will be taken of the poor. Other marginalized groups, by race or ethnicity or region, can also suffer through forced research participation. The classic examples are Tuskegee, the Nazi Experiments and Willowbrook. Persons who voluntarily participate in research can choose to give their time and their bodies for such, but researchers should also be willing to provide compensation as if paying an employee—an employee participating in a high risk activity. This includes paying for any negative consequences—additional treatment and lost opportunity costs.

Who has interests in the research is another way to differentiate between who is giving and who is getting. A simple list of potential recipients of benefits includes

- The individual patient or volunteer
- All others sick with this disorder
- Students
- Future patients
- Researchers (including professors of student "volunteers")
- The community at large

Researchers and physicians asking humans to participate in research are always fulfilling multiple roles. They are attempting to gain information and serve patients (current or future), but also to gain profit or prestige. Similarly, communities—academic communities, cities that provide not-for-profit tax relief or other incentives—seek not only patient well-being but more money, power and honor. Disease advocacy groups often provide important assistance to individuals as they confront a disorder, but also seek benefits for those same people, sometimes apparently willing to ask others to participate in research to those people's possible detriment.

While organs and blood and, to a lesser extent, research participation, are obtained as gifts, when moving from procurement to transplant or transfusion, a shift occurs in the moral language from that of gift-giving to distributive justice (how the goods of a society or community are distributed among claimants). The best distribution mechanism begins with just procedures but includes consideration of utility—who can pay for the operation, who has a postsurgical support network, and who is most likely to benefit (very sick, but not too sick). This shift is ethically awkward, but seems to work better than most of the proposed alternatives and would work much better if ability to pay was somehow addressed.

A fourfold increase in demand for solid organs occurred between 1990 and 2000, which probably has much more to do with improved technical skills than with a change in the actual need. The demand continues to rise, meaning either more "gifts" must be obtained or they must be increasingly rationed. Possible means of rationing organs, tissues and blood include lottery; first come, first served; social worth; ability to pay; medical criteria (best recipient or most needy recipient); affirmative action; and geographic location of recipient and donor.

Though the current distribution methods vary with the disorder, the liver distribution mechanism is indicative of the general direction in the United States.

> Current liver allocation policy categorizes liver patients into four urgency categories, with waiting time as a tiebreaker. The revised system would [does] replace all but the highest medical urgency category (Status 1) with a continuous score calculated by MELD [Model for End-Stage Liver Disease] or PELD [Pediatric End-Stage Liver Disease] [both based on a "continuous scale of urgency"]. Those with higher scores are at higher risk of death without a transplant within three months and would receive first consideration for liver offers. Waiting time would still be used as a tiebreaker, but as there are a larger range of values (from 6 to 40 under MELD), these tiebreakers would be needed less often.[16]

The precise wording for different agencies and regions of the country varies, but the method is supposed to be determination by medical criteria within each region (both distribution categories combined in the scaling systems) with first come, first served being used as a tertiary criterion. Of course, questions arise as to whether this is actually the case, since it does appear less likely that someone who is poor has the same access to the health-care system which in turn is manifest in the medical criteria (especially likelihood of survival).

Donation is, after all is said, a function of the demand for the procured

[16]"Liver Allocation Policy Refinements Approved by OPTN/UNOS Board," UNOS News Release, November 15, 2001 <www.thetransplantnetwork.com/What's New/National News/LiverAllocation.shtml>.

organs, tissues and cells. If such things were readily available, that is, if supply exceeded demand, then donation would not be valued nor, conceivably, necessary. Gift-giving always is based on the idea that the gift is somehow precious. Likewise the market depends on some degree of scarcity. In addition, the just distribution of organs and (to a lesser extent) blood is a matter of rationing but with socially acceptable criteria.

If the process of giving and receiving the gift is deemed balanced or appropriate for the gift-giving relationship, then donations as gifts remain legitimate. If it is imbalanced—if the gift receiving is manipulative or benefits one group inappropriately over another—then it is unfair. Fairness can be defined as a combination of equitable sourcing, equitable distribution and maximizing efficiency of organs or other items used. If the process is biased in favor of the wealthy or powerful, then the morality of donating is contaminated. At best, donations would be given in the cynical hope that one of those close to the donor might be among the select. At worst, donations would end. If there is not real gift-giving and receiving, then there is no reason not to consider other, fairer approaches, including the market (if health care remains a market) and presumed donation (if health care is a right).

Selling in the case of some blood donation and reimbursement for participation in research is currently tolerated and is now being actively considered for solid organs and tissues. If the distribution of organs and tissues continues to be determined to a substantial degree by market value, then the ones who give could share in the profits. If the choice is to force more "donation" to relieve demand, then far more just methods of using the organs, tissues and research results must be developed.

One additional kind of giving warrants specific consideration. Increasingly, there is a social debate about the giving and getting of nonhuman animal research. Some argue that nonhuman higher animals should be as strongly protected as humans. This would assume some distinction among animals on the basis of sentience or relationship to humans. Like preborn humans, young children, the very sick or the otherwise incompetent, nonhuman animals cannot give informed consent, but indeed do warrant concern.

Evangelical doctrine and the U.S. social contract assumptions do not allow that nonhumans are bearers of the image of God or contract members. Even so, there is no reason for Christians to not protect those creatures as an expression of the virtue of the faithful and because they are part of God's good creation. Those of the world should do so simply to avoid risk for vulnerable human beings. As with humans who cannot convey rationality or easily interact, the default should be to protect life—human or nonhuman. Nonhuman animals do not have rights and cannot give gifts, but they do deserve welfare protection, which not only helps them as individuals but also protects the social order.[17]

To make the evaluation of welfare required, it is necessary to consider the purpose of the research and the impact on the animal. A list of purposes include

- Basic biological
- Applied basic biological/psychological
- Development of drugs/therapeutic chemicals
- Food and fiber research
- Testing of consumer goods
- Use in education
- Extraction of drugs/biological products

As justifiable coercion criteria were used for human donations, so they can be used for nonhumans research; however, a better model may be the "5 Rs." Assuming animals do not have rights and that under certain circumstances research on nonhuman animals for the sake of humans is acceptable, animal welfare can be improved through:

1. Refinement: *to lessen degree of pain/distress*
2. Reduction: *of number to the minimum scientifically required*
3. Replacement: *of animal models with non-animal when possible*
4. Reproduction protection: *of species as part of ecosystem*
5. Revise downward: *toward lower and more common animals when possible*[18]

CONCLUSION

Christians can accept giving as a moral obligation for believers, but should insist that giving not be required in the broader society. Believers give in re-

---

[17]The nonhuman animal equivalent of the IRB is the Institutional Animal Care and Use Committee.

[18]Numbers 1-3 are modified from William S. Russell and Rex L. Burch, *The Principles of Humane Experimental Technique* (London: Methuen, 1959) <http://altweb.jhsph.edu/publications/humane_exp/het-toc.htm>. Numbers 4 and 5 are my addition.

sponse to the greater gift given. On the other hand, the state should not mandate the giving of organs or risky research participation. This may mean the shortage will continue and other means of procuring organs need to be promoted (perhaps even growing organs on demand, as the technology develops). Though it would not strengthen the society through the valuing of giving, the sale of organs and more pay for research participation might allow a more honest portrayal of the organ procurement and distribution process and human research. Certainly, institutions, administrators and practitioners make a substantial amount of money when their networks and expertise are used. The argument is made, and accurately, that what is being paid for is not the organ. Yet, without that organ—a limited resource—the expertise would be meaningless. Similar arguments can be made when researchers use "donated" atypical tissues to produce a product or information from research endeavors that in turns yields money to researcher, company and/or research institution or university. Given that costs accrue, the donor of cadaver organs should minimally gain the benefit of lowered health-care costs for the final stay in the hospital. Perhaps such could be prospectively obtained in a kind of prepurchase that would put the donor (now seller) in no more of a dangerous situation than being designated a donor now would do. However, substantial protections would need to exist to prevent such preselling from becoming the selling of organs from live donors or sales arranged at the time of treatment decisions. Christians, as noted above, should never accept the intentional damaging of the gift of God (earthly existence) for money. Further, Christians can and should support the social contract state in its protection of contract members from death and injury, including self-inflicted death and injury for profit. Concern would also extend to those outside the social contract (in other countries) who might be victims of organ "entrepreneurs" who would import solid organs into the United States or who would encourage medical tourism for organ transplantation.

Since the actual implantation of organs is part of a market exchange, then there is no good reason why the poor should provide a limited resource for health-care centers and physicians to obtain prestige and wealth without profiting from the process. This is not the ideal, but is a concession to the current system and would require strict and proper constraints against importation and/or decisions to kill for profit. It is hoped that the threat of organ sales could push the health-care system into including the poor as genuinely eligible for receiving organs (in much the same way that the blood donation system functions in most locations). Given the current imbalance of the American health-care system, the toleration or even participation in postdeath cadaveric organ sales might be acceptable for the society from a Christian perspective.

One advantage of selling and charging for organs, more so than with research participation, might be that the real costs of the transplant process would be more transparent. The supposed heroic status of donors and the microallocation question of who gets the organ would no longer hide the macroallocation question of the costs of high technology medicine and who is profiting. Certainly this is not meant as a condemnation of organ transplant procedures. Kidney transplants, for instance, are far preferable to dialysis, when possible. And heart transplants seem to be efficient at keeping people alive for decades when successful. Also, reasonable costs for research ultimately lead to far lower costs—not only in transplants but also in other kinds of procedures which are improved by virtue of the knowledge gained. Yet, these costs should be compared to other costs, not only in preventative care but other expenditures the society makes.

To believers, who should have a sense of duty inclining them toward donation, selling organs or participation in research may well seem crass, even if not immoral. Yet, it can be legitimated as a matter of distributive and commutative justice—distributive in that the goods (money, prestige and health) that accrue in the procurement/transplantation and research processes are currently aligned away from the donor and should be, at least slightly, rearranged; commutative in that in can be easily argued that the real costs and benefits of the process are only partially revealed to the persons who have the most precious resource—the donor and the donor family. Though organs once removed no longer belong to the surgeon or hospital (they now "officially" belong to the community and are held in trust by various agencies) and research once published is public information, still the benefit is not proportionately distributed to the community. The market might allow those who are least likely to benefit—even though they are asked to donate to, accrue some credit or other profit from the process. The greatest danger in such arguments is that this commodifies the human body, especially with preborns; also, vulnerable persons (especially individuals with mental disabilities) become more vulnerable to greedy family members. Having said this, regardless of any market development, generally believers should recognize that it is their calling to donate resources.

Arguably, Christians themselves should give rather than sell. Christians can accept giving as a moral obligation for believers, but should insist that giving not be required in the broader society. Believers give in response to the greater gift given—the body and the blood of Jesus Christ.

17

Death and the Christian

HUMANS AS FINITE

Humans are finite. This reality does not intimidate mature Christians. The believer recognizes the opportunity to serve others is limited but nonetheless significant. The faithful follower seeks to live a temporary life for an eternal purpose. Even dying itself can serve this end.

> Woe to you, blind guides! You say, "If anyone swears by the temple, it means nothing; but if anyone swears by the gold of the temple, he is bound by his oath." You blind fools! Which is greater: the gold, or the temple that makes the gold sacred? You also say, "If anyone swears by the altar, it means nothing; but if anyone swears by the gift on it, he is bound by his oath." You blind men! Which is greater: the gift, or the altar that makes the gift sacred? Therefore, he who swears by the altar swears by it and by everything on it. And he who swears by the temple swears by it and by the one who dwells in it. And he who swears by heaven swears by God's throne and by the one who sits on it.
>
> Woe to you, teachers of the law and Pharisees, you hypocrites! You give a tenth of your spices—mint, dill and cummin. But you have neglected the more important matters of the law—justice, mercy and faithfulness. You should have practiced the latter, without neglecting the former. You blind guides! You strain out a gnat but swallow a camel. (Mt 23:16-24)

> The chief priests and the whole Sanhedrin were looking for false evidence against Jesus so that they could put him to death. But they did not find any, though many false witnesses came forward.
>
> Finally two came forward and declared, "This fellow said, 'I am able to destroy the temple of God and rebuild it in three days.'"
>
> Then the high priest stood up and said to Jesus, "Are you not going to answer? What is this testimony that these men are bringing against you?" But Jesus remained silent.
>
> The high priest said to him, "I charge you under oath by the living God: Tell us if you are the Christ, the Son of God."
>
> "Yes, it is as you say," Jesus replied. "But I say to all of you: In the future you

will see the Son of Man sitting at the right hand of the Mighty One and coming on the clouds of heaven."

Then the high priest tore his clothes and said, "He has spoken blasphemy! Why do we need any more witnesses? Look, now you have heard the blasphemy. What do you think?"

"He is worthy of death," they answered. (Mt 26:59-66)

PART ONE: THE TEXT

Death is real.[1] The Roman authorities and Jewish leaders destroyed the earthly Temple that was Jesus the Nazarene. He died. To the evangelical Christian the death of Jesus had to be the actual termination of existence in space and time. The body completely ceased to function. This was not a beaten man who lapsed into a coma nor was there a surrogate hanging on the cross nor was there some form of mass hysteria or spiritual illusion that allowed the real Christ to remain laughing at a distance from the specter of supposed suffering. Jesus was dead by the setting of the sun before the Sabbath evening began.

The leaders thought him worthy of execution. Earlier Caiaphas had made a simple utilitarian calculation and determined that Jesus should die to save the people—he thought from the Roman oppressors. Little did he know that God had made a similar calculation when he offered himself—to save humanity from eternal death. God's calculation was correct, while Caiaphas's was not, but then God can see all the costs and all the benefits. He has no difficulty determining what shall be valued as utility—it is his love for us and our love for him.

Still, the reality of the death did not mean that the death was the final expression of the reality of Jesus, and this is what fundamentally shapes evangelical ethics. Morality must account for finitude, for vulnerability. The physical body of every individual morally matters. Death matters. Yet the physical body is not everything and, consequently, death is not the ultimate evil. And, consequently, morality must direct one beyond this life in considering the concerns of this life. Jesus had a complete physical existence—yet the complete physical existence was not the complete existence of Jesus.

Jesus predicted he would die and that his body would be physically resur-

[1]Sections of this chapter were drawn from my paper presented at Mind, Bodies, Souls Conference, sponsored by the Templeton Foundation and Asbury Theological Seminary, 2003, Wilmore, Kentucky.

rected—that the temple would be raised—and he was (Mt 26). This is, for evangelicals, the proof that there is something beyond death that gives significance to earthly life and its conclusion. The significance of Jesus' death and the opening to eternal life it provides, which in turn gives meaning to and defines good and bad, right and wrong for this life, is asserted throughout the New Testament. As an example:

> Once you were alienated from God and were enemies in your minds because of your evil behavior. But now he has reconciled you by Christ's physical body through death to present you holy in his sight, without blemish and free from accusation—if you continue in your faith, established and firm, not moved from the hope held out in the gospel. This is the gospel that you heard and that has been proclaimed to every creature under heaven, and of which I, Paul, have become a servant. (Col 1:21-23)

This existence is a blessing from God, but one that should always be enjoyed with just the slightest melancholy as it is a place of shadows and sorrows in comparison to that to which the believer goes—a place through which we sojourn on the way to our home. A blessing, but only as a reflection of what is to come, a foreshadowing. As Paul said, "For to me, to live is Christ and to die is gain" (Phil 1:21).

Evangelicals and the Protestants immediately preceding the rise of revivalism insisted on this two-tiered understanding of death. The position was not only proclaimed from pulpits and asserted by theologians, it was woven throughout the life of congregations. Bunyan's *Pilgrim's Progress*, one of the most popular devotional books of the early evangelical movement, and hymns such as "Jordan's Stormy Banks," which still appears in most evangelical hymnals, declared a confidence meant to encourage. Suffering is real, the winds are stormy and the last stretch of the road can be hard and long, but death is now under the control of God and of the believer who submits to him.

> On Jordan's stormy banks I stand,
> And cast a wishful eye
> To Canaan's fair and happy land,
> Where my possessions lie.
>
> I am bound for the promised land,
> I am bound for the promised land;
> Oh who will come and go with me?

I am bound for the promised land.

O the transporting, rapturous scene,
That rises to my sight!
Sweet fields arrayed in living green,
And rivers of delight!

There generous fruits that never fail,
On trees immortal grow;
There rocks and hills, and brooks and vales,
With milk and honey flow.

O'er all those wide extended plains
Shines one eternal day;
There God the Son forever reigns,
And scatters night away.

No chilling winds or poisonous breath
Can reach that healthful shore;
Sickness and sorrow, pain and death,
Are felt and feared no more.

When I shall reach that happy place,
I'll be forever blest,
For I shall see my Father's face,
And in His bosom rest.

Filled with delight my raptured soul
Would here no longer stay;
Though Jordan's waves around me roll,
Fearless I'd launch away.

I am bound for the promised land,
I am bound for the promised land;
O who will come and go with me?
I am bound for the promised land.

The evangelical Christian understanding of death, then, is twofold. It is of extraordinary importance as it is the one moment by which all previous moments will be judged, yet it is not the ultimate end. Death remains evil, an enemy, but as a conquered enemy it must do the bidding of the Master. The sting of death is gone for the Christian, while the sadness of separation and the experience of physical pain remain. Biological death is the cessation of biological function, but it is not spiritual death for those who are faithful followers. The Christian position is unlike those of religions that view death as one moment on a near everlasting set of cycles, thus lowering its importance, or the secular assertion that death is the final termination of the individual. To the faithful, death defines life, but only because there is a deeper reality that makes it so.

Early in the movement, believers were literally taught how to die well and that they should live well in preparation for death.

> In fact, death proved a great leveller as even the poorest soul could assume authority on the basis of dying revelation. Perceived both as the first and last opportunity for men and women to communicate a genuine insight into life and afterlife, the words of dying persons were invested with profound significance. For Christians then, death was not solely the event of physical cessation but the portal to a new level of existence that was to last for eternity. Given the magnitude of this transition, the circumstances of death assumed monumental importance.[2]

Jeremy Taylor, whose work influenced the Wesleys and George Whitefield, in *The Rules and Exercises of Holy Dying*, said:

> Of all the evils of the world which are reproached with an evil character, death is the most innocent of its accusation. For when it is present, it hurts nobody, and when it is absent, it is indeed troublesome, but the trouble is owing to our fears, not to the affrighting and mistaken object: and besides this, if it were an evil, it is so transient that it passes like the instant or undiscerned portion of the present time; and either it is past, or it is not yet; for just when it is, no man hath reason to complain of so insensible, so sudden, so undiscerned a change.[3]

John Wesley was reported to have said, "Our people die well," implying that their deaths were indicators of lives well-lived and that the reality of death called them to live well to the end.

> Wesley once remarked upon hearing of his followers' persecution: "Our people die well." On another occasion a physician said to Charles Wesley, "most people die for fear of dying; but I never met with such people as yours. They are none of them afraid of death, but calm and patient and resigned to the last."[4]

---

[2]Richard J. Bell, "'Our People Die Well': Deathbed Scenes in John Wesley's Arminian Magazine," *Mortality* 10, no. 3 (2005): 210-23

[3]Jeremy Taylor, "The Second Temptation Proper to the State of Sickness, Fear of Death, with Its Remedies," *Rules and Exercises of Holy Dying*, chap. 3, sec. 7:5.

[4]Kenneth W. Osbeck, *101 More Hymn Stories* (Grand Rapids: Kregal, 1985), p. 14.

Evangelicals look back to Jesus, who as he stood before the Sanhedrin and later Pontius Pilate, did not seek the agony of death, but did not fear it either. In Jesus' prayers he wished not to drink the cup, presumably of betrayal and death, but accepted the Father's will (Mk 14:36). The author of Hebrews calls individual believers to follow the same path through death.

> Therefore, since we are surrounded by such a great cloud of witnesses, let us throw off everything that hinders and the sin that so easily entangles, and let us run with perseverance the race marked out for us. Let us fix our eyes on Jesus, the author and perfecter of our faith, who for the joy set before him endured the cross, scorning its shame, and sat down at the right hand of the throne of God. Consider him who endured such opposition from sinful men, so that you will not grow weary and lose heart. (Heb 12:1-4)

For the believer, the reality of death is empowering because it means that this life actually has significance as the finite that will be remembered infinitely. The recognition of finitude for the believer ought not to lead to the exasperated acquiescence of defeat more properly belonging to the despairing aesthete, the defiantly excessive denial of the reality of finitude by atheistic existentialists, or the posturing arrogance of the false indifference of reductionists. It should lead believers to recognize, in the midst of sorrow and pain, an opportunity to conform into the image of Christ. For this reason, believers should help the sick and suffering, should pray for miracles and accept them as they come or endure their absence, and—most importantly, though perhaps not as clearly recognized as well as in the earlier days of the movement—evangelicals should die well.

PART TWO: CHRISTIAN BIOETHICS

If heaven is so wonderful, why not hasten to enter? Tertullian claimed that the real birthday of a martyr was the day of death.[5] That actually makes some sense to evangelicals. It is not unusual to hear an evangelical knowingly and with some confident satisfaction, though not pleasure, say, "More Christians have died as martyrs in the last one hundred years than all the years before, and they are a witness to me." But the argument can go too far, as with the Circumcellions, a subset of the Donatists, who lived in North Africa.[6] They would attempt to violently (though without swords in a legalistic obedience to

[5] *De Corona* 3; *De resurrectione carnis* 13

[6] Donatist Circumcellion suicides are not of one sort with those at Jonestown in Guyana, a personality cult or the New Age sect Heaven's Gate suicides, but do bear similarities.

Christ's command to Peter) correct anything they thought was injustice while hoping to provoke others into killing them or would even fling themselves from cliffs in order to be pure martyrs. This was appropriately deemed immoral and heretical. First, it seemed to deny the power of God to forgive and, second, denied the penultimate goodness of the physical life God had given.

While no group of evangelicals favors suicide to hasten entry into heaven, different reasons are given as to why that is so. Generally, evangelicals accept all of the reasons, though with variation in emphasis. A position emphasized by those in Holiness churches is that physical existence is a temporary stopping place; people facing difficulty must view life and, then, dying as an opportunity to simply persevere and be shaped into the likeness of Christ. Certain Pentecostal groups emphasize this life is an opportunity for blessings, albeit not as wondrous as those to come. Some in the more extreme groups will declare that disease or death before the allotted time ("three score and ten" or maybe four score according to Psalm 90:10) is an indicator of sin or weak faith; still, they acknowledge that life itself is but a moment. Fundamentalists tend to use language that describes this life as an opportunity for obedience. Acknowledging subtle differences, most if not all evangelicals assert that this is a place through which all sojourn, journeying to heaven or to hell, but for believers it can be, under many circumstances, a pleasant place through which to travel.

The possibilities for good in this sojourn, both enjoyment of the blessings God provides and the many chances to do good and thereby glorify God in service to others, are—or should be—obvious to any mature evangelicals. Indeed, for bioethics this is especially important; there is no good reason for a Christian community or individual to base his or her moral claims on extensive deductions about the nature of persons when the Scripture itself speaks more directly to the goodness of this life and helping others as they live this life. Caring for the suffering is commanded and should be done. For Christians in particular, to engage in discussions about what defines the real individual human for the sake of "discussions" of bioethics without starting with consideration of the possible negative consequences on "real" people in hospitals, nursing facilities or in homes is morally irresponsible. If the Text provides a moral imperative, and repeats it over and over, then the philosophy of personhood must fit the morality, not the other way around. Regardless of debates about what is a "whole person," the Scriptures implore believers to help the sick and suffering.

What is asserted by believers about "person" or, more properly, ontological identity, must be compatible with this moral position. What is claimed about theodicy and who deserves what must likewise coincide with the moral claims of the gospel to respond to the suffering. The attitude of Jesus toward finitude and death did not distance him from grief and brokenness, but made him willing to bear sorrow and bind up wounds. This must be clearly asserted; then it can be explained with theological terms and arguments.

Any evangelical who fails to acknowledge an obligation, or does not demonstrate a willingness, to serve those who suffer physically is (to offer the most charitable interpretation) immature, and perhaps not of the faithful at all. The physical person is, one way or another, part of the real human individual, created in the image of God from the dust of the earth. This was the nature assumed by Christ; therefore, care for physical existence is a moral imperative.

Bioethics should matter to Christians because the mortal frame of each individual matters to God. To ignore the needs of the sick, broken and disabled will inevitably lead to the eternal sorrow of those who claim they follow Christ but do not seek to conform their lives to his—in life and death.

PART THREE: CHRISTIAN BIOETHICS AND THE WORLD

If it is true that this is all there is, then it is logical to exit early and easily or to cling with a death grip, literally, to biological life. One might refuse to abandon even the most clearly futile treatments or might spend, as the saying goes, the child's inheritance seeking the latest quack therapy. Others, in the face of such inevitability might declare themselves the determiners of meaning and masters of their own dying. Deceiving themselves the best they can with superficial assurance, they might proclaim their self-generated moral authority. In a sense, in spite of their sad errors, they have a right to services and a right to refuse them. Yet they do not have the right to kill innocents or ask others to do so.

With the harsh words of their intellectual orthodoxy, but a tepid commitment (thankfully) to seeing the logic of their philosophy played out, those who believe that there is no God (or at least not one who cares), proclaim their own righteousness and good intentions while denying the final reality of any right and good. Some seek to become the arbiters of what others do—but, to use the image of the fairy tale, the emperor has no clothing. Needless to say, to Christians, this seems like the apex of arrogance. Arrogance is a moral concern, but something that believers should tolerate. More immediately, it is a desperate problem for the social contract if such cultured elite actually do obtain control—through assertion or insinuation—and move from tepid to fervent in promoting their morality. The implications for the most vulnerable would be devastating. And it should not need repeating, but the well-worn cries about the Crusades and creation museums are muffled by the cries of the victims of Hitler, Stalin, Mao and Pol Pot—the orchestrators of butchery far more recent and far greater. They did not do these things in the name of Jesus, but in the name of science and history—perhaps bad science and bad history, but then the Crusades and Inquisition were bad Christianity.

Evangelicals, at least those who are not complete separatists like conservative Anabaptists and strict Holiness groups, should not be afraid of politics when their participation can help promote the value of human life. Death may not be the ultimate evil, but when the killing is of the sick, disabled or otherwise "unfit," then death is an egregious evil with both temporal, political and eternal consequences that should be prevented if possible. This will require that believers individually become such good witnesses in their service to those in need—including the sick, those with significant physical anomalies, and persons with developmental and mental disabilities—that those of the world will not be able to casually disregard Christian words offered in defense of the value of life when spoken on the public square.

> You are the light of the world. A city on a hill cannot be hidden. Neither do people light a lamp and put it under a bowl. Instead they put it on its stand, and it gives light to everyone in the house. In the same way, let your light shine before men, that they may see your good deeds and praise your Father in heaven. (Mt 5:14-16)

> But you are a chosen people, a royal priesthood, a holy nation, a people belonging to God, that you may declare the praises of him who called you out of darkness into his wonderful light. Once you were not a people, but now you are the people of God; once you had not received mercy, but now you have received mercy. Dear friends, I urge you, as aliens and strangers in the world, to abstain from sinful desires, which war against your soul. Live such good lives among the pagans that, though they accuse you of doing wrong, they may see your good deeds and glorify God on the day he visits us. (1 Peter 2:9-12)

Believers will have to address bioethical issues, especially in non-Western parts of the earth, in conversation with those of other religions. Sometimes that will mean responding to injustice in a society in which Christians are a small minority. That, though, is not the case in the West and especially not in the United States. In the United States, particularly among intellectuals in bioethics, the main contrary worldview is that of scientism and the second most prevalent anti-Christian position is privatized therapeutic syncretism.

Attempting to avoid the question of eternity and the significance of finitude, those practicing scientism refuse to acknowledge the real implications of life being infinitely insignificant. If the human individual is no more than an accidental speck on a miniscule planet in a momentary solar system that is part of a galaxy spinning toward oblivion in a deteriorating universe, then she or he has little upon which to assert significance and, therefore, little upon which to claim moral meaning. The question that evangelicals finally must ask those holding to scientism is, how can there be a basis for common discussion and at least some common conclusion on social ethics, bioethics in particular? The answer is in the social contract, and the social contract requires the acceptance of the concept that all human beings are endowed with fundamental worth and have a right to life that cannot be reduced.

Those others who claim worldview is purely a private matter and so, then, are good and evil, nonetheless demand their rights. They assert subjective authority and deny the social necessity of accountability. Of course, they can believe what they want, but not they nor anyone else can do whatever he or she or they "feel like." There is a limit to tolerance defined by the thin shared morality of the social contract, which provides social stability and, thereby, safeguards freedom. In bioethics, toleration is perfectly appropriate even when believers and nonbelievers disagree on significant moral issues, except in those cases in which toleration would mean the termination of the innocent. The way to negotiate this boundary is with the social contract, not moral subjectivism.

The social contract is an agreement for now—not for eternity. It therefore depends on persons having biological life. It protects the individual from the state, other states and other individuals (including corporations, etc.). First, life is to be protected, then liberty and the pursuit of the individual life purpose or *telos* are to be allowed and even, to a limited degree through common resources, facilitated. Happily, social contract standards for the protection of the individual's life, liberty and opportunity to seek one's own good within the limits generated by other people's rights coincide well with the evangelical valuing of this life as the opportunity for accepting Christ.

The social contract requires that one be deemed simply a person, a human being. Of course, no one personally considers him- or herself to be simply a person. People have sexuality, age, social location, personal history and so on.

Each is an individual and a being in unique relationships. People, at least the vast majority, experience themselves as physical bodies and something more—mind and soul being the terms usually used. This can and should be accepted by Christians and non-Christians alike, at least for legal purposes.

A question raised in bioethics repeatedly, though with little resolution, is, what actually constitutes a person? What should be asked first is, what is the obligation? Or, to put this another way, what relationships matter and how are they altered so as to change or terminate obligation? When the question of personhood is the subject of a debate in bioethics, one can be almost certain that those who are unquestionably biologically alive but at the edge (e.g., as defined by conditions of prenatality, increased likelihood of death or significant disabling conditions) are at risk of having care ended or even of facing active termination of their lives. The social shift of the boundary of life and death is often an effort to deprive someone of rights by redefinition.[7]

Reidentification or redefinition of the person often creates new obligations—even to the point that society shifts from protecting individuals to granting a right to die for persons with significant disabilities finally to asserting a "duty" to die. The definition becomes the description becomes the prescription. When the people with serious illnesses or disabling conditions declare that they are not dead yet, they are actually demanding that they not be degraded, for that simultaneously deprives them of rights (in this social contract society) and relieves others of their familial and cultural obligations. Note—and this should not be downplayed—the decision-makers seek to assuage their consciences as much as resolve dilemmas.

Moral precision is certainly problematic when people live in ICUs, when new humans can be engineered, and when people are born with or survive with serious disabilities. Or, at least, this is what bioethicists and philosophers have asserted—the society needs more precision in its language about who is what and, therefore, who or what is that something that deserves something (the convoluted language is representative). But perhaps the measurement cannot be any more precise. Perhaps the measurement has such uncertainties that the effort to construct and use a moral measuring machine to minutely determine humanness or personhood misses the point that all are obligated to one another under the social contract. Perhaps much in bioethics is deceptive.

[7]See John F. Kavanaugh, *Who Counts as Persons?: Human Identity and the Ethics of Killing* (Washington, D.C.: Georgetown University Press, 2001); Mary Douglas and Steven Ney, *Missing Persons: A Critique of Personhood in the Social Sciences* (Berkley: University of California Press, 1998).

Though seemingly esoteric, the philosophical and bioethical arguments about personhood become powerful as they are accepted as political claims for or against a right to continue to exist. The most inclusive definition of the human should be used, namely that any individual who is biologically human is a person. Otherwise, when threatened by the power of the state, insurers which are often primarily interested in cost, health-care providers who interpret persons with disabilities as professional failures, or family members who lack necessary models for understanding radical change yet are confronting a sudden, tragic situation, people will die.[8]

If the very sick and those with disabilities are treated as normal in a political sense even while the uniqueness of each individual in his or her roles and with his or her own narrative is recognized, then others may have to be inconvenienced or even discomforted. It is a price society must pay so that precedents are not set and laws not established that would serve to deprive people of those rights. The possibility of death is the reality that creates the need for rights. Finitude of biological life and limited earthly resources generate demands and necessitate protections, including negative rights as endorsed by the social contract.

Asserting a right to life is most difficult when, at an emotional level, families seemingly cannot endure the suffering of someone they love. Though it seems harsh when considering the family member who feels overwhelmed by tragedy, the right to kill is not intrinsic and should not be asserted. The family members need support and they need economic and social resources to respond to the changes that occur.

This leaves room, too, for the state to expand by the people's authority positive rights or what might be more clearly referred to as entitlements. After all, as technological options increase and the reasonable demand that the state protect the vulnerable takes on new meaning, efforts to prevent morally precarious situations seem reasonable. Expanding a positive right to basic health care, including catastrophic coverage, can be viewed as a protection of the common good (air, water, etc.). Those entitlements that are accepted, such as education and apparently health care, should be delivered more efficiently and in a manner that maximizes freedom. In other words, no one is entitled to the finest care or the finest university education, but to a basic minimum so that there is true fair opportunity. The state can facilitate, and may need to provide some basic minimum entitlements to do so, but cannot set the standards for

---

[8]See above, chapter 4, note 15.

how one uses liberty and pursues happiness (the individual *telos*).

Political power must be met with political power if the powerful choose to disregard the weakest and most marginal, pushing them into death. The arguments that de-identify or "de-person" require a political response. The similarity of justifications (read, psychologically soothing rationalizations for people in professional classes) for the termination of those defined as unworthy of life to terms like *Lebenunwertes Leben* and *Dasein ohne Leben* is not accidental, for the similarity of the conclusions such reasonings reach is evident.

While this should be obvious, it sometimes is not; the real question for bioethics is a moral one: not what is the identity of persons, but rather, how will the individual be identified in day-to-day activities? Logical deductions about the body/soul in Christianity or the body/mind in Enlightenment-based thought are important, but they do not provide moral truth. Likewise, empirical findings drawn from neurological studies or from opinion surveys cannot finally resolve what constitutes a person nor whether or not she or he will have his or her rights or be treated respectfully. Though the U.S. social contract does not require that everyone accept that biological life and daily living have eternal significance, it does require that everyone act as if such significance exists and to respect the right of the individual to exist and be treated decently. No one is legally required to die well in the Christian sense; all are required, though, to not cause the innocent to die prematurely.

CONCLUSION

Biological life, in a sense, is an analogue for the life to come. For the Christian believer, the necessary truth about the body and soul is not a philosopher's discourse, but the simple assertion that we do not know what we will be after death, but we know that finally we will be like him (1 Jn 3:2). This life, then, is a time to shape ourselves into what we will be after death.

This hope does not mean that the stages-of-grief model should be discarded.[9] Individual believers often go through denial, anger, bargaining, depression and, ideally, acceptance. Christians, though, should want to move through preparatory grief about this existence, be prepared to die, and, in recognizing and accepting their own finitude, offer purpose and hope to others for this life and the next.

The Christian who desires biological healing for himself or herself or for

[9]Elisabeth Kübler-Ross, *On Death and Dying* (New York: Macmillan, 1969).

another truly wants the good—yet, even better is to want the eternal healing that requires genuine acceptance of the inevitability of biological death. Therefore, evangelicals should not make an argument for life at any price, as if vitalism should guide ethics. That is a reductionism similar (though less threatening for sick and injured individuals) to those who try to describe human existence or personhood in terms of an intellectual characteristic they happen to value. Instead, this life is to matter and be defined because it is yielding to a life to come that gives value to the moments we live. Life should be lived as if it is an analogue of life in heaven—though the analogy is imperfect, it is close enough to guide the believer's morality.

Caiaphas for all of history is remembered as one who conspired to kill an innocent man. Did Jesus deserve to die? Contrary to what Caiaphas implied in asking the question, no. But, even if Jesus was not worthy of death, what of everyone else? Is not everyone, one way or another, worthy of such? This is a harsh question that is, perhaps, better addressed with its inverse. Is everybody worthy of eternal life? To evangelicals the answer is simple—no. Yet, by grace, God opens eternity and in that offers renewed significance to this life.

Nobody is worthy of eternal life, but the infinite One offers it anyway—because he is not value neutral, but is loving and seeks to be loved. Perhaps too no one deserves biological life—at least if that requires intellectual perfection worked out in an ideal physical body—but God has determined that this life matters. Happily, the U.S. social contract and evangelism agree on this point.

Name Index

Subject Index

Scripture Index